MW00714715

Neuro-Ophthalmology

Section 5

2009–2010

BASIC AND CLINICAL SCIENCE COURSE

LEO

LIFELONG
EDUCATION FOR THE
OPHTHALMOLOGIST®

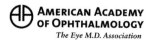

AMERICAN ACADEMY
OF OPHTHALMOLOGY
The Eye M.D. Association

The Basic and Clinical Science Course is one component of the Lifelong Education for the Ophthalmologist (LEO) framework, which assists members in planning their continuing medical education. LEO includes an array of clinical education products that members may select to form individualized, self-directed learning plans for updating their clinical knowledge. Active members or fellows who use LEO components may accumulate sufficient CME credits to earn the LEO Award. Contact the Academy's Clinical Education Division for further information on LEO.

The American Academy of Ophthalmology is accredited by the Accreditation Council for Continuing Medical Education to provide continuing medical education for physicians.

The American Academy of Ophthalmology designates this educational activity for a maximum of 40 *AMA PRA Category 1 Credits*™. Physicians should only claim credit commensurate with the extent of their participation in the activity.

The Academy provides this material for educational purposes only. It is not intended to represent the only or best method or procedure in every case, nor to replace a physician's own judgment or give specific advice for case management. Including all indications, contraindications, side effects, and alternative agents for each drug or treatment is beyond the scope of this material. All information and recommendations should be verified, prior to use, with current information included in the manufacturers' package inserts or other independent sources, and considered in light of the patient's condition and history. Reference to certain drugs, instruments, and other products in this course is made for illustrative purposes only and is not intended to constitute an endorsement of such. Some material may include information on applications that are not considered community standard, that reflect indications not included in approved FDA labeling, or that are approved for use only in restricted research settings. **The FDA has stated that it is the responsibility of the physician to determine the FDA status of each drug or device he or she wishes to use, and to use them with appropriate, informed patient consent in compliance with applicable law.** The Academy specifically disclaims any and all liability for injury or other damages of any kind, from negligence or otherwise, for any and all claims that may arise from the use of any recommendations or other information contained herein.

Copyright © 2009
American Academy of Ophthalmology
All rights reserved
Printed in Singapore

Basic and Clinical Science Course

Gregory L. Skuta, MD, Oklahoma City, Oklahoma, *Senior Secretary for Clinical Education*

Louis B. Cantor, MD, Indianapolis, Indiana, *Secretary for Ophthalmic Knowledge*

Jayne S. Weiss, MD, Detroit, Michigan, *BCSC Course Chair*

Section 5

Faculty Responsible for This Edition

Lanning B. Kline, MD, *Chair,* Birmingham, Alabama
M. Tariq Bhatti, MD, Durham, North Carolina
Sophia Mihe Chung, MD, St. Louis, Missouri
Eric Eggenberger, DO, East Lansing, Michigan
Rod Foroozan, MD, Houston, Texas
Karl C. Golnik, MD, Terrace Park, Ohio
Aki Kawasaki, MD, *Consultant,* Lausanne, Switzerland
Harold E. Shaw, MD, Greenville, South Carolina
Practicing Ophthalmologists Advisory Committee for Education

The authors state the following financial relationships:

Dr Bhatti: BayerHealth Care, consultant, lecture honoraria recipient; EMD Serono, consultant, lecture honoraria recipient; Pfizer, lecture honoraria recipient

Dr Eggenberger: Allergan, lecture honoraria and grant recipient; Berlex, consultant, lecture honoraria recipient; Biogen, consultant, lecture honoraria and grant recipient; EMD Serono, consultant, grant recipient; Teva Pharmaceutical, consultant, lecture honoraria and grant recipient

Dr Golnik: Allergan, consultant

The other authors state that they have no significant financial interest or other relationship with the manufacturer of any commercial product discussed in the chapters that they contributed to this publication or with the manufacturer of any competing commercial product.

Recent Past Faculty

Anthony C. Arnold, MD
Joseph F. Rizzo, III, MD

In addition, the Academy gratefully acknowledges the contributions of numerous past faculty and advisory committee members who have played an important role in the development of previous editions of the Basic and Clinical Science Course.

American Academy of Ophthalmology Staff

Richard A. Zorab, *Vice President, Ophthalmic Knowledge*

Hal Straus, *Director, Publications Department*

Carol L. Dondrea, *Publications Manager*

Christine Arturo, *Acquisitions Manager*

D. Jean Ray, *Production Manager*

Stephanie Tanaka, *Medical Editor*

Steven Huebner, *Administrative Coordinator*

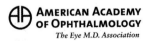

**AMERICAN ACADEMY
OF OPHTHALMOLOGY**
The Eye M.D. Association

655 Beach Street
Box 7424
San Francisco, CA 94120-7424

Contents

General Introduction

The Basic and Clinical Science Course (BCSC) is designed to meet the needs of residents and practitioners for a comprehensive yet concise curriculum of the field of ophthalmology. The BCSC has developed from its original brief outline format, which relied heavily on outside readings, to a more convenient and educationally useful self-contained text. The Academy updates and revises the course annually, with the goals of integrating the basic science and clinical practice of ophthalmology and of keeping ophthalmologists current with new developments in the various subspecialties.

The BCSC incorporates the effort and expertise of more than 80 ophthalmologists, organized into 13 Section faculties, working with Academy editorial staff. In addition, the course continues to benefit from many lasting contributions made by the faculties of previous editions. Members of the Academy's Practicing Ophthalmologists Advisory Committee for Education serve on each faculty and, as a group, review every volume before and after major revisions.

Organization of the Course

The Basic and Clinical Science Course comprises 13 volumes, incorporating fundamental ophthalmic knowledge, subspecialty areas, and special topics:

1 Update on General Medicine
2 Fundamentals and Principles of Ophthalmology
3 Clinical Optics
4 Ophthalmic Pathology and Intraocular Tumors
5 Neuro-Ophthalmology
6 Pediatric Ophthalmology and Strabismus
7 Orbit, Eyelids, and Lacrimal System
8 External Disease and Cornea
9 Intraocular Inflammation and Uveitis
10 Glaucoma
11 Lens and Cataract
12 Retina and Vitreous
13 Refractive Surgery

In addition, a comprehensive Master Index allows the reader to easily locate subjects throughout the entire series.

References

Readers who wish to explore specific topics in greater detail may consult the references cited within each chapter and listed in the Basic Texts section at the back of the book. These references are intended to be selective rather than exhaustive, chosen by the BCSC faculty as being important, current, and readily available to residents and practitioners.

Related Academy educational materials are also listed in the appropriate sections. They include books, online and audiovisual materials, self-assessment programs, clinical modules, and interactive programs.

Study Questions and CME Credit

Each volume of the BCSC is designed as an independent study activity for ophthalmology residents and practitioners. The learning objectives for this volume are given on page 1. The text, illustrations, and references provide the information necessary to achieve the objectives; the study questions allow readers to test their understanding of the material and their mastery of the objectives. Physicians who wish to claim CME credit for this educational activity may do so by mail, by fax, or online. The necessary forms and instructions are given at the end of the book.

Conclusion

The Basic and Clinical Science Course has expanded greatly over the years, with the addition of much new text and numerous illustrations. Recent editions have sought to place a greater emphasis on clinical applicability while maintaining a solid foundation in basic science. As with any educational program, it reflects the experience of its authors. As its faculties change and as medicine progresses, new viewpoints are always emerging on controversial subjects and techniques. Not all alternate approaches can be included in this series; as with any educational endeavor, the learner should seek additional sources, including such carefully balanced opinions as the Academy's Preferred Practice Patterns.

The BCSC faculty and staff are continuously striving to improve the educational usefulness of the course; you, the reader, can contribute to this ongoing process. If you have any suggestions or questions about the series, please do not hesitate to contact the faculty or the editors.

The authors, editors, and reviewers hope that your study of the BCSC will be of lasting value and that each Section will serve as a practical resource for quality patient care.

Objectives

Upon completion of BCSC Section 5, *Neuro-Ophthalmology*, the reader should be able to

- describe a symptom-driven approach to patients with common neuro-ophthalmic complaints in order to formulate an appropriate differential diagnosis

- select the most appropriate tests and imaging, based on symptomatology, to diagnose and manage neuro-ophthalmic disorders in a cost-effective manner

- review anatomical structures relevant to the neuro-ophthalmologist (including the skull and orbit, brain, vascular system, and cranial nerves) in order to localize lesions

- assess eye movement disorders and the ocular motor system

- describe the association between pupil and eyelid position and ocular motor pathology

- review the pathophysiology and management of diplopia and central eye movement disorders

- identify the effects of systemic disorders on visual and ocular motor pathways

- explain the possible systemic significance of ophthalmic disorders

Introduction

The Basic and Clinical Science Course has undergone continuous evolution since its inception. These volumes originated as a topic outline with suggested reading lists, including primary and secondary sources for each topic. In recent years, the books have grown into far more detailed reviews of each of the ophthalmic subspecialties, taking on many of the attributes of textbooks.

Section 5, *Neuro-Ophthalmology,* has likewise evolved. With the revision published in 2001, we introduced a relatively major change in format. To increase clinical relevance, the text was reorganized to take a symptom-driven approach, focusing on how to approach patients with neuro-ophthalmic complaints. The emphasis here is on the examination—both basic and extended—and the appropriate use of adjunctive studies to determine the status of the visual system as a whole. With this edition, we have simplified some of the diagnostic approaches, revised much of the illustrative material, and updated references.

This book is in no way comprehensive; thus, we have included a list of some of the more useful secondary sources of information, as well as references with primary source material. We have endeavored to make this book more readable as well as clinically relevant and hope that it will help to instill confidence in approaching patients with common clinical neuro-ophthalmic problems.

In several chapters throughout the book, you will see links to the NOVEL (Neuro-Ophthalmology Virtual Education Library) website of NANOS (Neuro-Ophthalmology Society of North America). This is a web-accessible collection of images, video, lectures, and other digital media, containing open-access, copyrighted resources. Once you have accessed the collections, you can navigate through to the relevant resource. See the website for more information: http://library.med.utah.edu/NOVEL/.

CHAPTER 1

Neuro-Ophthalmic Anatomy

Medicine in general and surgical subspecialties in particular are exercises in applied anatomy. Although an adequate understanding of physiology and, increasingly, molecular genetics is important in understanding disease and potential treatments, anatomy is the foundation. Important anatomical topics for the neuro-ophthalmologist include the anatomy of the globe (both the anterior and posterior segments), the orbit and adnexal structures, and the afferent and efferent visual pathways with their intracranial projections. The anatomy of the globe and adnexal structures is covered in more detail in BCSC Section 2, *Fundamentals and Principles of Ophthalmology,* Section 7, *Orbit, Eyelids, and Lacrimal System,* and Section 8, *External Disease and Cornea.* The material in this book is not intended to substitute for detailed anatomy texts; rather, it focuses on tracing the important anatomical connections that underlie visual function. Accordingly, we outline the intracranial pathways subserving the afferent and efferent visual pathways. We also briefly discuss the sensory and motor anatomy of the face and the autonomic nervous system as it applies to the eye and visual system.

Bony Anatomy

Skull Base

Understanding the anatomy of the visual pathways should start with the bony anatomy of the head. The skull base in particular has an intimate relationship with visually critical structures (Fig 1-1). The *sella turcica,* located posterior and medial to the 2 orbits, is a skull-based depression within the body of the *sphenoid bone.* The orbit (discussed in the following section) is connected posteriorly to the parasellar region and makes up the anterior aspect of the skull; it is composed of 7 craniofacial bones (Fig 1-2):

1. maxilla
2. zygomatic
3. frontal
4. lacrimal
5. sphenoid
6. palatine
7. ethmoid

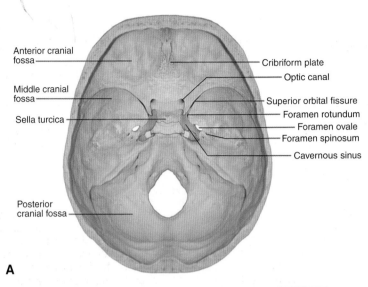

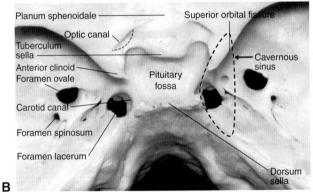

Figure 1-1 Bony anatomy of the skull base. **A,** General view of the skull base. The cavernous sinuses are located on each side of the sella turcica. Several important openings to be aware of within the skull base are the cribriform plate (transmits branches of the olfactory nerve, CN I), optic canal (transmits the optic nerve, CN II), foramen ovale (transmits the mandibular division [V₃] of the trigeminal nerve, CN V), foramen rotundum (transmits the maxillary division [V₂] of CN V), superior orbital fissure (transmits the oculomotor, CN III; trochlear, CN IV; abducens, CN VI; and CN V [ophthalmic division, V₁]), and the foramen spinosum (transmits the middle meningeal artery, a branch of the external carotid artery). **B,** View of the parasellar bony anatomy demonstrates the relationship of the pituitary fossa to the cavernous sinus, including the foramina of the skull base. The foramen lacerum is filled with cartilage and contains the artery of pterygoid canal, nerve of pterygoid canal, and venous drainage structures. The carotid artery enters the skull base through the carotid canal. *(Courtesy of Albert L. Rhoton, Jr, MD.)*

The lesser wing of the sphenoid bone is pierced by the *optic canals,* which allow the optic nerves to exit from the orbit. The *superior orbital fissure,* which transmits the ocular motor nerves (CNs III, IV, and VI), the sensory trigeminal nerve (CN V₁), the sympathetic fibers, and the superior ophthalmic vein (Fig 1-3), represents the gap between the lesser and greater wings of the sphenoid. The parasellar region is connected laterally to the

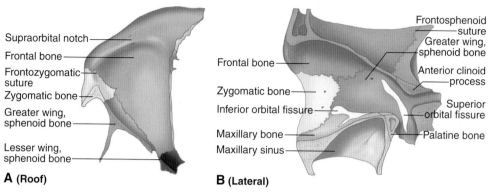

A (Roof)   **B (Lateral)**

Figure 1-2 Bony anatomy of the right orbit. **A,** The orbital roof is composed of the frontal bone and the lesser wing of the sphenoid bone. Laterally, the anterior orbital roof connects to the zygomatic bone at the frontozygomatic suture. The frontal sinus lies within the anterior orbital roof. The supraorbital notch, located within the medial one third of the superior orbital rim, transmits the supraorbital nerve, a terminal branch of the frontal nerve of the ophthalmic division (V_1) of CN V. Posteriorly, the orbital roof becomes the anterior clinoid process, which lies just temporal to the intracranial entrance of the optic canal. The vast majority of the roof is formed by the frontal bone. Medially, the frontal bone forms the roof of the ethmoidal sinus and extends to the cribriform plate. **B,** The lateral orbital wall is formed by the zygomatic bone and the greater wing of the sphenoid bone. The junction between the lateral orbital wall and the roof is represented by the frontosphenoid suture. Posteriorly, the wall is bordered by the inferior and superior orbital fissures. The sphenoid wing makes up the posterior portion of the lateral wall and separates the orbit from the middle cranial fossa. Medially, the lateral orbital wall ends at the inferior and superior orbital fissures. Two small openings within the zygomatic bone of the lateral orbital wall allow the exit of the zygomaticotemporal and zygomaticofacial nerves (branches of the zygomatic nerve), which innervate the lateral orbit and zygomatic prominence.

(continued)

petrous and *temporal bones* and inferiorly to the *clivus*, extending to the *foramen magnum* and the exit of the spinal cord. The posterior skull base is enclosed by the *occipital bones.*

The skull base is connected to the lower facial skeleton by 3 sets of pillars formed by the *maxillary* and *zygomatic bones* anteriorly and the *pterygoid process* of the sphenoid bone posteriorly. Superiorly, the vault of the skull is made up of the *parietal bones,* which meet at the *sagittal suture* and adjoining the *frontal bone* at the *coronal suture,* and the occipital bone at the *lambdoid suture.*

The Orbit

The orbit is surrounded by several important structures. The 4 *paranasal sinuses* surround the floor *(maxillary sinus)* and the medial wall *(ethmoidal and sphenoid sinuses)* of the orbit (Fig 1-4). The *frontal sinus* has a variable relationship to the anterior orbital roof. The other major structures around the orbit are the *anterior cranial fossa* superiorly (containing the frontal lobe) and the *temporal fossa* laterally (containing the temporalis muscle). The roof of the *ethmoidal complex,* delineated by the *frontal ethmoidal suture* (top of the ethmoidal bone, or *lamina papyracea*), marks the inferior boundary of the anterior cranial

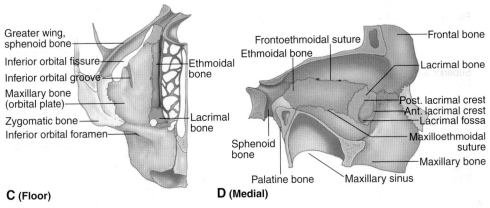

Figure 1-2 C, The orbital floor is triangular in shape and slopes slightly upward as it extends posteriorly and medially toward the inferior orbital fissure and medial orbital wall, respectively. The floor is composed mainly of the orbital plate of the maxillary bone but also of the maxillary process of the zygomatic bone, as well as a small area, posteriorly, of the palatine bone. The inferior orbital nerve, a branch of the maxillary division (V₂) of CN V, enters the orbit through the inferior orbital fissure and into the inferior orbital groove. Once in the groove, the nerve travels medially to laterally through a canal to exit the facial skeleton via the inferior orbital foramen. The nasolacrimal duct sits in the anterior middle area of the orbital floor, medial to the origin of the inferior oblique muscle. The duct then travels within a canal bounded by the maxillary and ethmoidal bones and runs in front of the middle turbinate and medial wall of the ethmoidal air cells to empty tears into the inferior meatus 30–35 mm posterior to the nares. **D,** The medial orbital wall is formed by 4 bones: maxilla (frontal process), lacrimal, sphenoid, and ethmoid. The largest component of the medial wall is the lamina papyracea of the ethmoidal bone. Superiorly, the anterior and posterior foramina at the level of the frontoethmoidal suture transmit the anterior and posterior ethmoidal arteries, respectively. This important transition area between the ethmoidal and frontal bones also represents the roof of the ethmoidal air cells and anterior cranial fossa (frontal lobe of the brain). Inferiorly, the medial orbital wall is bordered by the maxilloethmoidal suture line. The anterior medial orbital wall includes the frontal process of the maxillary bone and lacrimal sac fossa, which is formed by both the maxillary and lacrimal bones. The lacrimal bone is divided by the posterior lacrimal crest. The anterior part of the lacrimal sac fossa is formed by the anterior lacrimal crest of the maxillary bone. The posterior medial orbital wall, which comprises the sphenoid bone, continues to below the optic canal. *(Illustration by Dave Peace.)*

fossa. It is important to note that surgical intervention—for example, during endoscopic sinus surgery—above this anatomical landmark will result in entrance to the anterior cranial fossa and a likely cerebrospinal fluid (CSF) leak.

The sphenoid sinus forms the medial wall of the optic canal (Fig 1-5). Surgery within the sphenoid sinus has the potential to damage the optic nerve; alternatively, the sphenoid sinus is a surgical route facilitating decompression of the chiasm. In approximately 4% of patients, the bone may be incomplete, leaving only mucosa separating the sinus from the optic nerve. The *pterygomaxillary area*, which contains the sphenopalatine ganglion and the internal maxillary artery, underlies the apex of the orbit. This area communicates posteriorly through the *foramen rotundum* and the *vidian canal* to the *middle cranial fossa*, anteriorly through the *infraorbital canal* to the cheek and lower eyelid, and superiorly through the *inferior orbital fissure* to the orbit.

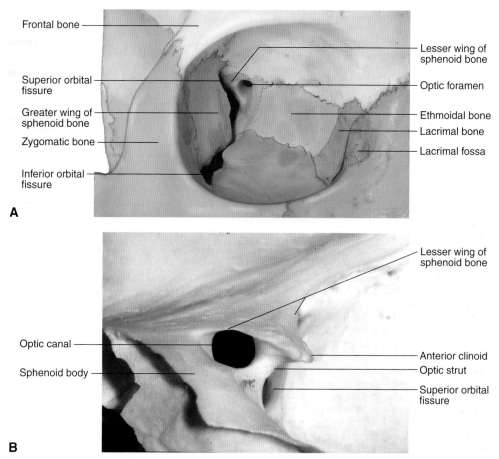

Figure 1-3 A, Bony anatomy of the right orbital apex. The optic foramen transmits the optic nerve, ophthalmic artery, and oculosympathetic nerves. The superior orbital fissure, a gap between the greater and lesser wings of the sphenoid bones, transmits CNs III, IV, VI, V_1, and the superior ophthalmic vein. **B,** Intracranial view of the left optic canal. Within the lesser wing of the sphenoid bone is the optic foramen, which leads to the optic canal. The optic strut separates the optic canal from the superior orbital fissure.

(continued)

The orbit is approximately 45 mm wide and 35 mm in maximal height. The total volume of the orbit is approximately 30 cm³. The medial wall is approximately 40 mm from the rim to the optic canal. The medial walls are roughly parallel, whereas the lateral walls form an angle of almost 90°. The orbital rim is made up of the frontal bone superiorly, which connects to the zygomatic bone (at the *frontozygomatic suture*) laterally. The inferior orbital rim is made up of the zygomatic bone inferolaterally and the maxillary bone inferonasally (meeting at the *zygomaticomaxillary suture*). Medially, the orbital rim consists of the maxillary and *lacrimal bones,* which join the frontal bone superiorly. Three additional bones contribute to the orbit: the *ethmoidal bone* medially, the *palatine bone*

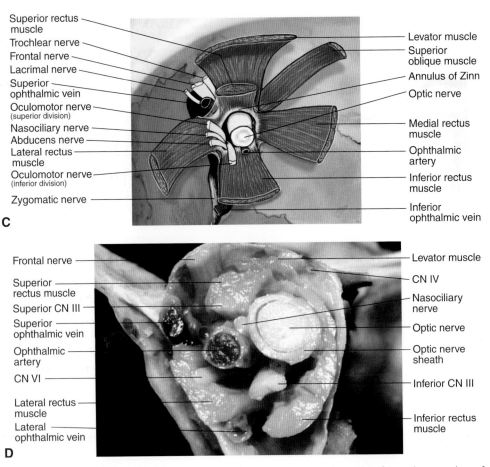

Superior rectus muscle
Trochlear nerve
Frontal nerve
Lacrimal nerve
Superior ophthalmic vein
Oculomotor nerve (superior division)
Nasociliary nerve
Abducens nerve
Lateral rectus muscle
Oculomotor nerve (inferior division)
Zygomatic nerve

Levator muscle
Superior oblique muscle
Annulus of Zinn
Optic nerve
Medial rectus muscle
Ophthalmic artery
Inferior rectus muscle
Inferior ophthalmic vein

C

Frontal nerve
Superior rectus muscle
Superior CN III
Superior ophthalmic vein
Ophthalmic artery
CN VI
Lateral rectus muscle
Lateral ophthalmic vein

Levator muscle
CN IV
Nasociliary nerve
Optic nerve
Optic nerve sheath
Inferior CN III
Inferior rectus muscle

D

Figure 1-3 **C,** Anatomy of the orbital apex. The 4 rectus muscles arise from the annulus of Zinn. CNs II, III (superior and inferior branches), VI, and the nasociliary nerve all course through the annulus of Zinn. CN IV and the frontal and lacrimal nerves and the ophthalmic veins are located outside the annulus. **D,** Anatomical dissection just anterior to the superior orbital fissure. *(Parts A and C illustrations by Dave Peace; parts B and D courtesy of Albert L. Rhoton, Jr, MD.)*

inferiorly in the posterior orbit, and the sphenoid bone laterally and superiorly in the orbital apex (see Fig 1-2).

Canals and fissures

The orbit communicates with the surrounding areas through several bony canals and fissures. Posteriorly, the orbit is contiguous with the *cavernous sinus* through the superior orbital fissure, which transmits the ocular motor nerves (CNs III, IV, and VI), the trigeminal nerve (V_1), and the orbital venous drainage via the superior ophthalmic vein (see Fig 1-3). The medial wall of the orbit continues as the lateral wall of the sphenoid bone, marking the medial extent of the cavernous sinus. Therefore, when sharp objects enter the medial orbit, they are directed through the superior orbital fissure, where they can lacerate the carotid artery.

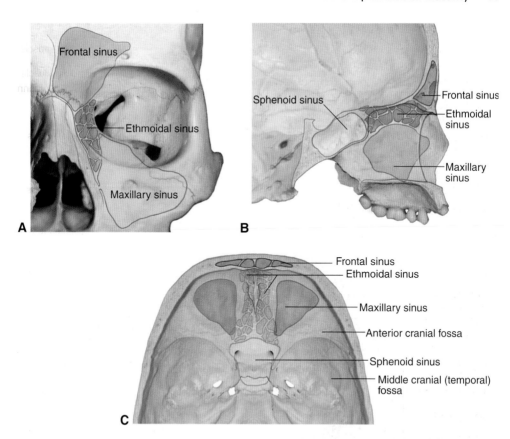

Figure 1-4 Coronal **(A)**, sagittal **(B)**, and axial **(C)** views of the anatomical relationship of the 4 paranasal sinuses to the orbit. *(Illustration by Dave Peace.)*

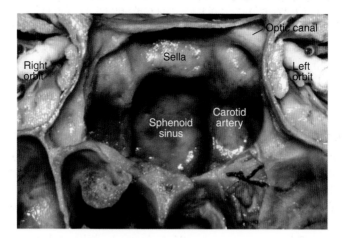

Figure 1-5 Coronal section, anterior view into the sphenoid sinus demonstrating the relationship of the internal carotid artery and optic nerve within the lateral wall of the sinus. *(Courtesy of Albert L. Rhoton, Jr, MD.)*

The orbit is connected superiorly and posteriorly to the anterior cranial fossa by way of the optic canal (see Fig 1-3B), which transmits the optic nerve, ophthalmic artery, and sympathetic fibers. Inferiorly at the apex, the orbit is connected to the *pterygopalatine area*—and thus the temporal and inferotemporal regions—through the inferior orbital fissure. This fissure, formed by the greater wing of the sphenoid, maxillary, zygomatic, and palatine bones, carries the maxillary nerve (V_2), infraorbital vessels, the inferior ophthalmic vein, branches from the pterygopalatine ganglion, parasympathetic fibers that innervate the lacrimal gland, and collateral meningeal arteries that help connect the external and internal carotid circulation.

Anteriorly, the orbit connects to the *inferior meatus* of the nose (beneath the inferior turbinate) through the *nasolacrimal duct,* which carries tears to the nose. In addition, multiple variable bony canals carry blood vessels that travel to and from the orbit and surrounding structures. Some of the most constant of these canals include the *anterior* and *posterior ethmoidal foramina,* which carry blood vessels connecting the internal carotid circulation (ophthalmic artery) to the external carotid (terminal branches of the ethmoidal arteries) at the level of the roof of the ethmoidal complex. Additional supraorbital and *zygomaticotemporal foramina* carry blood vessels between the orbit and corresponding vessels of the forehead and temple.

Dutton JJ. *Atlas of Clinical and Surgical Orbital Anatomy.* Philadelphia: Saunders; 1994.

Rhoton AL, Natori Y. *The Orbit and Sellar Region: Microsurgical Anatomy and Operative Approaches.* New York: Thieme; 1996.

Zide BM, Jelks GW. *Surgical Anatomy of the Orbit.* New York: Raven; 1985.

Vascular Anatomy

Arterial System

Knowledge of the vascular anatomy of the head is critical to understanding the potential for ischemic damage to the visual system. Such ischemic damage is one of the most common pathophysiologic causes of visual dysfunction (including visual loss and double vision). The common *carotid arteries,* arising from the *innominate artery* on the right and directly from the aorta on the left, supply most of the blood to the skull and its contents. The remainder comes from the 2 vertebral arteries, which enter the skull through the foramen magnum after traversing foramina in the cervical vertebral segments. Once the vertebral arteries penetrate the dura, they join near the pontomedullary junction to form the *basilar artery,* which ascends along the anterior surface of the pons to terminate in the *posterior cerebral arteries* at the level of the midbrain.

The carotid artery divides into internal and external branches at the C2 level near the angle of the jaw (Fig 1-6). The *external carotid artery (ECA)* supplies blood to the face through its major branches of the *facial artery.* The scalp is supplied via branches of the *occipital artery* posteriorly and the *superficial temporal artery* anteriorly. The paranasal sinuses receive their blood supply from branches of the *maxillary artery* (sphenopalatine, infraorbital), which terminates in the pterygopalatine fossa. The coverings of the brain are supplied by branches of the middle *meningeal artery*—a major branch of the maxillary

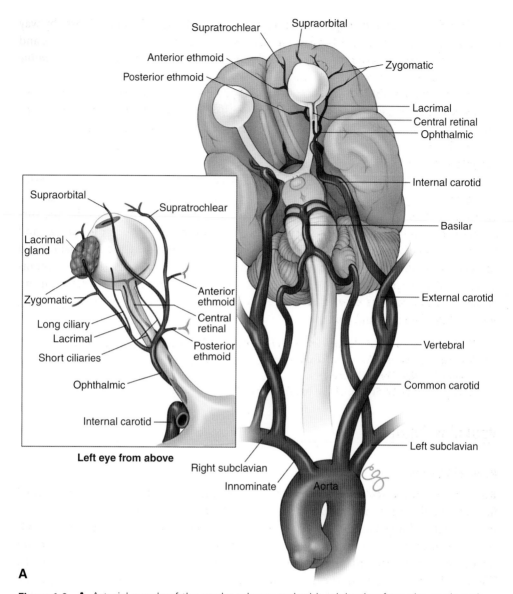

A

Figure 1-6 **A,** Arterial supply of the ocular adnexa and orbit originating from the aortic arch.

(continued)

artery—which enters the middle cranial fossa through the foramen spinosum, lateral to the foramen ovale. Branches of the middle meningeal artery supply the parasellar area, including the lateral wall of the cavernous sinus (containing CNs III, IV, and VI), and terminate in the arteries of the foramen rotundum and ovale. Variable meningeal branches may enter the superior orbital fissure.

Ophthalmologists are sometimes concerned about encountering branches of the ECA, particularly when performing a temporal artery biopsy or during orbital (ethmoidal

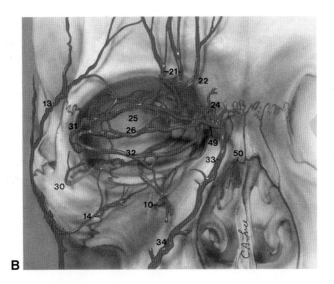

B

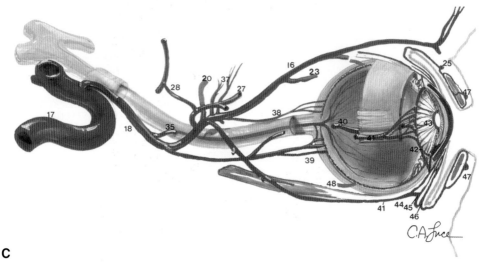

C

Figure 1-6 B, Anterior view of the superficial arterial supply to the eyelids and anterior orbit. **C,** The ophthalmic artery and its branches in the muscle cone. **Key:** *10,* infraorbital; *13,* superficial temporal artery; *14,* transverse facial; *16,* frontal branch; *17,* internal carotid artery; *18,* ophthalmic; *20,* posterior ethmoidal branch of ophthalmic; *21,* supraorbital artery; *22,* supratrochlear; *23,* anterior ethmoidal branch of ophthalmic; *24,* infratrochlear; *25,* superior peripheral arcade; *26,* superior marginal arcade; *27,* lacrimal; *28,* recurrent meningeal; *30,* zygomaticofacial; *31,* lateral palpebral; *32,* inferior marginal arcade; *33,* angular; *34,* facial; *35,* central retinal; *37,* muscular branches (SR, SO, levator); *38,* medial posterior ciliary; *39,* short ciliary; *40,* long ciliary; *41,* anterior ciliary; *42,* greater circle of the iris; *43,* lesser circle of the iris; *44,* episcleral; *45,* subconjunctival; *46,* conjunctival; *47,* marginal arcade; *48,* vortex vein; *49,* medial palpebral; *50,* dorsal nasal. *(Part A illustration by Christine Gralapp; parts B and C reproduced with permission from Zide BM, Jelks GW. Surgical Anatomy of the Orbit. New York: Raven; 1985.)*

branches) or lacrimal surgery. Terminal branches of the facial artery supply the marginal arcades of the eyelids. With regard to the ECA, it is extremely important to understand the extent of the collateral connections between the external and internal circulations (Fig 1-7). This point is particularly critical to interventional neuroradiologists, who may inadvertently embolize distal *internal carotid artery (ICA)* branches—including the *central retinal artery*—while placing particles into the ECA. This event is most likely in the treatment of arteriovenous malformations, but it can also occur when tumors of the skull base are being embolized prior to surgical resection.

The most important collaterals between the internal and external circulations traverse the orbit. They include the *anterior* and *posterior ethmoidal arteries* in the medial

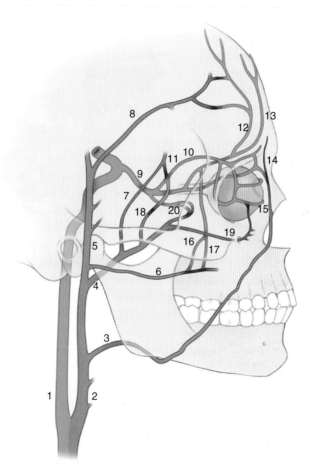

Figure 1-7 Internal carotid artery and external carotid artery collateral anatomy. **Key:** *1,* internal carotid; *2,* external carotid; *3,* facial; *4,* maxillary; *5,* superficial temporal; *6,* transverse facial; *7,* middle meningeal; *8,* frontal branch of superficial temporal; *9,* ophthalmic; *10,* lacrimal; *11,* recurrent meningeal; *12,* supraorbital; *13,* supratrochlear; *14,* angular; *15,* palpebral; *16,* zygomaticotemporal; *17,* zygomaticofacial; *18,* deep temporal; *19,* infraorbital; *20,* muscular.
(Modified with permission from Kline LB. Neuro-Ophthalmology Review Manual. *6th ed. Thorofare, NJ: Slack; 2008:213, by Christine Gralapp.)*

orbit, the *infraorbital* and *supraorbital arteries* (including distal connections to the lacrimal artery) anteriorly, and the zygomaticotemporal branch laterally. The facial arteries join distal branches of the *supra-* and *infratrochlear arteries* around the *angular artery* in the area of the medial orbit. In addition, variable collateral dural branches traverse the superior and inferior orbital fissures. In rare instances, the *ophthalmic artery* may also arise as a branch off the meningeal system and thus the ECA.

The major blood supply to the head and certainly to the intracranial contents is carried by the internal carotid arteries (Fig 1-8). They enter the bone at the base of the skull laterally in the petrous portion of the temporal bone running anteromedially. Within the petrous bone, the carotid is in close proximity to the middle and inner ear, as well as the intrapetrosal portion of the facial nerve. The carotid is also paralleled superficially by the *greater superficial petrosal nerve*, which supplies the parasympathetic fibers to the lacrimal gland. As the carotid reaches the parasellar area, it turns superiorly just above the foramen lacerum. Sympathetic fibers that continue within the intrapetrous carotid sheath exit to run through the vidian canal to reach the pterygomaxillary area. The carotid then enters the cavernous sinus, where it first gives off the *meningohypophyseal trunk* and then turns anteriorly to run horizontally parallel to the body of the sphenoid. The meningohypophyseal trunk subsequently divides into the *inferior hypophyseal artery* of the tentorium (the *artery of Bernasconi-Cassinari*), and the *dorsal meningeal artery* (extending to the tip of the petrous bone and clivus). These arteries supply the dura at the back of the cavernous sinus and the nerves entering the cavernous sinus (CNs III, IV, V, and VI). They also variably supply the lateral aspect of the sella turcica, including the pituitary capsule and a large portion of the gland itself. More anteriorly along the horizontal course of the carotid artery within the cavernous sinus, the *inferolateral trunk* supplies the cranial nerves before they enter the superior orbital fissure and forms anastomoses with branches of the middle meningeal artery.

At the anterior aspect of the cavernous sinus, the carotid makes a loop to reverse its direction under the anterior clinoid and the optic nerve, which is exiting the optic canal. This loop of the carotid passes through 2 dural rings, both in relationship to the anterior clinoid (the terminal portion of the lesser wing of the sphenoid). As the carotid passes through the second ring, it becomes intradural (Fig 1-9). Just after the artery becomes intradural, the carotid gives off the ophthalmic artery, which enters the orbit along with the optic nerve through the optic canal.

Within the orbit, the ophthalmic artery (see Fig 1-6) may anastomose with recurrent meningeal branches that enter through the superior orbital fissure. The ophthalmic artery gives off the central retinal artery. The central retinal artery enters the substance of the optic nerve approximately 10–12 mm posterior to the globe. Within the eye, the central retinal artery divides into superior and inferior arcades. Like vessels within the central nervous system, these arteries and arterioles have tight junctions that form a blood–retina barrier, similar to the blood–brain barrier. The intraretinal arterioles run within the substance of the nerve fiber layer to supply the inner two thirds of the retina. Capillaries run in 4 planes, bracketing the inner nuclear layer (bipolar cells) and the ganglion cells.

The *lacrimal artery* runs parallel to the lacrimal branch of V_1 in the superior lateral orbital roof to reach the lacrimal gland. It also gives off a branch that forms the *anterior*

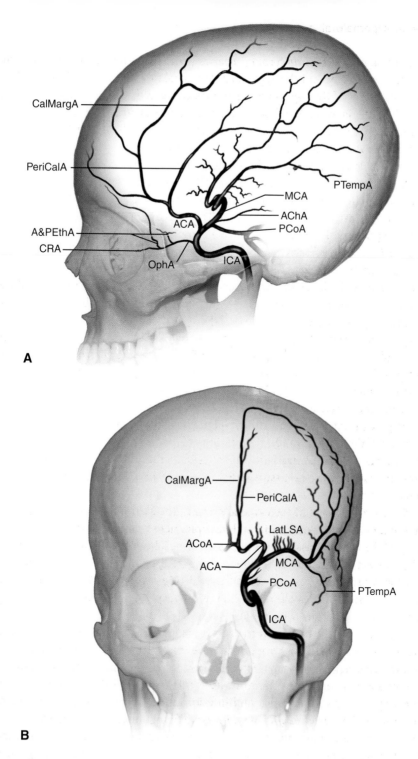

Figure 1-8 Branches of the internal carotid artery *(ICA)*. **A,** Lateral view. **B,** Anteroposterior view. Proximal ICA branches: ophthalmic artery *(OphA)* and its branches (anterior and posterior ethmoidal arteries *[A&PEthA]* and central retinal artery *[CRA]*); posterior communicating artery *(PCoA)*; anterior choroidal artery *(AChA)*; anterior communicating artery *(ACoA)*; anterior cerebral artery *(ACA)* and its branches (callosomarginal artery *[CalMargA]* and pericallosal artery *[PeriCalA]*); middle cerebral artery *(MCA)* and its branches (lateral lenticulostriate *[LatLSA]* and posterior temporal artery *[PTempA]*). *(Illustration by Dave Peace.)*

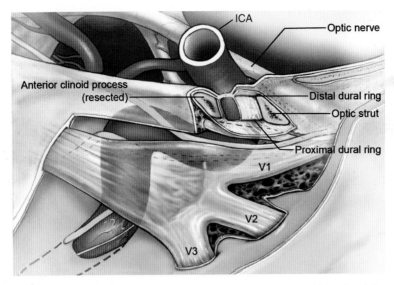

Figure 1-9 Lateral view of the bend of the internal carotid artery within the right cavernous sinus. The anterior clinoid process has been resected to show the proximal and distal dural rings. *(Illustration by Dave Peace.)*

ciliary artery of the lateral rectus muscle and reaches the anterior segment at the muscle's insertion. The *frontal artery* runs within the superior orbit, paralleling the frontal branch of V_1 to branch and terminate as the supraorbital and supratrochlear arteries, which, along with the lacrimal artery, supply the eyelid.

The next branches leaving the ophthalmic artery are the *superior* and *inferior muscular arteries.* They supply the anterior ciliary arteries of the medial and inferior rectus (inferior muscular artery) and the superior rectus and superior oblique (superior muscular branch). They enter the extraocular rectus muscles (usually 2 arterial branches within the medial, inferior, and superior rectus muscles) and supply the extraocular muscles and the anterior segment. They are responsible for the major blood flow to the ciliary body (producing aqueous). The *medial* and *lateral long posterior ciliary arteries* variably anastomose with penetrating branches of the anterior ciliary arteries (within the rectus muscles) to form the *greater arterial circle* near the anterior part of the ciliary body. Branches from this circle extend radially within the iris to form a second anastomotic circle (the *lesser arterial circle*) near the collarette of the iris.

The terminal ophthalmic artery supplies additional branches that collateralize with the *anterior* and *posterior ethmoidal arteries* and form the *short* (up to 20 small branches supplying the optic disc and posterior choroid) and *long posterior ciliary arteries* (running horizontally to help supply the anterior segment and the anterior choroid) (Fig 1-10). Together, these arteries supply blood to the choroid; the retinal pigment epithelium; and approximately one third of the outer retina, including the photoreceptors. In approximately 30% of individuals, branches of the posterior ciliary arteries directly supply a portion of the inner retina *(cilioretinal arteries)*; this blood supply may protect the macula in the setting of a central retinal artery occlusion. Approximately 4 short posterior ciliary arteries

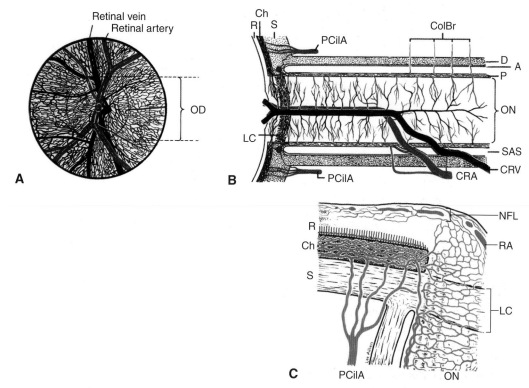

Figure 1-10 Schematic drawing of the vascular supply to the optic nerve and optic nerve head: Intraocular view **(A)**, lateral view **(B)**, and sagittal view **(C)** of optic nerve head. Short posterior ciliary arteries supply centripetal capillary beds of the anterior optic nerve head. The central retinal artery *(CRA)* contribution is restricted to nerve fiber layer capillaries and capillaries of the anterior intraorbital optic nerve. Capillary beds at all levels drain into the central retinal vein *(CRV)*. **Key:** *A*= arachnoid, *Ch* = choroid, *ColBr* = collateral branches, *D* = dura, *LC* = lamina cribrosa, *NFL* = surface nerve fiber layer of disc, *OD* = optic disc, *ON* = optic nerve, *P* = pia, *PCilA* = posterior ciliary artery, *R* = retina, *RA* = retinal arteriole, *S* = sclera, *SAS* = subarachnoid space. *(Reproduced from Hayreh SS. The blood supply of the optic nerve head and the evaluation of it—myth and reality. Prog Retin Eye Res. 2001;20(5):563–593.)*

form a variably complete anastomotic ring (known as the *circle of Zinn-Haller*) around the optic disc, which is also supplied from the peripapillary choroid and the terminal branches of the pial network.

Collateral branches from terminal branches of the infraorbital artery and the superficial temporal artery help to supply the lower and upper eyelids and may also provide collateral supply to the anterior segment. These collaterals may be interrupted if the conjunctiva and Tenon capsule are removed from the limbus during ocular surgery.

Distal to the origin of the ophthalmic artery, the intradural supraclinoid ICA gives off the *anterior choroidal artery* and anastomoses with the proximal *posterior cerebral artery* through the *posterior communicating arteries*. The anterior choroidal artery supplies blood to the optic tract and distally to the lateral geniculate (Fig 1-11). Injury to the anterior choroidal artery can produce the optic tract syndrome, consisting of contralateral

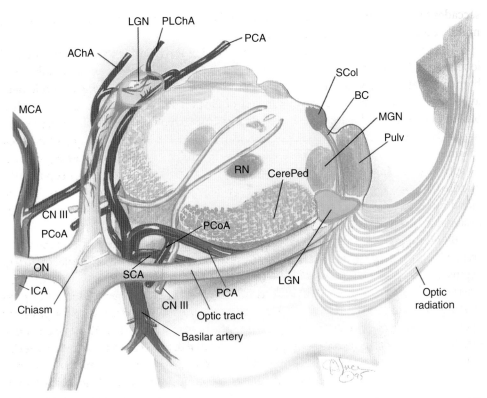

Figure 1-11 The relationship of the lateral geniculate nucleus to nearby structures and its blood supply. **Key:** *AChA* = anterior choroidal artery, *BC* = brachium conjunctivum, *CerePed* = cerebral peduncles, *ICA* = internal carotid artery, *LGN* = lateral geniculate nucleus, *MCA* = middle cerebral artery, *MGN* = medial geniculate nucleus, *ON* = optic nerve, *PCA* = posterior cerebral artery, *PCoA* = posterior communicating artery, *PLChA* = posterior lateral choroidal artery, *Pulv* = pulvinar, *RN* = red nucleus, *SCA* = superior cerebellar artery, *SCol* = superior colliculus. *(Illustration by Craig A. Luce.)*

homonymous hemianopia, contralateral band atrophy of the optic disc, and a contralateral relative afferent pupillary defect (see Chapter 4). The ICA gives off the *anterior cerebral artery* and terminates as branches of the *middle cerebral artery*. The proximal anterior cerebral arteries (A1 segment) cross over the optic nerves and join via the *anterior communicating artery*. The combination of the anterior and posterior communicating arteries makes up the *circle of Willis*, which permits collateral flow between the carotid and vertebrobasilar systems when there is vascular compromise. Small perforating branches arising from the proximal anterior cerebral artery (as well as the anterior communicating artery) supply the intracranial optic nerves and the chiasm. More distally, the anterior cerebral artery divides into frontal, frontopolar, paracallosal, and pericallosal branches. Although the afferent visual pathways are spared with distal anterior cerebral artery occlusion, the premotor areas of the frontal lobes responsible for initiating saccades are supplied by branches of the anterior cerebral artery. Thus, patients with acute occlusion of the anterior cerebral artery may have a transient gaze preference and difficulty initiating saccades to the contralateral side, although this is more commonly encountered following middle cerebral artery territory lesions.

The middle cerebral artery divides into several branches, which supply the temporal lobe, parietal lobe, and superficial portions of the frontal lobe and occipital lobe. The branches that are important to the visual pathways include those supplying the optic radiations as they traverse the deep white matter of the parietal and temporal lobes. Terminal branches of the middle cerebral artery also variably supply the occipital tip representing the macula. This supply is chiefly responsible for the perimetric finding of macular sparing in the setting of posterior cerebral or calcarine artery occlusion (see Fig 4-35, in Chapter 4). In addition to the afferent pathways, the middle cerebral artery supplies the middle temporal region, which is critical in visually guided pursuit movements. Lack of blood supply can thus cause problems with ipsilateral pursuit or asymmetry in optokinetic nystagmus (OKN) as the drum is rotated toward the side of the infarct.

Blood supply to the posterior aspect of the intracranial contents begins with the aortic arch. The *right vertebral artery* arises from the innominate artery; the *left vertebral artery* begins as a branch off the proximal *subclavian artery*. The vertebral arteries travel through a series of foramina in the lateral aspects of the cervical vertebral processes. After penetrating the dura at the foramen magnum, the vertebral arteries give rise to the *posterior inferior cerebellar artery* before joining to form the basilar artery (Fig 1-12). The posterior inferior cerebellar arteries represent the most caudal of the major circumferential arteries that wrap around the brainstem. Proximally, the posterior inferior cerebellar and basilar arteries first give off branches that perforate the medial portion of the brainstem at the medullary level; the paramedian branches that follow supply the lateral aspects of the brainstem. Distally, the posterior inferior cerebellar artery supplies the inferior cerebellum, including the flocculus and nodulus, which (together as the vestibulocerebellum) are intimately involved in eye movements. Vertebral artery or posterior inferior cerebellar artery occlusion is associated with Wallenberg lateral medullary syndrome, which manifests as ipsilateral Horner syndrome; skew deviation; CNs V, IX/X paresis; and contralateral body numbness (see Chapter 2, Fig 2-5). There is no extremity weakness with the syndrome.

The second set of circumferential arteries is the *anterior inferior cerebellar arteries*. These arteries arise from the caudal basilar artery and supply the area of the pontomedullary junction of the brainstem, as well as the cerebellum, distally. A large proximal branch of the anterior inferior cerebellar arteries, the *internal auditory artery*, supplies the CN VIII complex in the subarachnoid space and follows it into the internal auditory canal. Terminally, the internal auditory artery branches into the *anterior vestibular artery* (supplying the anterior and horizontal semicircular canals and the utricle), the *posterior vestibular artery* (supplying the posterior semicircular canal and the saccule plus part of the cochlea), and the *cochlear artery*.

Along the course of the basilar artery, small perforators arise directly to supply portions of the pons and midbrain. The branches off the basilar are divided into median or paramedian vessels and short circumferential branches. The median perforators are particularly important, as they supply the medial longitudinal fasciculus, the paramedian pontine formation, and the medially located nuclei of CNs III, IV, and VI. Interruption

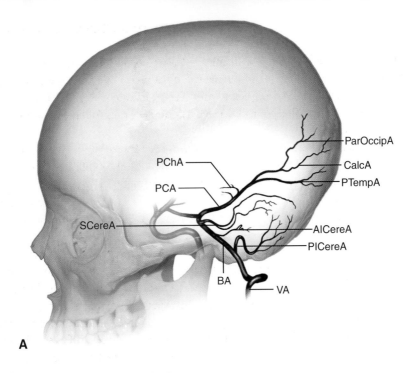

A

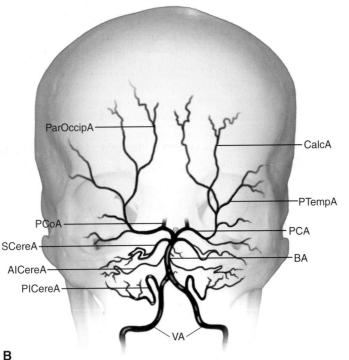

B

Figure 1-12 Vertebrobasilar arterial system and major arteries with common variations of the cortical branches of the posterior cerebral artery. **A,** Lateral view. **B,** Anteroposterior view. Vertebral artery *(VA)* and basilar artery *(BA)* branches: anterior inferior cerebellar artery *(AICereA)*, posterior inferior cerebellar artery *(PICereA)*, superior cerebellar artery *(SCereA)*. Posterior cerebral artery *(PCA)* and its branches: calcarine artery (CalcA), parieto-occipital artery *(ParOccipA)*, posterior choroidal artery *(PChA)*, posterior temporal *(PTempA)*, posterior communicating artery *(PCoA)*. *(Illustration by Dave Peace.)*

of these branches (which occurs commonly with vertebrobasilar atherosclerotic disease or emboli to these endarteries) often affects these pathways, producing variable ophthalmoplegia, internuclear ophthalmoplegia, and skew deviation. Pontine branches of the basilar artery also supply the proximal portions of the cranial nerves (particularly the trigeminal) as they exit.

The distal 2 sets of circumferential arteries consist of the *superior cerebellar arteries* followed by the posterior cerebral arteries, representing the terminal branches of the basilar artery at the level of the midbrain. Perforators from the proximal superior cerebellar arteries partially supply the third nerve nucleus and its fascicles. In addition, small branches often supply the trigeminal root. The tentorium, separating the posterior cranial fossa below, opens to pass the midbrain between these 2 arteries. The third nerve exits between the superior cerebellar arteries and the posterior cerebral arteries, where it may be compressed.

Proximally (P1 segment), perforators from the posterior cerebral arteries (including the median thalamostriate branches and the lateral choroidal arteries) supply rostral portions of the midbrain involved in vertical gaze and part of the lateral geniculate. A large branch, the *artery of Percheron,* often supplies both sides of the midbrain from 1 posterior cerebral artery. Because *thalamostriate arteries* originate from P1, infarcts related to the internal carotid–middle cerebral artery spare the thalamus. The P1 segment ends with the posterior communicating artery, which joins the vertebrobasilar circulation to the carotid anteriorly. The connecting artery parallels the course of CN III, which explains the high frequency of third nerve palsy with aneurysms of the posterior communicating artery (see Chapter 8). As the distal posterior cerebral artery courses around the brainstem, it gives off a *parieto-occipital branch* before terminating in the calcarine branch, which supplies the primary visual cortex (Fig 1-13).

Venous System

Although discussed less often, the venous system is also critical to normal functioning of the visual pathways. Ocular venous outflow begins in the *arcade retinal veins,* which exit into

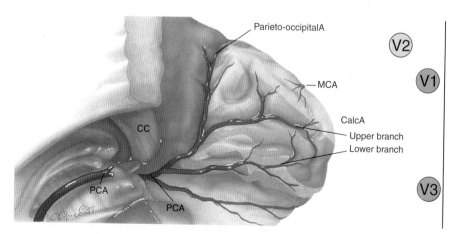

Figure 1-13 The occipital cortex and its blood supply. Areas V1, V2, and V3 keyed by color. *CalcA* = calcarine artery, *CC* = corpus callosum, *MCA* = middle cerebral artery, *PCA* = posterior cerebral artery. *(Illustration by Craig A. Luce.)*

the *central retinal vein* and in the *choroidal veins,* which exit the sclera through the *vortex veins.* Anteriorly, the episcleral venous plexus collects both blood from the anterior uveal circulation and aqueous percolating through the Schlemm canal. These 3 primary venous drainage pathways (Fig 1-14) empty mainly into the *superior ophthalmic vein,* which runs

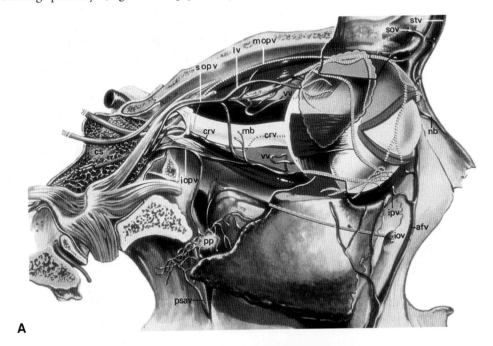

A

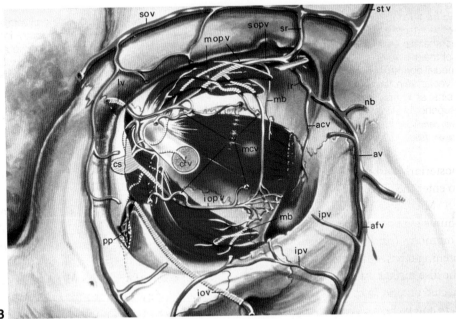

B

Figure 1-14 Venous drainage of the orbit. **A,** Lateral view of venous drainage of the orbit and adjacent plexus. **B,** Anterolateral view.

(continued)

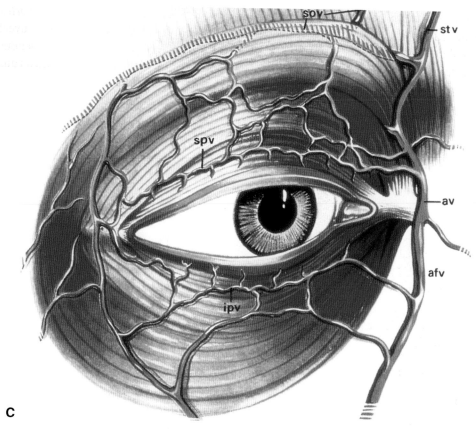

C

Figure 1-14   C, Superficial venous structures of the eyelid. **Key:** *acv* = anterior collateral vein, *afv* = anterior facial vein, *av* = angular vein, *crv* = central retinal vein, *cs* = cavernous sinus, *iopv* = inferior ophthalmic vein, *iov* = infraorbital vein, *ipv* = inferior palpebral vein, *ir* = inferior root of superior ophthalmic vein, *lv* = lacrimal vein, *mb* = muscular branch, *mcv* = medial collateral vein, *mopv* = medial ophthalmic vein, *nb* = nasal branch, *pp* = pterygoid venous plexus, *psav* = posterior superior alveolar vein, *sopv* = superior ophthalmic vein, *sov* = supraorbital vein, *spv* = superior palpebral veins, *sr* = superior root of superior ophthalmic vein, *stv* = supratrochlear vein, *vv* = vena vorticosa (superior lateral and medial vorticose veins; inferior lateral and medial vorticose veins). *(Reproduced with permission from Rootman J, Stewart B, Goldberg RA. Orbital Surgery: A Conceptual Approach. Philadelphia: Lippincott-Raven; 1995.)*

posteriorly within the superior medial orbit to the orbital apex, where it crosses laterally to enter the cavernous sinus posterior to the superior orbital fissure.

Microscopic collaterals variably exist between these venous beds. In rare instances, shunts connecting retinal veins to choroidal veins may be seen within the retina. More commonly (usually in association with central retinal vein occlusion or optic nerve sheath meningioma), optociliary shunt vessels (retinochoroidal collateral vessels) may appear on the disc surface. At a more macroscopic level, the superior ophthalmic vein is variably connected anteriorly to the *angular* and *facial veins* and inferiorly to the *inferior ophthalmic vein* and *pterygoid venous plexus*. These collaterals may become important, particularly in the setting of elevated venous pressure (usually related to a carotid cavernous fistula).

Intracranially, the superficial cortical venous system drains mainly superiorly and medially to the *superior sagittal sinus* running in the sagittal midline (Fig 1-15). In addition

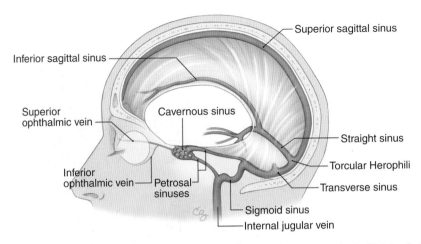

Figure 1-15 Illustration of the cerebral venous sinus system. *(Illustration by Christine Gralapp.)*

to the cortical drainage, the superior sagittal sinus absorbs CSF through the arachnoid villi and the pacchionian granulations. Thus, obstruction to venous outflow results in decreased CSF absorption and elevated intracranial pressure. The superior sagittal sinus runs posteriorly to terminate at the *torcular Herophili* (confluence of the venous sinuses) at the level of the tentorium separating the cerebellum from the occipital lobes. The *transverse sinuses* run anteriorly from the connection of the tentorium and the skull to the petrous pyramid, where they turn to run caudally as the *sigmoid sinus* down to the *jugular bulb,* where the *internal jugular vein* exits the skull.

Inferior superficial cortical venous drainage is carried directly down to the transverse and sigmoid sinuses through the *vein of Labbé* and the *basilar vein of Rosenthal.* The deep drainage of the supratentorial diencephalon and mesencephalon begins as deep draining veins (often in relationship to the ventricular system). These drain together to form the *vein of Galen,* which runs posteriorly to drain into the straight sinus. This runs within the tentorium to drain, along with the superior sagittal sinus, into the torcular Herophili.

Some anterior cerebral venous drainage may access the cavernous sinus. The 2 cavernous sinuses are joined by variable connections through the sella and posteriorly through a plexus of veins over the clivus. The cavernous sinus drains primarily caudally into the jugular bulb via the *inferior petrosal sinus,* which traverses the Dorello canal with CN VI under the petroclinoid ligament. Alternatively, drainage may be lateral along the petrous apex through the *superior petrosal sinus* to the junction of the transverse and sigmoid sinuses (Fig 1-16). Small veins may drain through the foramen rotundum and foramen ovale as well as through the pterygoid plexus to anastomose with the *facial venous system (external jugular vein).*

Veins of the eyelids anastomose medially between the *angular vein* and branches of the superior ophthalmic vein (particularly at the superior medial orbit in the region of the trochlea). Facial veins drain inferiorly and laterally to form the external jugular vein, which eventually joins the internal jugular in the neck.

Kupersmith MJ. *Neurovascular Neuro-Ophthalmology.* New York: Springer-Verlag; 1993.

Lasjaunias P, Berenstein A, ter Brugge KG. *Surgical Neuroangiography.* 2nd ed. Vol 1. *Clinical Vascular Anatomy and Variations.* New York: Springer; 2001.

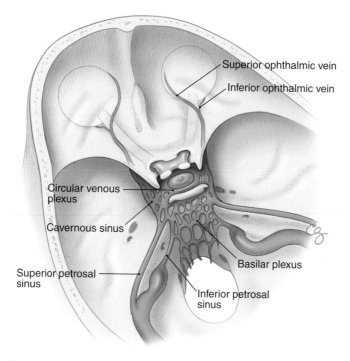

Figure 1-16 Anatomy of the cavernous sinus drainage system. *(Illustration by Christine Gralapp.)*

Nolte J. *The Human Brain: An Introduction to Its Functional Anatomy.* 5th ed. St Louis: Mosby; 2002.

Rootman J, Stewart B, Goldberg RA. *Orbital Surgery: A Conceptual Approach.* Philadelphia: Lippincott; 1995.

Afferent Visual Pathways

It is important to recognize that any disturbance in afferent function may result in the same complaints of visual loss seen with pathology affecting the retina, optic nerve, and visual pathways (Fig 1-17).

Retina

The posterior segment transduces the focused electromagnetic image photochemically into a series of impulses. (The anatomy of the retina is covered in more detail in BCSC Section 2, *Fundamentals and Principles of Ophthalmology,* and Section 12, *Retina and Vitreous.*) Photochemical transduction takes place within the outer segments of the rods (approximately 80–120 million, distributed uniformly over the retina except at the fovea) and cones (approximately 5–6 million, with a peak distribution at the fovea and approximately 50% within 30°). The absence of retinal receptors over the optic disc creates a *physiologic scotoma* (the *blind spot*), located approximately 17° from the fovea and measuring approximately 5° × 7°. Cones are divided into 3 subgroups according to the presence of

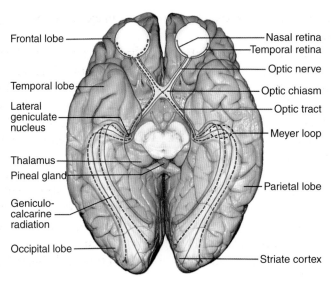

Frontal lobe

Nasal retina

Temporal retina

Optic nerve

Temporal lobe

Optic chiasm

Lateral geniculate nucleus

Optic tract

Meyer loop

Thalamus

Pineal gland

Geniculo-calcarine radiation

Parietal lobe

Occipital lobe

Striate cortex

Figure 1-17 Basal view of the brain showing the anterior and posterior visual pathways. *(Illustration by Dave Peace.)*

pigments, with peak sensitivity to red, green, or blue wavelengths. The blue cones (the smallest subpopulation) are, like the rods, absent at the fovea. The fovea (approximately 1.5 mm or 1 disc diameter) is located approximately 4 mm (or 2.5 disc diameters) from and 0.8 mm lower than the optic disc. The retina measures approximately 2500 mm² in surface area and is between 100 and 250 μm thick.

The choroid, the extremely vascular posterior extension of the uvea, lines the sclera and supports the single-cell-layer retinal pigment epithelium (RPE). The RPE is in direct contact with the retinal photoreceptors and is responsible for metabolic support as well as regeneration of the chromophore 11-*trans*-retinal to the *cis* form to restore receptor sensitivity. The impulses that make up the optical signal originate in the ganglion cells within the inner retina. Between the outer and inner retinal layers, the retinal signal starting in the rods and cones is processed primarily through the bipolar cells that connect the photoreceptors to the ganglion cells. Most ganglion cells can be subdivided into small *P cells* (*parvocellular,* accounting for 80%) and larger *M cells* (*magnocellular,* approximately 5%–10%). The P cells are concerned with color perception and have small receptor fields and low contrast sensitivity. The M cells have larger receptor fields and are more responsive to luminance contrast and motion. A newly described subset of retinal ganglion cells (RGCs) are melanopsin-containing, intrinsically photosensitive retinal ganglion cells (ipRGCs), which have very large receptive fields and project to extrastriate areas.

Horizontal, amacrine, and *interplexiform cells* (which communicate horizontally between neighboring cells) permit signal processing within the retinal layer. Physiologically, this processing includes the center-surround system that underlies response preferentially to dots of light, edges of light, oriented edges, and moving oriented edges at progressively more complicated levels of interaction. In addition, the color-opponent system (red and green, blue and "yellow") permits color appreciation across the visible spectrum. The glial support cells—*Müller cells* and *astrocytes*—also affect image processing and probably play a metabolic role as well.

One of the primary anatomical features of retinal organization in the primate is the variable ratio of photoreceptor cells to ganglion cells. The ratio is highest in the periphery (at more than 1000:1) and lowest at the fovea (where a ganglion cell may receive a signal from a single cone). This ratio underlies the increase in receptor field with increasing eccentricity and the maximal spatial resolution at the fovea. Ganglion cell density in the macula is approximately 60 times that in the periphery. This "central weighting" of neural tissue continues throughout the afferent visual system. In the cortex, the number of cells responding to foveal stimulation may be 1000 times the number associated with peripheral activity. Because of the increased density of ganglion cells centrally (69% within the central 30°), the bipolar cells are oriented radially within the macula. This radial arrangement of the axons of the bipolar cells (the *Henle layer*) is responsible for fluid accumulation in a star-shaped pattern. Multiple neurotransmitters are present in the retina, including primarily glutamate but also gamma-aminobutyric acid (GABA), acetylcholine, and dopamine.

The other critical anatomical feature of the retina is the location of the optic disc and the beginning of the optic nerve nasal to the fovea. Thus, although ganglion cell fibers coming from the nasal retina can travel uninterrupted directly to the disc, those coming from the temporal retina must avoid the macula by anatomically separating to enter the disc at either the superior or the inferior pole (Fig 1-18). This unique anatomy means that some of the nasal fibers (nasal within the macula) enter the disc on its temporal side *(papillomacular bundle)*. Focal loss of the nerve fiber layer may be seen as grooves or slits or as reflections paralleling the retinal arterioles where the internal limiting membrane drapes over the vessels, whereas diffuse nerve fiber layer loss is often more difficult to detect and brings the retinal vessels into sharp relief.

Optic Nerve

The optic nerve begins anatomically at the optic disc but physiologically and functionally within the ganglion cell layer that covers the entire retina. The first portion of the optic nerve, representing the confluence of approximately 1.0–1.2 million ganglion cell axons, traverses the sclera through the lamina cribrosa, which contains approximately 200–300 channels. The combination of small channels and a unique blood supply (largely from branches of the posterior ciliary arteries) probably plays a role in several optic neuropathies. The axons of the optic nerve depend on metabolic production within the ganglion cell bodies in the retina. Axonal transport—both anterograde and retrograde—of molecules, subcellular organelles, and metabolic products occurs along the length of the optic nerve and is an energy-dependent system requiring high concentrations of oxygen. The anterograde axonal transport system can be divided into slow, intermediate, and fast speeds. Components of the axonal cytoskeleton (microtubules, neurofilaments, and microfilaments) are important for slow and fast anterograde transport. Different motor proteins are needed for anterograde and retrograde axonal transport. The axonal transport system is sensitive to ischemic, inflammatory, and compressive processes. Interruption of axonal transport, from whatever cause, produces swelling, or disc edema, at the optic disc.

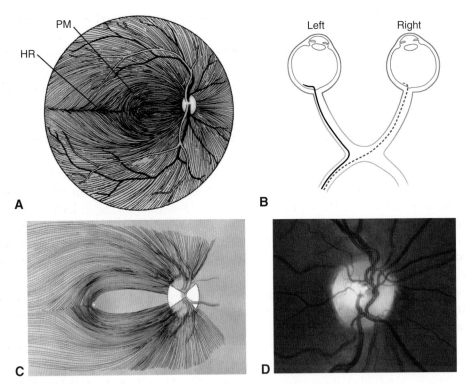

Figure 1-18 A, Pattern of the nerve fiber layer of axons from ganglion cells to the optic disc. Superior, inferior, and nasal fibers take a fairly straight course. Temporal axons originate above and below horizontal raphe *(HR)* and take an arching course to the disc. Axons arising from ganglion cells in the nasal macula project directly to the disc as the papillomacular bundle *(PM).* **B,** Lesions involving the decussating nasal retinal fibers, represented by the *dashed red line,* can result in bow-tie atrophy. **C,** Artist's schematic depiction of damage to nasal and macular fibers of the retina and patterns of nasal and temporal optic nerve atrophy (represented by *red outlined triangles)* corresponding to damage to crossing nasal fibers. Therefore, band, or bow-tie, atrophy occurs with loss of nasal macular and peripheral fibers in the contralateral eye of a patient with a pregeniculate homonymous hemianopia or a bitemporal hemianopia. **D,** Clinical photograph of a right optic nerve demonstrating bow-tie atrophy. *(Part A reprinted from Kline LB, Foroozan R, eds. Optic Nerve Disorders. 2nd ed. Ophthalmology Monograph 10. New York: Oxford University Press, in cooperation with the American Academy of Ophthalmology; 2007:5; part B illustration by Christine Gralapp; part C courtesy of Neil Miller, MD; part D courtesy of Lanning Kline, MD.)*

Just posterior to the sclera, the optic nerve acquires a dural sheath that is contiguous with the periorbita of the optic canal and an arachnoid membrane that supports and protects the axons and is contiguous with the arachnoid of the subdural intracranial space through the optic canal. This arrangement permits a free circulation of CSF around the optic nerve up to the optic disc. Just posterior to the lamina cribrosa, the optic nerve also acquires a myelin coating, which increases its diameter to approximately 3 mm (6 mm in diameter, including the optic nerve sheaths) from the 1.5 mm of the optic disc. The myelin investment is part of the membrane of oligodendrocytes that join the nerve posterior to the sclera.

The intraorbital optic nerve extends approximately 28 mm to the optic canal. The extra length of the intraorbital optic nerve allows unimpeded globe rotation as well as axial shifts within the orbit. The central retinal artery and vein travel within the anterior 10–12 mm of the optic nerve. The central retinal artery supplies only a minor portion of the optic nerve circulation; most of the blood supply comes from pial branches of the surrounding meninges, which is in turn supplied by small branches of the ophthalmic artery (see Fig 1-10). Topographic (retinotopic) representation is maintained throughout the optic nerve. Peripheral retinal receptors are found more peripherally, and the papillomacular bundle travels temporally and increasingly centrally within the nerve.

As the optic nerve enters the optic canal, the dural sheath fuses with the periorbita. It is also surrounded by the *annulus of Zinn,* which serves as the origin of the 4 rectus muscles and the superior oblique muscle. Within the canal, the optic nerve is accompanied by the ophthalmic artery inferiorly and separated from the superior orbital fissure by the optic strut (the lateral aspect of the lesser wing of the sphenoid), which terminates superiorly as the anterior clinoid. Medially, the optic nerve is separated from the sphenoid sinus by bone that may be thin or even dehiscent. The optic canal normally measures approximately 8–10 mm in length and 5–7 mm in width but may be elongated and narrowed by processes that cause bone thickening (fibrous dysplasia, intraosseous meningioma). The canal runs superiorly and medially. Within the canal, the optic nerve is relatively anchored and can easily be injured by shearing forces transmitted from blunt facial trauma (see Chapter 4).

At its intracranial passage, the optic nerve passes under a fold of dura (the falciform ligament) that may impinge on the nerve, especially if it is elevated by lesions arising from the bone of the sphenoid (tuberculum) or the sella. Once it becomes intracranial, the optic nerve no longer has a sheath. The anterior loop of the carotid artery usually lies just below and temporal to the nerve, and the proximal anterior cerebral artery passes over the nerve. The gyrus rectus, the most inferior portion of the frontal lobe, lies above and parallel to the optic nerves. The 8–12 mm intracranial portion of the optic nerve terminates in the optic chiasm.

Optic Chiasm

The optic chiasm measures approximately 12 mm wide, 8 mm long in the anteroposterior direction, and 4 mm thick (Fig 1-19). It is inclined at almost 45° and is supplied by small branches off the proximal anterior cerebral and anterior communicating arteries. The chiasm is located just anterior to the hypothalamus and the anterior third ventricle (forming part of its anterior wall and causing an invagination) and approximately 10 mm above the sella. The exact location of the chiasm with respect to the sella is variable. Most of the time it is directly superior, but in approximately 17% of individuals it is anterior (prefixed), and in approximately 4% it is posterior (postfixed) (Fig 1-20).

Within the chiasm, the fibers coming from the nasal retina (approximately 53% of total fibers) cross to the opposite side to join the corresponding contralateral fibers. The inferior fibers (subserving the superior visual field) are first to cross. Evidence suggests that the anterior loop of fibers into the contralateral optic nerve (Wilbrand knee) may be an artifact; however, the finding of a superior temporal visual field defect contralateral to a central scotoma is helpful clinically in localizing pathology to the junction of the optic nerve and chiasm. The macular fibers tend to cross posteriorly within the chiasm; this

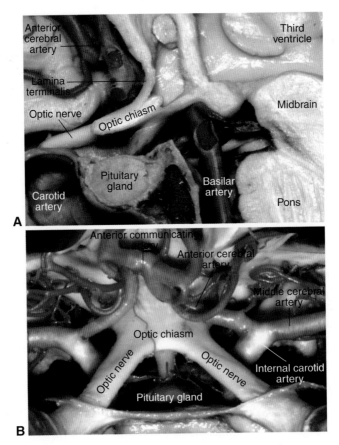

Figure 1-19 Anatomical dissection of the optic chiasm and surrounding structures. **A,** Sagittal view. **B,** Superior view. *(Courtesy of Albert L. Rhoton, Jr, MD.)*

arrangement underlies the bitemporal scotomatous field defects seen with posterior chiasmatic compression.

Optic Tract

The fibers exiting from the chiasm proceed circumferentially around the diencephalon lateral to the hypothalamus and in contact with the ambient cistern (see Fig 1-11). Just prior to the lateral geniculate, the fibers involved in pupillary pathways exit to the pretectal nuclei; other fibers exit to the superficial layers of the superior colliculus via the brachium of the superior colliculus. These fibers originate from intrinsically photosensitive retinal ganglion cells (ipRGC) and are likely the sole source of pupillomotor input from the retina to the midbrain. These ipRGCs also project to the suprachiasmatic nucleus of the hypothalamus, which is probably responsible for light-induced diurnal rhythms.

The incongruous nature of optic tract visual field defects is explained by the lack of close proximity between corresponding fibers from the right and left eyes. Most

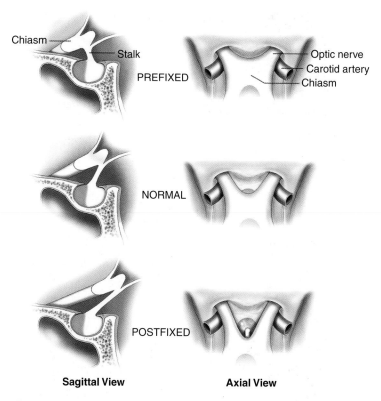

Figure 1-20 Position of the optic chiasm in relationship to the tuberculum sella. *(Illustration by Dave Peace.)*

of the axons that originated in the retinal ganglion cells terminate within the lateral geniculate.

The *lateral geniculate nucleus* is located in the posterior thalamus below and lateral to the pulvinar and above the lateral recess of the ambient cistern. This peaked, mushroom-shaped structure is divided into 6 levels. The 4 superior levels are the termini of P-cell axons, which are the ganglion cells with smaller receptive fields that are responsible for mediating maximal spatial resolution and color perception. The 2 inferior layers receive input from the M-cell fibers, which are the ganglion cells with larger receptive fields that are more sensitive to detecting motion. Axons originating in the contralateral eye terminate in layers 1, 4, and 6; the ipsilateral fibers innervate 2, 3, and 5. As the fibers approach the lateral geniculate, the superior fibers move superomedially and the inferior fibers swing inferolaterally. Overall, the retinal representation rotates almost 90°, with the superior fibers moving medially and the inferior fibers laterally. The macular fibers tend to move superolaterally. Cortical and subcortical pathways may modulate activity in the lateral geniculate. In addition, the cortex, superior colliculus, and pretectal nuclei project back to the lateral geniculate.

Cortex

Following a synapse in the lateral geniculate nucleus, the axons travel posteriorly as the optic radiations to terminate in the primary visual (calcarine) cortex in the occipital lobe (Fig 1-21). The most inferior of the fibers first travel anteriorly, then laterally and posteriorly to loop around the temporal horn of the lateral ventricles (Meyer loop) (see Fig 1-17). More superiorly, the fibers travel posteriorly through the deep white matter of the parietal lobe. The macular (central) fibers course laterally, with the peripheral fibers concentrated more at the superior and inferior aspects of the radiations. Injury to fibers within the radiations produces a homonymous hemianopia, a contralateral visual field defect that respects the vertical midline. If the corresponding fibers from the 2 eyes are in close proximity, the field defect is identical in each eye (congruous). Congruous field defects occur with lesions involving the calcarine cortex. More anterior involvement often produces incongruous field defects, suggesting that the corresponding fibers lie farther apart more anteriorly in the visual pathways.

The *primary visual cortex* (known variously as *V1, striate cortex,* or *Brodmann area 17*) is arrayed along the horizontal calcarine fissure, which divides the medial surface of the occipital lobe. Fibers of the optic radiations terminate in the fourth of the 6 layers in the primary visual cortex. This layer, the *lamina granularis interna,* is further subdivided into 3 layers: 4A, 4B, and 4C (4C, also known as the *line of Gennari,* gives rise to the name *striate cortex*). P-cell input terminates mainly in 4Cβ (the lower half of 4C), whereas M-cell fibers project mainly to 4Cα. The macular fibers terminate more posteriorly. Fibers from the most lateral (temporal crescent) visual field (originating only in the contralateral eye) terminate most anteriorly.

The cortex is heavily weighted to central retinal activity, with 50%–60% of the cortex responding to activity within the central 10° and approximately 80% of the cortex devoted to macular activity (within 30°). The superior portion of the cortex continues to receive information from the inferior visual field in a retinotopic distribution. This retinotopic mapping throughout the afferent visual pathways allows lesions to be localized on the basis of visual field defects.

Neurons within the striate cortex may be separated into 3 types: simple, complex, and end-stopped, based on their receptive field properties. The simple cells respond optimally to specifically oriented light–dark borders. The complex cells respond maximally to oriented motion of the light–dark interface. The end-stopped cells decrease firing when the stimulus reaches the end of the cell's receptive field. Some simple cells may receive input from 1 eye, whereas complex cells, end-stopped cells, and other simple cells receive binocular information (from corresponding retinal ganglion cells from both eyes). The preference for information coming from 1 eye or the other may be seen as ocular dominance columns, which run perpendicularly to the cortical surface within the calcarine cortex. In addition to eye-specific columns, the cortex is also marked by orientation-preference columns.

The *parastriate cortex* (also called *V2,* or *Brodmann area 18*) is contiguous with the primary visual cortex and receives its input from V1. Area V3 lies primarily in the posterior parietal lobe and receives direct input from V1. V3 has no sharp histologic delineation

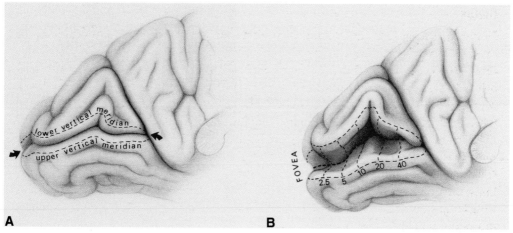

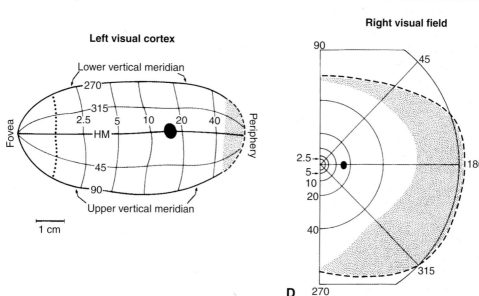

Figure 1-21 **A,** Left occipital cortex showing the location of striate cortex within the calcarine fissure *(running between arrows)*. The boundary *(dashed line)* between striate cortex (V1) and extrastriate cortex (V2) contains the representation of the vertical meridian. **B,** View of striate cortex after the lips of the calcarine fissure are opened. *Dashed lines* indicate the coordinates of the visual field map. The representation of the horizontal meridian runs approximately along the base of the calcarine fissure. *Vertical dashed lines* mark the isoeccentricity contours from 2.5° to 40°. Striate cortex wraps around the occipital pole to extend about 1 cm onto the lateral convexity of the hemisphere, where the fovea is represented. **C,** Schematic flattened map of the left striate cortex shown in part **B** representing the right hemifield. The *row of dots* shows where striate cortex folds around the occipital tip. The *black oval* marks the region of striate cortex corresponding to the contralateral eye's blind spot. *HM* = horizontal meridian. **D,** Right visual hemifield, plotted with a Goldmann perimeter. The *stippled area* corresponds to the monocular temporal crescent, which is mapped in the most anterior ~8% of striate cortex. *(Reprinted with permission from Horton JC, Hoyt WF. The representation of the visual field in human striate cortex: a revision of the classic Holmes map. Arch Ophthalmol. 1991;109:822. Copyright 1991, American Medical Association.)*

from V2 and sends efferent information to the basal ganglia (pulvinar) and the midbrain. Cells in this area are thought to be capable of responding to more than one stimulus dimension, suggesting that visual integration occurs in this region. V3a, identified as having a separate retinotopic representation, receives its input from V3. Cells in this area are mostly binocularly driven and are sensitive to motion and direction. V4, located within the lingual and fusiform gyrus, seems to be particularly sensitive to color. Damage to this area is probably responsible for most cases of cerebral achromatopsia. Anterior and lateral to area V4, V5 (posterior and within the superior temporal sulcus and gyrus subangularis) is very sensitive to movement and direction (Fig 1-22). The underlying white matter is heavily myelinated. The V5 area, which corresponds to the medial temporal visual region, receives ipsilateral input from V1 and direct input from the M-cell layers of the lateral geniculate. The neurons here encode the speed and direction of moving stimuli. This sensory area is likely the origin of pursuit movements and thus links the afferent and efferent pathways. Compared with those of V1, the receptive fields are larger. One additional associative area, V6 (located medially in the parietal cortex adjacent to V3a), is thought to have representation of "extrapersonal space." The superior colliculus receives afferent input both directly from the anterior visual pathways and secondarily from the calcarine

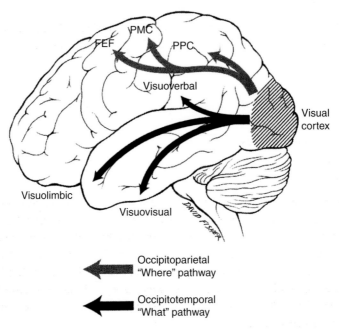

Figure 1-22 Parallel visual processing pathways in the human. The occipitotemporal, or "what," pathway begins in the striate cortex (V1) and projects to the angular gyrus for language processing, the inferior temporal lobe for object identification and limbic structures. The occipitoparietal, or "where," pathway begins in the striate cortex and projects to the posterior parietal and superior temporal cortex, dealing with visuospatial analysis. *FEF* = frontal eye field, *PMC* = premotor cortex, *PPC* = posterior parietal cortex. *(Modified from Kline LB. Neuro-Ophthalmology Review Manual. 6th ed. Thorofare, NJ: Slack; 2008:235.)*

cortex. The superficial layers contain a retinotopic map that overlies the deeper layers, which are primarily concerned with saccadic generation.

Horton JC. Wilbrand's knee of the primate optic chiasm is an artifact of monocular enucleation. *Trans Am Ophthalmol Soc.* 1997;95:579–609.

Trobe JD. *The Neurology of Vision.* New York: Oxford University Press; 2001.

Efferent Visual System (Ocular Motor Pathways)

Our understanding of the anatomical pathways of the ocular motor system is incomplete. Nevertheless, detailed anatomical, physiologic, and pathologic knowledge of the ocular motor system has increased dramatically over the past several years due to results derived from primate model experiments, human electrophysiology testing, functional magnetic resonance imaging (fMRI) studies, and the clinical-pathologic-radiologic correlation of patients with documented eye movement abnormalities.

The ultimate purpose of the ocular motor system is to establish clear, stable, and binocular vision. To perform these tasks, 2 basic human eye movements exist:

1. gaze shift
2. gaze stabilization

These can be further divided into 7 functional systems or classes (see Anatomy and Clinical Testing of the Functional Classes of Eye Movements in Chapter 7):

1. vestibular
2. visual fixation
3. optokinetic
4. smooth pursuit
5. nystagmus quick phases
6. saccades
7. vergence

Each system appears to be under the control of—and modulated by—different regions of the brain (cortex) and brainstem, with considerable anatomical and functional overlap. This section provides an overview of the ocular motor system, with a detailed discussion of particularly clinically relevant structures. For interested readers, a comprehensive description of the ocular motor system can be found in the outstanding textbook by Leigh and Zee (Leigh RJ, Zee DS. *The Neurology of Eye Movements.* 4th ed. New York: Oxford University Press; 2006.) To facilitate learning, the discussion is organized following a top-to-bottom approach:

- cortical control of eye movements, including basal ganglion (BG), thalamus, and superior colliculus (SC)
- brainstem or premotor coordination of conjugate eye movements, including the vestibular-ocular system and cerebellum

- ocular motor cranial nerves (oculomotor nerve [CN III], trochlear nerve [CN IV] and abducens nerve [CN VI])
- extraocular muscles (EOMs)

Cortical Input

The efferent visual system spans a large segment of the central nervous system, with many areas of the brain generating eye movements (Fig 1-23).

The following list of major anatomical structures and their functions helps set a foundation for discussion of the pathways for coordinating conjugate eye movements (Fig 1-24):

- *rostral interstitial nucleus of the medial longitudinal fasciculus (riMLF)*: excitatory burst neurons that generate vertical and torsional saccades
- *interstitial nucleus of Cajal (INC)*: inhibitory burst neurons for vertical saccades and neural integrator for vertical and torsional gaze
- *region of riMLF and INC*: inhibitory burst neurons for vertical and torsional saccades
- *posterior commissure (PC)*: projecting axons from INC to contralateral CNs III, IV, and VI, and the INC
- *medial longitudinal fasciculus (MLF)*: major pathway for relaying signals within the brainstem
- *nucleus raphe interpositus (RIP)*: omnipause cells
- *nucleus reticularis tegmenti pontis (NRTP)*: long-lead burst cells
- *dorsolateral pontine nuclei (DLPN)*: neurons for smooth pursuit
- *nucleus prepositus hypoglossi (NPH)*: neural integrator for horizontal gaze

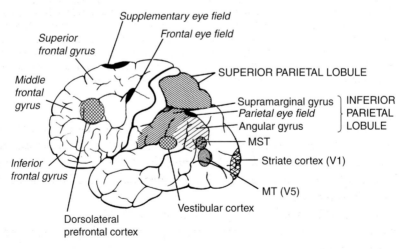

Figure 1-23 Overview of the cortical centers involved in the control of human eye movements. *MST* = medial superior temporal visual area, *MT* = medial temporal visual area. *(Used with permission from Leigh RJ, Zee DS. The Neurology of Eye Movements. 4th ed. New York: Oxford University Press; 2006.)*

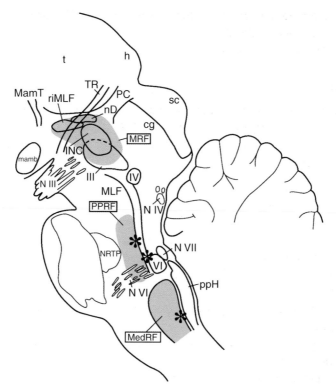

Figure 1-24 Sagittal section of monkey brainstem showing the location of the rostral interstitial nucleus of the medial longitudinal fasciculus *(riMLF)* and other structures important in the control of vertical and horizontal gaze. The *shaded areas* indicate the mesencephalic reticular formation *(MRF)*, paramedian pontine reticular formation *(PPRF)*, and medullary reticular formation *(MedRF)*. *Asterisks* indicate the location of cell groups of the paramedian tracts, which project to the flocculus. **Key:** *III* = oculomotor nucleus, *IV* = trochlear nucleus, *VI* = abducens nucleus, *cg* = central gray, *h* = habenular complex, *INC* = interstitial nucleus of Cajal, *mamb* = mamillary body, *MamT* = mammillothalamic tract, *MLF* = medial longitudinal fasciculus, *N III* = rootlets of the oculomotor nerve, *N IV* = trochlear nerve, *N VI* = rootlets of the abducens nerve, *N VII* = facial nerve, *nD* = nucleus of Darkschewitsch, *NRTP* = nucleus reticularis tegmenti pontis, *PC* = posterior commissure, *ppH* = nucleus prepositus hypoglossi, *sc* = superior colliculus, *t* = thalamus, *TR* = tractus retroflexus. *(Modified from Leigh RJ, Zee DS.* The Neurology of Eye Movements. *3rd ed. New York: Oxford University Press; 1999. Modified by C. H. Wooley.)*

- *pontine paramedian reticular formation (PPRF)*: excitatory burst neurons that generate horizontal saccades and inhibitory burst neurons for horizontal saccades
- *medullary reticular formation (MedRF)*: inhibitory burst cells for horizontal gaze
- *cell groups of paramedian tracts (PMTs)*: neurons that project from the CN VI nucleus to the cerebellum
- *CNs III, IV and VI*: neurons that project directly to EOMs
- *vestibular nuclei (CN VIII)*: neurons that project to saccade generators and ocular motor cranial nerves
- *y-group cells*: cells that project to CN III and IV nuclei for vertical smooth pursuit and vertical vestibular eye movements

Saccadic system

The cortical, or supranuclear, input for generating saccadic eye movements is divided into 2 parallel and interconnected descending pathways: visually reflexive (parietal lobe) movements and memory-guided and volitional (frontal lobe) movements. In general, these cortical fibers project to the following structures in an organized framework (Fig 1-25):

- *subcortical structures:* SC, BG, and thalamus
- *brainstem neural network or premotor neurons:* several types of pontine neurons, including omnipause cells of the RIP and long-lead burst cells of the NRTP
- *brainstem saccade generators:* PPRF and riMLF
- *motoneurons of the ocular motor cranial nerves:* CNs III, IV, and VI

(Note that few cortical fibers project directly to the PPRF and riMLF.)

Visually guided movements require afferent system information either from the primary visual system and cortex or from the accessory afferent system. The visually guided (to seen or remembered targets) and volitional saccadic supranuclear input comes largely from the *frontal eye fields (FEFs,* or *Brodmann area 8).* Cortical cells discharge prior to all voluntary and visually guided contralateral saccades. *Supplementary eye fields (SEFs)*— located on the dorsomedial surface of the superior frontal gyrus—receive input from the FEFs and are responsible for programming saccades, particularly as part of learned behavior. The FEF projects to the ipsilateral SC and many other areas, including the contralateral FEF, SEF, BG, NRTP, and RIP. Cortical projections to the SC also arise from

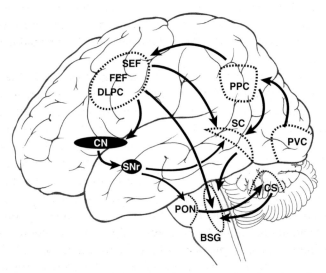

Figure 1-25 Schematic illustration of the saccadic system showing the relevant cortical centers for generating saccades. Note that this illustration is not meant to show all the hypothetical supranuclear pathways for the saccadic system. **Key:** *BSG* = brainstem saccadic generator, *CN* = caudate nucleus of the basal ganglia, *CS* = cerebellar structures, *DLPC* = dorsolateral prefrontal cortex, *FEF* = frontal eye field, *PON* = precerebellar pontine nuclei, *PPC* = posterior parietal cortex, *PVC* = primary visual cortex, *SC* = superior colliculus, *SEF* = supplementary eye field, *SNr* = substantia nigra pars reticulata. *(Used with permission from Kline LB.* Neuro-Ophthalmology Review Manual. *6th ed. Thorofare, NJ: Slack; 2008:49.)*

the *posterior parietal cortex (PPC)*, which is equivalent to the lateral intraparietal area in rhesus monkeys. The PPC is important in visually guided reflexive saccades.

The SC is divided into a superficial (dorsal) and deep (ventral) part. The sensory signal (input from the visual cortex and retina) is mainly processed by the superficial SC. The motor signal originates within the deeper layers (the stratum griseum profundum and stratum album profundum) that receive position information from the more superficial layers. The SC projects contralaterally to multiple locations throughout the brainstem, most particularly to the RIP, NRTP, and DLPN.

Both the parietal and frontal lobe supranuclear pathways travel mainly to the SC; few fibers connect directly to brainstem premotor neurons. The supranuclear pathways also go through the BG (caudate nucleus, putamen nucleus, and substantia nigra pars reticulate). The BG appears to have several roles in the saccadic system, including inhibiting unnecessary reflexive saccades during fixation and helping in the control of voluntary saccades.

Another important structure involved in the programming of saccades is the thalamus (internal medullary lamina and pulvinar). The thalamus receives information from the cortex and brainstem and projects only to the cortex and BG. Therefore, the thalamus appears to relay messages from the brainstem to the cortical eye fields.

For clinical disorders of saccadic dysfunction, see Clinical Disorders of the Ocular Motor System in Chapter 7.

Smooth pursuit system

It was once felt that saccadic and smooth pursuit eye movements each derived from a distinct supranuclear pathway. However, it now appears that considerable overlap exists between these systems. In addition, there are 2 major visual pathways, one for the movement of images (magnocellular: M cells) and the other for discrimination of images (parvocellular: P cells).

The smooth pursuit system for visual targets originates in V5—the human homologue of the *medial temporal (MT)* visual area in the rhesus monkey—where it receives input from the primary visual system, both from the cortex (striate and extrastriate areas) and likely from magnocellular input directly from the geniculate (Fig 1-26). Retinal image slip serves as a stimulus to tonically alter ocular drift. The *medial superior temporal (MST)* area is also involved in generating pursuit signals in response to moving stimuli. The area appears to be supplied with information about head movement as well as eye movement commands (efference copy) and thus is critical in generating pursuit movements to follow a target while the head is moving. Target recognition and selection probably receive additional input through the reciprocal connections to the posterior parietal cortex (human homologue of area 7a in the rhesus monkey). Information from the MT and MST projects via the posterior portion of the internal capsule to the DLPN and lateral pontine nuclei, including the NRTP. From these pontine nuclei, projections are sent to the cerebellum (paraflocculus and dorsal vermis), with outflow signals to the vestibular nuclei and the y-group—a collection of cells at the inferior cerebellar peduncle (Fig 1-27).

For clinical disorders of the pursuit function, see Clinical Disorders of the Ocular Motor System in Chapter 7.

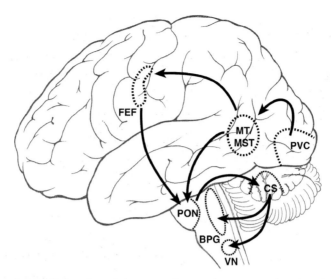

Figure 1-26 Schematic illustration of the smooth pursuit system, showing the relevant cortical centers and their pathways for generating smooth pursuit eye movements. Note that this illustration is not meant to show the hypothetical scheme for the smooth pursuit system. **Key:** *BPG* = brainstem pursuit generator, *CS* = cerebellar structures, *FEF* = frontal eye field, *MT/MST* = middle temporal area/medial superior temporal area, *PON* = precerebellar pontine nuclei, *PVC* = primary visual cortex, *SC* = superior colliculus, *VN* = vestibular nucleus. *(Used with permission from Kline LB. Neuro-Ophthalmology Review Manual. 6th ed. Thorofare, NJ: Slack; 2008:54.)*

Brainstem

The supranuclear pathways for saccades and smooth pursuits eventually reach the brainstem neural network (via the SC and BG), which allows for conjugate eye movements. Following is a description of the important structures within the brainstem that allow for controlling gaze. As a general guideline, the midbrain is concerned with vertical eye movements and the pons with horizontal eye movements. Vertical and torsional saccades are generated from excitatory burst cells of the riMLF within the midbrain. In contrast, the pathways for vertical vestibular and vertical smooth pursuit ascend from the medulla and pons to the midbrain via the MLF. Horizontal saccades are generated from excitatory burst cells within the PPRF and horizontal smooth pursuit eye movements arise from the CN VI nucleus, which receives input from the vestibulocerebellum (see "Cerebellum" later in the chapter).

Vertical gaze is controlled through the midbrain. The primary gaze center is located in the riMLF (Fig 1-28). This area receives input from the medial and superior vestibular nuclei via the MLF and other internuclear connections. Other areas in the rostral midbrain, including the INC and the *nucleus of Darkschewitsch,* also modulate vertical motility. Burst cell input may come in part from the PPRF caudally but also locally within the riMLF. The INC (neural integrator for vertical and torsional gaze) receives signals from the riMLF and from the vestibular nuclei and projects to the motoneurons of the CN III

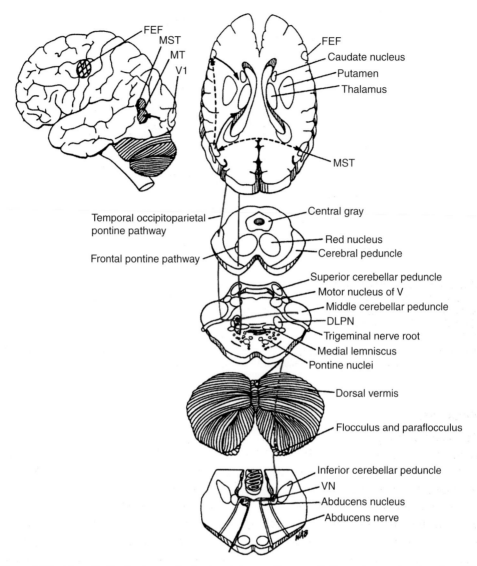

Figure 1-27 Hypothetical scheme for horizontal smooth pursuit. The primary visual cortex *(V1)* projects to the homologue of the middle temporal visual area *(MT)*, which, in humans, lies at the temporal-occipital-parietal junction. The MT projects to the homologue of the medial superior temporal visual area *(MST)* and also to the frontal eye field *(FEF)*. The MST also receives inputs from its contralateral counterpart. The MST projects through the retrolenticular portion of the internal capsule and the posterior portion of the cerebral peduncle to the dorsolateral pontine nucleus *(DLPN)*. The DLPN also receives inputs important for pursuit from the FEF; these inputs descend in the medial portion of the cerebral peduncle. The DLPN projects, mainly contralaterally, to the flocculus, paraflocculus, and ventral uvula of the cerebellum; projections also pass to the dorsal vermis. The flocculus projects to the ipsilateral vestibular nuclei *(VN)*, which in turn project to the contralateral abducens nucleus. Note that the sections of the brainstem are in different planes from those of the cerebral hemispheres. *(Used with permission from Leigh RJ, Zee DS.* The Neurology of Eye Movements. *4th ed. New York: Oxford University Press; 2006.)*

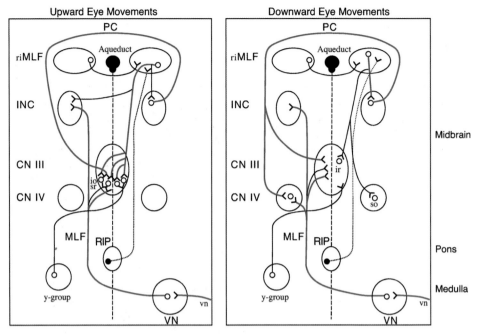

Figure 1-28 Anatomical schemes for the synthesis of upward and downward movements *(in red)*. From the vertical semicircular canals, primary afferents on the vestibular nerve *(vn)* synapse in the vestibular nuclei *(VN)* and ascend into the medial longitudinal fasciculus *(MLF)* and brachium conjunctivum (not shown) to contact neurons in the trochlear nucleus *(CN IV)*, oculomotor nucleus *(CN III)*, and interstitial nucleus of Cajal *(INC)*. (For clarity, only excitatory vestibular projections are shown.) The rostral interstitial nucleus of the medial longitudinal fasciculus *(riMLF)*, which lies in the prerubral fields, contains saccadic burst neurons. It receives an inhibitory input from omnipause neurons of the nucleus raphe interpositus *(RIP)*, which lies in the pons (for clarity, this projection is shown only for upward movements). Excitatory burst neurons in the riMLF project to the motoneurons of CN III and CN IV and send axon collaterals to the INC. Each riMLF neuron sends axon collaterals to yoke-pair muscles (Hering's law). Projections to the elevator subnuclei (innervating the superior rectus and inferior oblique muscles) may be bilateral because of axon collaterals crossing at the level of the CN III nucleus. Projections of inhibitory burst neurons are less well understood and are not shown here. Signals contributing to vertical smooth pursuit and eye–head tracking reach CN III from the *y-group* via the brachium conjunctivum and a crossing ventral tegmental tract. **Key:** io = inferior oblique subnucleus, *ir* = inferior rectus subnucleus, *PC* = posterior commissure, *so* = superior oblique nucleus, *sr* = superior rectus subnucleus. *(Modified from Leigh RJ, Zee DS.* The Neurology of Eye Movements. *4th ed. New York: Oxford University Press; 2006.)*

and CN IV nuclei through the PC. Activity from the vertical gaze center is distributed to the CN III and CN IV nuclei. Information involved in upgaze crosses in the posterior commissure. Damage to this pathway results in the dorsal midbrain syndrome, which clinically includes vertical gaze difficulty (most commonly impaired supraduction), skew deviation, light–near pupillary dissociation, lid retraction, and convergence-retraction nystagmus (CRN). CRN, which is usually elicited by having the patient follow a downward rotating optokinetic (OKN) drum, represents simultaneous co-contraction of the medial and lateral rectus muscles (see Chapter 9).

Horizontal gaze is coordinated through the CN VI nucleus in the dorsal caudal pons (Fig 1-29). This nucleus receives tonic input from the contralateral horizontal semicircular

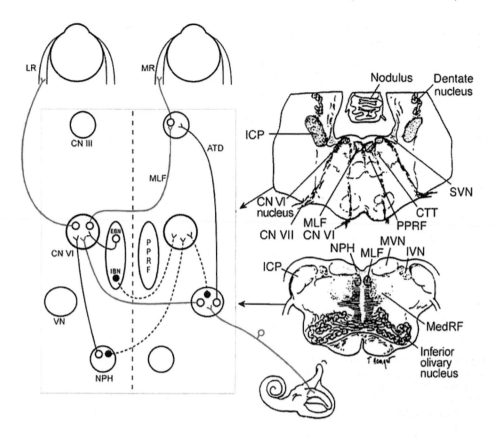

Figure 1-29 Anatomical scheme for the synthesis of signals for horizontal eye movements. The abducens nucleus *(CN VI N)* contains abducens motoneurons, which innervate the ipsilateral lateral rectus muscle *(LR)*, and abducens internuclear neurons, which send an ascending projection in the contralateral medial longitudinal fasciculus *(MLF)* to contact medial rectus *(MR)* motoneurons in the contralateral third nerve nucleus *(CN III N)*. From the horizontal semicircular canal, primary afferents on the vestibular nerve project mainly to the vestibular nucleus *(CN VIII N)*, where they synapse and then send an excitatory connection to the contralateral CN VI N and an inhibitory projection to the ipsilateral CN VI N. Saccadic inputs reach CN VI N from ipsilateral excitatory burst neurons *(EBN)* and contralateral inhibitory burst neurons *(IBN)*. The EBN and IBN are housed in the pontine paramedian reticular formation *(PPRF)*. Specifically, the PPRF is composed of 3 nuclei, from the caudal pons to rostral medulla: (1) the nucleus reticularis pontis caudalis (containing the EBN), (2) the nucleus raphe interpositus (containing pause cells), and (3) the nucleus paragigantocellularis dorsalis or medullary reticular formation *(MedRF)* (containing the IBN). Eye position information (the output of the neural integrator) reaches the abducens from neurons within the nucleus prepositus hypoglossi *(NPH)* and adjacent CN VIII N. The medial rectus motoneurons in CN III also receive a command for vergence eye movements. The anatomical sections on the right correspond to the level of the arrowheads on the schematic on the left. **Key:** *ATD* = ascending tract of Deiters, *CN VII* = facial nerve, *CTT* = central tegmental tract, *ICP* = inferior cerebellar peduncle, *IVN* = inferior vestibular nucleus, *MVN* = medial vestibular nucleus, *SVN* = superior vestibular nucleus. *(Modified from Leigh RJ, Zee DS.* The Neurology of Eye Movements. *4th ed. New York: Oxford University Press; 2006.)*

canal through the medial and lateral vestibular nuclei. Burst information is supplied from the PPRF that is directly adjacent to the CN VI nucleus and MLF. The burst cells are normally inhibited by omnipause neurons located in the RIP. It is now thought that saccades are initiated by supranuclear inhibition of the omnipause cells, which allows burst cell impulses to activate the horizontal and vertical gaze centers (Fig 1-30). To produce horizontal movement of both eyes, a signal to increase firing must be distributed to the ipsilateral lateral rectus and the contralateral medial rectus muscles. The lateral rectus muscle is supplied directly through ipsilateral CN VI. The contralateral medial rectus is stimulated by interneurons that cross in the pons and ascend in the contralateral MLF. Therefore, for example, pathology affecting the right MLF will result in a right (ipsilateral) adduction deficit with attempted left gaze, often accompanied by abducting nystagmus of the left (contralateral) eye. These findings are clinically known as an *internuclear ophthalmoplegia (INO)*. For further information on INO, see Internuclear Causes of Diplopia in Chapter 8.

The distribution of both infranuclear (ocular motor cranial nuclei and nerves) and supranuclear information requires internuclear communication within the brainstem. The most important of these pathways, the MLF, runs in 2 parallel columns from the spinal cord to an area of the midbrain PC that is located dorsomedial to the red nucleus and rostral to the INC. The bulk of the fibers contributing to the MLF have their origin in the vestibular nuclei. The projections from the superior vestibular nucleus are ipsilateral, and those from the medial vestibular nucleus are contralateral. The MLF also receives interneurons originating from the contralateral CN VI nucleus. Additional vertical pathways include the *brachium conjunctivum* and the *ascending tract of Deiters*. The latter pathway runs lateral to the MLF and conveys signals from the vestibular nuclei ipsilaterally to the

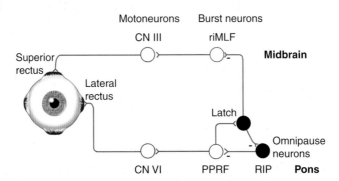

Figure 1-30 Schematic of the brainstem network for saccade generation. Motoneurons innervating horizontally acting extraocular muscles receive saccadic commands from burst neurons in the paramedian pontine reticular formation *(PPRF)*. Motoneurons innervating vertically acting extraocular muscles receive saccadic commands from burst neurons in the midbrain's rostral interstitial nucleus of the medial longitudinal fasciculus *(riMLF)*. Both sets of burst neurons are modulated by omnipause neurons that lie in the pontine nucleus raphe interpositus *(RIP)*. A saccade is initiated by a trigger signal that inhibits ominpause neurons; subsequently, hypothetical latch neurons, which receive input from burst neurons, inhibit omnipause neurons until the saccade is complete. *(Modified with permission from Leigh RJ, Zee DS. The Neurology of Eye Movements. 4th ed. New York: Oxford University Press; 2006.)*

medial rectus subnucleus in the midbrain, modulating the vestibular response during near fixation.

To maintain eccentric gaze, additional tonic input must be provided to the yoke muscles that hold the eye in position. This additional tonic input is provided by integrating the velocity signal provided by the burst neuron activity. For horizontal eye movements, integration takes place in the NPH, located adjacent to the medial vestibular nucleus at the pontomedullary junction, with input from the cerebellum. Neural integration for vertical eye movements involves the INC in addition to the cerebellum. Pathology affecting the neural integrator (often metabolic, associated with alcohol consumption or anticonvulsant medication) results in failure to maintain eccentric gaze, recognized clinically as gaze-evoked nystagmus.

Vestibular ocular system

The output of the vestibular nuclei provides both the major infranuclear input into ocular motility and the major tonic input into eye position. This system has one of the shortest arcs in the nervous system, producing a fast response with extremely short latency. The hair cells of the semicircular canals (Fig 1-31) alter their firing in response to relative movement of the endolymph. The signal is produced by a change in velocity (head acceleration) in any one of 3 axes. The information is then conveyed to the vestibular nuclei (located laterally in the rostral medulla) via the inferior and superior vestibular nerves. An

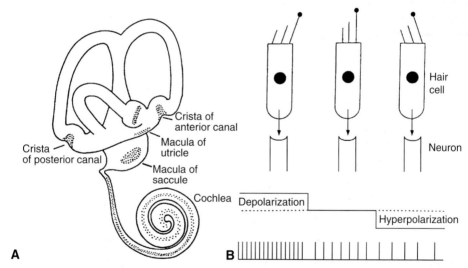

Figure 1-31 Vestibular system. **A,** Schematic of the mammalian labyrinth. The crista of the lateral semicircular canal is shown but not labeled (with the canal projecting forward). **B,** Motion transduction by the vestibular hair cells. At rest there is a resting rate of action potential discharge in the primary vestibular afferents *(center)*. Shearing forces on the hair cells cause depolarization *(left)* if the stereocilia are deflected toward the kinocilium (indicated by the longest cilium, with beaded end), or hyperpolarization *(right)* if the stereocilia are deflected away from the kinocilium. This modulates the discharge rate in the vestibular nerve neuron. *(Reproduced with permission from Leigh RJ, Zee DS. The Neurology of Eye Movements. 4th ed. New York: Oxford University Press; 2006.)*

additional contribution to the vestibular nerve is from hair cells in the macula acoustica of the utricle and saccule. Calcium carbonate crystals within the otoliths respond to linear acceleration (most important, gravity) to orient the body. The vestibular nerve and the output of the membranous labyrinth (the cochlear nerve) make up the eighth nerve complex and exit the petrous bone through the internal auditory meatus. CN VIII traverses the subarachnoid space within the cerebellopontine angle. Within the medulla, the vestibular information synapses in the medial, lateral, and superior vestibular nuclei. Tonic information from the horizontal canal crosses directly to the contralateral gaze center within the sixth nerve nucleus in the dorsal medial aspect of the caudal pons just under the fourth ventricle. Tonic information from the anterior and posterior canals (Fig 1-32) travels rostrally through several of the important internuclear connections to innervate the vertical gaze center in the rostral midbrain. Medial and inferior vestibular nuclei, as well as the NPH and the inferior olivary nucleus, project to the *nodulus* (a central nucleus of the cerebellum) and the *ventral uvula*. This pathway, which projects back to the vestibular nuclei, is responsible for the velocity storage mechanism (that is, the mechanism that maintains the vestibular signal beyond the output of the primary vestibular neurons).

For clinical disorders of vestibular ocular function, see Clinical Disorders of the Ocular Motor System in Chapter 7.

Cerebellum

The other major connection in the ocular motor system is to the *vestibulocerebellum*. The structures in this area, largely through the brachium conjunctivum, are responsible for adjusting the gain of all ocular movements. *Gain* may be defined as the output divided by the input. For example, keeping the eyes stable in space while the head rotates requires the eyes to move in a direction opposite that of head rotation at the same velocity and distance; this would be considered a gain of 1. The cerebellum is involved in gain adjustment to allow compensation after peripheral lesions (eg, vestibular nerve dysfunction such as vestibular neuritis). Disease processes directly affecting the cerebellum may increase or decrease the gain of eye movement systems such as the vestibular ocular reflex. The cerebellum can be divided into the *archaeocerebellum* (the most caudal and inferior portion, containing the paired flocculi and the midline nodulus), the *paleocerebellum* (consisting of the vermis, the pyramis, the uvula, and the paraflocculus), and the *neocerebellum* (including the remainder of the cerebellar hemispheres). The flocculonodular lobe plus parts of the paraflocculus make up the vestibulocerebellum. Two additional cerebellar nuclei of ocular motor importance located in the white matter of the cerebellar hemisphere are the *dentate* (most lateral) and *fastigial* (most medial) *nuclei.*

Efference copy information (regarding the position of the eyes) is supplied directly from the ocular motor pathways (possibly through cell groups of the paramedian tracts within the vestibular nuclei), whereas *afferent signal error* information arrives at the cerebellum via the climbing fibers from the inferior olivary nucleus. Additional cerebellar inputs to the paraflocculus and flocculus include *mossy fiber input* from the vestibular nuclei and the NPH. Purkinje cells within the paraflocculus discharge during smooth pursuit. An error signal (the difference between gaze velocity and retinal image velocity) results in discharge within the sixth and seventh lobules of the dorsal vermis; thus,

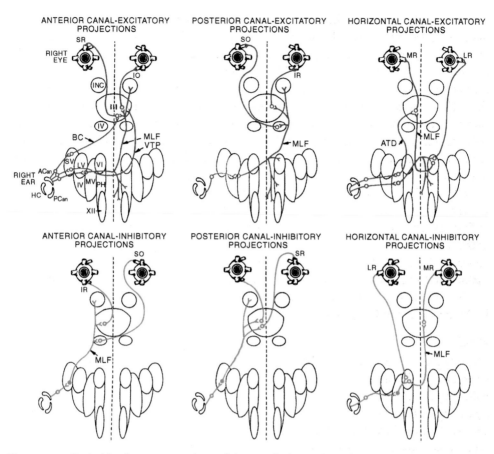

ANTERIOR CANAL-EXCITATORY PROJECTIONS

POSTERIOR CANAL-EXCITATORY PROJECTIONS

HORIZONTAL CANAL-EXCITATORY PROJECTIONS

ANTERIOR CANAL-INHIBITORY PROJECTIONS

POSTERIOR CANAL-INHIBITORY PROJECTIONS

HORIZONTAL CANAL-INHIBITORY PROJECTIONS

Figure 1-32 Probable direct connections of the vestibular ocular reflex. Excitatory neurons are indicated by open circles and inhibitory neurons by filled circles. **Key:** *III* = oculomotor nuclear complex, *IV* = trochlear nucleus, *VI* = abducens nucleus, *XII* = hypoglossal nucleus, *ACan* = anterior semicircular canal, *ATD* = ascending tract of Deiters, *BC* = brachium conjunctivum, *HC* = horizontal (or lateral) semicircular canal, *INC* = interstitial nucleus of Cajal, *IO* = inferior oblique muscle, *IR* = inferior rectus muscle, *IV* = inferior vestibular nucleus, *LR* = lateral rectus muscle, *LV* = lateral vestibular nucleus, *MLF* = medial longitudinal fasciculus, *MR* = medial rectus muscle, *MV* = medial vestibular nucleus, *PCan* = posterior semicircular canal, *PH* = prepositus hypoglossi nucleus, *SO* = superior oblique muscle, *SR* = superior rectus muscle, *SV* = superior vestibular nucleus, *VTP* = ventral tegmental pathway. *(Reproduced with permission from Leigh RJ, Zee DS.* The Neurology of Eye Movements. *3rd ed. New York: Oxford University Press; 1999.)*

the dorsal vermis, which projects to the fastigial nucleus, may play a role in initiating pursuit and saccades. The output from the flocculus projects to the superior and medial vestibular nuclei. The fastigial nucleus is responsible for overcoming a natural imbalance in the input from the vertically oriented semicircular canals. Thus, loss of fastigial function may be associated with development of downbeat nystagmus, as the imbalance in the vertical information causes constant updrift. See Chapter 9, The Patient With Nystagmus or Spontaneous Eye Movement Disorders, for further discussion of nystagmus and other disordered eye movements.

Ocular Motor Cranial Nerves

Without neural activity, the visual axes are usually mildly to moderately divergent. The major tonic input to ocular motility is supplied by 3 pairs of ocular motor cranial nerves— CNs III, IV, and VI—that innervate the 6 EOMs controlling ocular movement (Fig 1-33). In addition, CN III also innervates the levator palpebrae and the pupillary sphincter muscles.

Except for the inferior oblique, the innervation to each of the EOMs occurs approximately one third the distance from the apex. The inferior oblique receives its innervation at approximately its midpoint from a neurovascular bundle running parallel to the lateral aspect of the inferior rectus. All 6 EOMs receive their innervation on the inside surface, except for the superior oblique, where branches of CN IV terminate on the upper (outer) surface of the muscle.

See Chapter 8, The Patient With Diplopia, for clinical presentation of disorders due to infranuclear, fascicular, and peripheral ocular motor cranial nerve lesions.

Abducens nerve (CN VI)

CN VI originates in the dorsal caudal pons just beneath the fourth ventricle. Its nucleus is surrounded by the looping fibers (genu) of the facial nerve and is adjacent to the PPRF and the MLF (Fig 1-34). The nucleus contains both primary motoneurons and interneurons that cross to the contralateral MLF to reach the CN III nucleus. Thus, pathology affecting the CN VI nucleus produces an ipsilateral gaze palsy. The motor axons exiting the CN VI nucleus (approximately 4000–6000 axons) travel ventrally and slightly laterally, medial to the superior olivary nucleus, to exit on the ventral surface of the caudal pons. As the fascicles pass through the brainstem, they lie adjacent to the spinal tract of the trigeminal nerve and traverse the corticobulbar tracts. Exiting the brainstem, the nerves run rostrally within the subarachnoid space on the surface of the clivus from the area of the cerebellopontine angle to the posterior superior portion of the posterior fossa. The nerves pierce the dura approximately 1 cm below the petrous apex and travel beneath the petroclinoid ligament (Gruber ligament, which connects the petrous pyramid to the posterior clinoid) to enter the canal of Dorello. Within the canal, CN VI travels with the inferior petrosal sinus. Once it becomes extradural, the nerve is within the cavernous sinus (the only cranial nerve within the substance of the cavernous sinus), where it runs

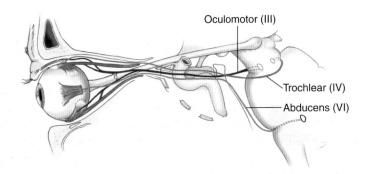

Oculomotor (III)

Trochlear (IV)

Abducens (VI)

Figure 1-33 Lateral view of the course of CNs III, IV, and VI. *(Illustration by Dave Peace.)*

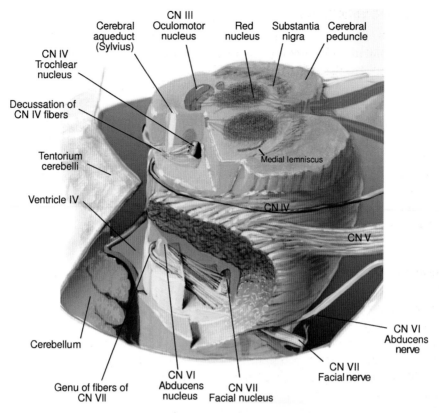

Figure 1-34 Intra-axial course of the ocular motor nerves at the level of the pons (below) and midbrain (above). Note the relationship to the surrounding cerebellum and CNs V and VII. *(Illustration by Craig A. Luce.)*

parallel to the horizontal segment of the carotid artery. It is also joined for a short segment by branches of the sympathetic chain lying within the wall of the intrapetrous carotid artery. Reaching the anterior portion of the cavernous sinus, CN VI traverses the superior orbital fissure (Fig 1-35) through the annulus of Zinn (see Fig 1-3C) to enter the medial surface of the lateral rectus muscle.

Trochlear nerve (CN IV)

The CN IV nucleus lies within the gray matter in the dorsal aspect of the caudal midbrain just below the aqueduct, directly contiguous with the more rostral third nerve nucleus (see Fig 1-34). The intra-axial portion (fascicle) of CN IV is very short, running dorsally around the periaqueductal gray to cross within the anterior medullary vellum just caudal to the inferior colliculi and below the pineal gland. CN IV is the only cranial nerve exiting on the dorsal surface of the brain and brainstem and has the longest unprotected intracranial course (which is probably responsible for its frequent involvement in closed head trauma). Within the subarachnoid space, CN IV (containing approximately 2000 fibers) swings around the midbrain, paralleling the tentorium just under the tentorial edge (where it is easily damaged during neurosurgical procedures that involve the tentorium).

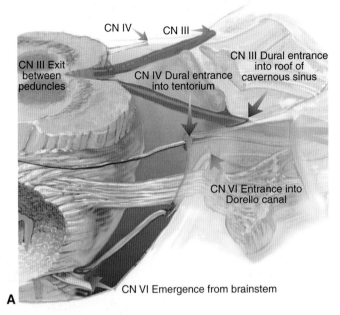

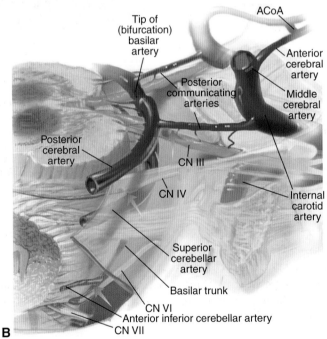

Figure 1-35 **A,** Subarachnoid course of the ocular motor nerves. Note the relationship to the surrounding dural structures, particularly the tentorium and the dura of the clivus. The nerves enter dural canals at the posterior aspect of the cavernous sinus for *CN III,* at the tentorial edge for *CN IV,* and along the clivus for *CN VI.* **B,** Major blood vessels and their relationships to the ocular motor nerves. Note the passage of CN III between the superior cerebellar artery below and posterior cerebral artery above. The vascular supply to CN III comes from branches off the posterior communicating artery, which is in close proximity. CN VI also runs by the anterior inferior cerebellar artery, which is a major branch off the basilar artery.

(continued)

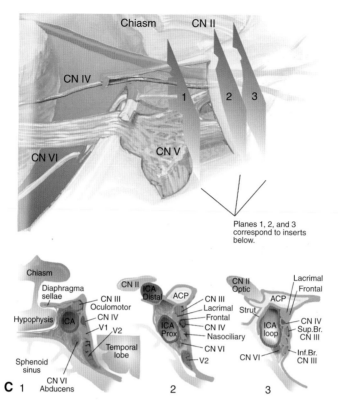

Figure 1-35 C, Intracavernous course of the ocular motor nerves. CN III and CN IV run in the lateral wall of the cavernous sinus along with *CN V* divisions V_1 and V_2. CN VI runs in close approximation to the carotid artery within the cavernous sinus itself. As the nerves course toward the anterior aspect of the cavernous sinus and the superior orbital fissure, V_1 (ophthalmic) divides into 3 branches: the lacrimal, frontal, and nasociliary nerves. The lacrimal and frontal nerves cross over the top of CN III and CN IV. CN III divides into superior and inferior divisions, which cross under CN IV to enter the orbital apex through the annulus of Zinn. **Key:** *ACoA* = anterior communicating artery, *ACP* = anterior clinoid process, *ICA* = internal carotid artery. *(Illustrations by Craig A. Luce.)*

Just below the anterior tentorial insertion, CN IV enters the posterior lateral aspect of the cavernous sinus just underneath CN III. Covered by a variable sheath, CN IV runs forward within the lateral wall of the cavernous sinus. Anteriorly, CN IV crosses over CN III to enter the superior orbital fissure outside and superior to the annulus of Zinn. CN IV crosses over the optic nerve to enter the superior oblique muscle within the superior medial orbit.

Oculomotor nerve (CN III)

The nucleus of CN III is located dorsally within the midbrain beneath the aqueduct connecting the third and fourth ventricles (see Fig 1-35). The nuclear complex itself represents a collection of subnuclei that have specific identifiable functions. Most dorsally, the *central caudal nucleus* is a midline structure that innervates both levator palpebrae muscles. Rostrally, the *Edinger-Westphal (EW) nucleus* is a paired structure that sends parasympathetic signals to the sphincter muscles of the pupil and the muscles of accommodation in the ciliary body. The *medial complex,* which lies most ventrally, has been shown to contain 3 subnuclei that play variable roles in medial rectus function. One of these subsets may receive input from the mesencephalic reticular formation, firing in response to retinal temporal disparity that indicates a near target. Additional connections include pathways that tie the NRTP to the cerebellar vermis and the flocculus and fastigial nucleus. The inferior rectus subnucleus lies dorsally and rostrally. The inferior oblique subnucleus is located laterally between the inferior rectus subnucleus and the ventral medial rectus subnucleus. The fibers exit ventrally, along with the fibers destined to innervate the medial rectus, inferior rectus, and the pupil and ciliary body. Fibers from the superior rectus subnucleus, which lies along the midline, cross before exiting ventrally to travel along with the fibers destined for the levator; recall that CN IV also crosses to innervate the contralateral superior oblique muscle. Within the midbrain, CN III is topographically organized into a superior division (supplying the superior rectus and levator) and an inferior division (supplying the medial and inferior rectus, inferior oblique, and pupillary sphincter and ciliary body), but the true anatomical division into 2 branches occurs at the level of the anterior cavernous sinus/superior orbital fissure.

The fascicles of CN III traverse the ventral midbrain tegmentum, passing near and possibly through the red nucleus, the substantia nigra, and the corticospinal tracts within the cerebral peduncle. Multiple fascicles, totaling approximately 15,000 fibers, exit on the ventral surface of the peduncles. Although seen as 1 structure within the subarachnoid space—as is the case in the midbrain—the nerve and its various fibers are topographically organized. Within the subarachnoid space, the nerve passes between the superior cerebellar artery below and the posterior cerebral artery above and receives its blood supply from branches off the proximal posterior cerebral artery and superior cerebellar artery and tentorial branches from the meningohypophyseal trunk. The nerve runs slightly oblique to the tentorial edge, parallel and lateral to the posterior communicating artery. The pupillary fibers are usually found on the dorsomedial surface of the nerve, where they are anatomically vulnerable to compression. The *uncus,* which is the most medial aspect of the temporal lobe, is located just above the tentorium and the subarachnoid third nerve. Unilateral supratentorial mass lesions may force the uncus through the tentorial notch (uncal herniation) to compress the ipsilateral CN III.

At the back edge of the dura of the clivus and cavernous sinus, the nerve enters its own dural canal just above CN IV. Running forward in the superior lateral wall of the cavernous sinus, the nerve separates into a superior and an inferior division. These divisions enter the orbit through the superior orbital fissure within the annulus of Zinn. The superior division runs forward intraconally to innervate first the superior rectus and then the levator above on its inferior surface. The inferior division sends parasympathetic fibers to the ciliary ganglion in the orbital apex approximately 10 mm anterior to the annulus of Zinn and lateral to the optic nerve. Within the ciliary ganglion, the fibers destined for the pupillary sphincter and the ciliary body synapse. The fibers subsequently accompany the branch destined for the inferior oblique muscle. There are approximately 9–10 times as many fibers associated with accommodation innervating the ciliary body as there are fibers reaching the pupillary sphincter muscle. This disparity is possibly one of the reasons for the development of light–near dissociation in Adie tonic pupil (see Chapter 10).

Bhatti MT, Eisenschenk S, Roper SN, Guy JR. Superior divisional third cranial nerve paresis: clinical and anatomical observations of 2 unique cases. *Arch Neurol.* 2006;63(5):771–776.

Leigh RJ, Zee DS. *The Neurology of Eye Movements.* 4th ed. New York: Oxford University Press; 2006.

Rhoton AI, Natori Y. *The Orbit and Sellar Region: Microsurgical Anatomy and Operative Approaches.* New York: Thieme; 1996.

Extraocular Muscles

The final common pathways that influence the position of the eye within the orbit are the multiple soft-tissue elements connected to the globe. In addition to the EOMs, these tissues include the optic nerve, Tenon capsule, blood vessels, and the conjunctiva anteriorly. (Orbital anatomy is discussed in BCSC Section 7, *Orbit, Eyelids, and Lacrimal System.*)

Of the 6 EOMs, 4 are *rectus muscles* (lateral, medial, superior, and inferior), and 2 are oblique (superior and inferior). The recti originate along with the levator at the annulus of Zinn, a condensation of tissue around the optic nerve at the orbital apex. They run forward within sheaths that are connected by intermuscular septa to pierce the posterior Tenon capsule and insert on the anterior sclera, at points variably posterior to the corneal limbus, increasing from the medial through the inferior and lateral to the superior *(spiral of Tillaux).* The recti are also maintained in position by septal attachments to the orbital periosteum that act as pulleys.

The 2 *oblique muscles* insert on the posterior lateral aspect of the globe. The origin of the inferior oblique muscle is in the anteromedial periorbita near the posterior margin of the lacrimal fossa. The effective origin of the superior oblique muscle is the trochlea, a pulleylike structure located at the notch in the superior medial orbit. The superior oblique muscle runs anteriorly in the superior medial orbit to the trochlea, where its tendon reverses its direction of action.

The EOMs are of variable mass and cross section: the inferior oblique is the thinnest, and the medial rectus is the largest. Thus, with normal tonic innervation, the somewhat stronger medial rectus reduces the divergent phoria.

Each of the EOMs has a series of repeating sarcomeres that make up each of the muscle fibers. The fibrils within the EOMs can be divided into at least 2 populations: *fast twitch fibers* and sparse *tonic,* or *slow twitch, fibers.* Tonic fibers are innervated by a series of grapelike neuromuscular junctions (en grappe); fast twitch fibers have a single neuromuscular junction for each fiber (en plaque). Ocular myofibrils and their attendant neuromuscular connections are unique. These specializations distinguish ocular muscle systems from cardiac, smooth, or skeletal muscles and help explain why certain diseases preferentially affect or spare the EOMs.

The lateral rectus moves the globe into abduction. Similarly, the medial rectus moves the eye into adduction. Each of the other muscles has a primary, secondary, and tertiary function that varies depending on the position of gaze (Fig 1-36). The superior rectus muscle primarily causes elevation. As the globe moves into adduction, it becomes increasingly an incyclotorter and adductor. Similarly, in abduction, the inferior rectus is primarily a depressor but becomes more and more an excyclotorter and adductor as the position moves medially. The superior oblique functions as an incyclotorter and abductor but becomes increasingly a depressor as it moves into adduction. The inferior oblique (also inserting

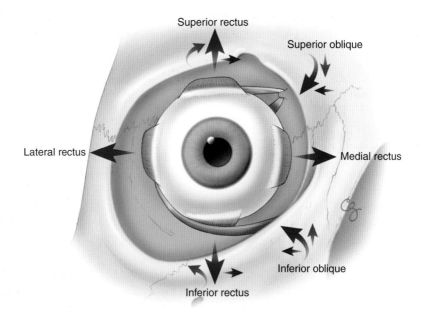

Figure 1-36 Primary, secondary, and tertiary functions of the extraocular muscles, right eye. *(Illustration by Christine Gralapp)*

Muscle	Primary	Secondary	Tertiary
Medial rectus	Adduction		
Lateral rectus	Abduction		
Inferior rectus	Depression	Excyclotorsion	Adduction
Superior rectus	Elevation	Incyclotorsion	Adduction
Inferior oblique	Excyclotorsion	Elevation	Abduction
Superior oblique	Incyclotorsion	Depression	Abduction

posteriorly on the sclera) acts primarily as an excyclotorter and abductor but becomes increasingly an elevator in adduction. The superior muscles (contralaterally innervated superior oblique and superior rectus) are thus incyclotorters, whereas the inferiors (ipsilaterally innervated) are excyclotorters. A helpful mnemonic is SIN (Superiors INcyclotort). The obliques are abductors, whereas the vertical rectus muscles are adductors. A helpful mnemonic is RAD (Recti ADduct). For further discussion and illustration of the EOMs and their actions, see BCSC Section 6, *Pediatric Ophthalmology and Strabismus.* Also see Chapter 8, The Patient With Diplopia, for the clinical etiologies of EOM dysfunction.

Sensory and Facial Motor Anatomy

Although the importance of CNs II, III, IV, and VI is obvious, the trigeminal (CN V) and facial (CN VII) nerves are also critical for normal ophthalmic function and are among those frequently involved in neuro-ophthalmic cases. For example, proper functioning of CN V is essential for preventing corneal damage. In addition, complete loss of corneal sensation may be accompanied by abnormal corneal epithelial growth (neurotrophic keratitis associated with loss of neural secreted growth factors).

Rhoton AI, Natori Y. *The Orbit and Sellar Region: Microsurgical Anatomy and Operative Approaches.* New York: Thieme; 1996.

Trigeminal Nerve (CN V)

The sensory nerve terminates within the *trigeminal nucleus.* The nuclear complex of CN V extends from the midbrain to the cervical spinal cord and includes a main sensory nucleus, a mesencephalic nucleus, and a spinal nucleus (Fig 1-37). The *main sensory nucleus* is located within the pons lateral to the motor nucleus (the most rostral portion of the trigeminal complex except for the mesencephalic nucleus) and receives light touch information from the skin of the face and the mucous membranes. It subsequently projects to the contralateral ventral posterior nucleus of the thalamus. From there, sensation is projected to the postcentral gyrus (Fig 1-38). The *mesencephalic nucleus* serves proprioception and deep sensation from the facial muscles, including those of mastication and the EOMs. In addition, a *spinal nucleus* extends caudally to the level of the C4 vertebra, receiving pain and temperature information. The spinal nucleus is arranged ventral-dorsally from V1 to V3 and rostral-caudally from the perioral region, peripherally involving all 3 divisions

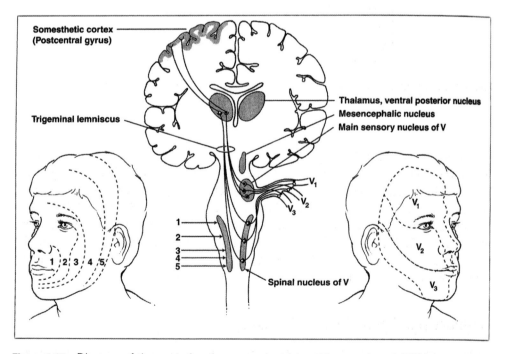

Figure 1-37 Diagram of the central pathways and peripheral innervation of CN V. *(Used with permission from Kline LB. Neuro-Ophthalmology Review Manual. 6th ed. Thorofare, NJ: Slack; 2008:174.)*

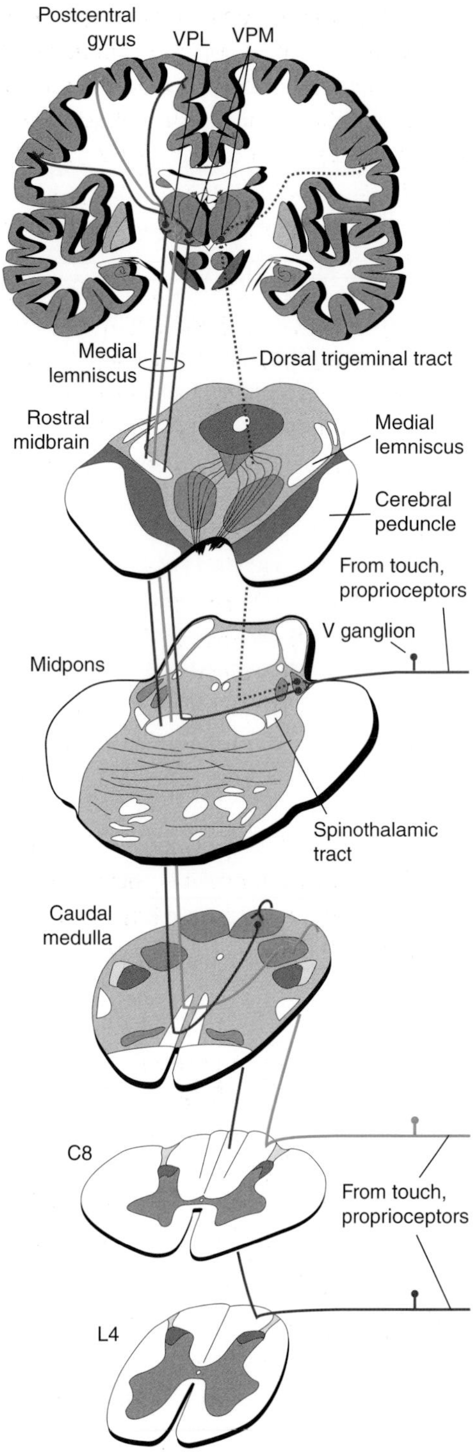

Figure 1-38 Ascending trigeminal pathways from the main sensory nucleus. *VPL* = ventral posterior lateral nucleus, *VPM* = ventral posterior medial nucleus. *(Reproduced with permission from Nolte J.* The Human Brain: An Introduction to Its Functional Anatomy. *4th ed. St Louis: Mosby; 1998.)*

(resulting in an onionskin pattern). The various sensory nuclei of the trigeminal nerve project to the contralateral thalamus and thence to the postcentral gyrus (primary sensory cortex). The *motor nucleus* of the trigeminal nerve lies in the pons, medial to the sensory nucleus. The motor nucleus sends signals to the muscles of mastication (temporalis, pterygoid, and masseter), the tensor tympani (which damps the eardrum within the middle ear as a reflex response to loud noises), the tensor veli palatini (which orients the uvula), the mylohyoid, and the anterior belly of the digastric muscle (both strap muscles in the neck).

The fascicles of CN V enter the brainstem ventrally in the pons and extra-axially traverse the subarachnoid space to penetrate the dura just over the petrous pyramid. Within the subarachnoid space, the trigeminal root often comes in contact with the superior cerebellar artery. This proximity may be a cause of trigeminal neuralgia (atypical facial pain, discussed in Chapter 12, The Patient With Head, Ocular, or Facial Pain) and is the anatomical basis for microvascular decompression. The blood supply to the trigeminal root comes from branches of the superior cerebellar, pontine, and anterior inferior cerebellar arteries.

The 3 divisions of CN V synapse in the trigeminal (gasserian) ganglion, located in an extradural space at the floor of the middle cranial fossa (Meckel cave) (Fig 1-39).

The *ophthalmic division (V₁)* is the most anterior branch exiting the trigeminal ganglion. It runs forward within the lateral wall of the cavernous sinus just below CN IV. As it extradurally approaches the superior orbital fissure, it divides into 3 major branches: lacrimal, frontal, and nasociliary. In addition, small branches innervate the dura of the anterior middle cranial fossa, including the cavernous sinus, the parasellar region, the tentorium, and the dura of the petrous apex. These branches also innervate the floor of the anterior cranial fossa, including the falx and the major blood vessels at the skull base.

The lacrimal and frontal nerves enter the orbital apex outside the annulus of Zinn. The frontal nerve passes slightly medially to run in the superior orbit just below the periorbita over the levator. At its terminus, the frontal nerve divides into supraorbital and

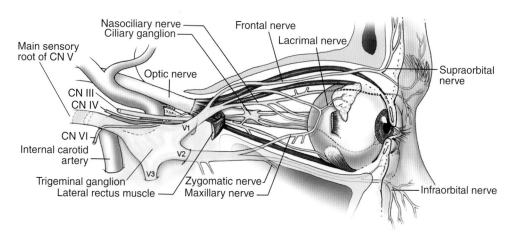

Figure 1-39 Lateral view of the orbit, showing its sensory nerves. *(Illustration by Dave Peace.)*

supratrochlear branches, which innervate the forehead, frontal sinus, and upper eyelid (including the conjunctiva). The lacrimal nerve also runs anteriorly in the superior lateral orbit just above the lateral rectus to innervate the lacrimal gland and some skin just superotemporal to the orbit. The nasociliary branch is the only branch entering the intraconal space through the annulus of Zinn. Before entering the orbit, the nasociliary branch becomes associated with the sympathetic fibers that originally accompanied CN VI after leaving the carotid sheath. The nasociliary branch runs through the ciliary ganglion and anteriorly to innervate the globe through the short and long posterior ciliary nerves. Prior to reaching the globe, branches from the nasociliary division pass through the anterior and posterior ethmoidal foramina to innervate part of the ethmoidal sinuses, the lateral wall of the nose, and the skin of the nose to the nasal tip. This co-innervation of the globe and the nasal skin is responsible for the Hutchinson sign. This may be seen with zoster ophthalmicus, in which a herpetic lesion at the tip of the nose carries an increased risk of corneal involvement due to the neurotrophic nature of this DNA virus.

The terminal branches of the nasociliary nerve within the cornea contain one of the highest concentrations of sensory nerve endings in the body. These bare fibrils insinuate between cells of the 4 basal layers of the epithelium and provide the anatomical basis for the extreme sensitivity of the cornea.

The *maxillary division (V₂)* runs forward at the inferior lateral base of the cavernous sinus to enter the foramen rotundum, located just below the superior orbital fissure. Just before entering the canal, V_2 gives off the middle meningeal nerve, which supplies the dura of the lateral middle cranial fossa. On the anterior end of the foramen rotundum, V_2 enters the pterygomaxillary area, located just below the inferior orbital fissure. Two large pterygopalatine nerves supply sensation to the nasopharynx, hard and soft palate, and portions of the nasal cavity. Posterior alveolar nerves supply sensation to the upper gums and molars. The zygomatic nerve enters the orbit through the inferior orbital fissure and divides into the zygomaticofacial and the zygomaticotemporal nerves, which supply sensation to the lateral face (see Fig 1-39). The maxillary nerve continues anteriorly within a canal between the orbit above and the maxillary sinus below to exit through the infraorbital foramen (as the infraorbital nerve) just below the inferior orbital rim. It subsequently divides into palpebral, nasal, and labial branches. The sensation of the cheek as well as the lower lid and upper teeth and gums is provided by this division.

The *mandibular division (V₃)* enters through the foramen ovale, lateral to the foramen lacerum and medial to the foramen spinosum (carrying the middle meningeal artery). Division V_3 innervates the skin of the jaw and also carries the motor division of the trigeminal nerve to the muscles of mastication and neck. Motor paralysis results in contralateral deviation of the jaw when it is closed (weakness of the temporalis) and ipsilateral deviation when protruded (because of weakness in the lateral pterygoid).

Facial Nerve (CN VII)

CN VII is responsible for the movement of the facial muscles. Voluntary facial movements originate along with other motor activity in the *precentral gyrus*. White matter tracts pass through the internal capsule and cerebral peduncles along with the other corticobulbar fibers. The motor neurons destined for the upper face receive information from both sides (bilateral innervation), whereas the lower facial musculature receives information only from the contralateral cortex. The facial nuclei receive additional information from basal ganglia extrapyramidal connections, which are largely responsible for involuntary blinking, as well as for the abnormal blinking seen in basal ganglia diseases such as Parkinson, probably mediated through alteration in inhibition of the blink reflex. Projections from the superior colliculus through the nucleus raphe magnus that reduce the excitability of spinal trigeminal neurons associated with the blink reflex have been identified. The superior colliculus, in turn, receives inhibitory (GABA) input from the pars reticulata of the substantia nigra.

The motor fibers of the CN VII nucleus originate in the tegmentum of the caudal pons ventrolateral to the sixth nerve nucleus and medial to the spinal nucleus of the trigeminal nerve (Fig 1-40). The dorsal subnucleus receives bilateral innervation and supplies the upper face; the lateral subnucleus (contralateral innervation) supplies the lower face. The fascicles of CN VII pass dorsomedially to surround the sixth nerve nucleus, creating a bump on the floor of the fourth ventricle (the genu of the facial nerve intra-axially and the colliculus of the facial nerve on the floor of the fourth ventricle). CN VII exits the ventrolateral surface of the pons along with fascicles of the nervus intermedius, which contains the facial nerve sensory fibers and the visceral efferent fibers (see Parasympathetic Pathways later in the chapter). The subarachnoid seventh nerve runs anteriorly and laterally to enter the internal auditory meatus along with the superior and inferior vestibular nerves and the cochlear, or auditory, nerve (CN VIII).

Within the petrous bone, CN VII enters the fallopian canal and traverses 3 segments (the labyrinthine, the tympanic, and the mastoid) that run in close proximity to the semicircular canals. The parasympathetic fibers destined for the lacrimal gland separate from CN VII in the region of the geniculate ganglion to accompany the greater superficial petrosal nerve. The stapedial nerve exits to innervate the stapedius muscle, and the chorda tympani conducts parasympathetic innervation to the submaxillary gland and afferent fibers from the anterior two thirds of the tongue. These special afferent fibers are responsible for taste in the anterior tongue and synapse in the geniculate ganglion.

The main branch of CN VII exits the stylomastoid foramen just behind the styloid process at the base of the mastoid. The extracranial trunk of the nerve passes between the superficial and deep lobes of the parotid gland, where it divides into 2 trunks: the temporofacial superiorly and the smaller cervicofacial inferiorly. These further variably divide into 5 major branches: the temporal, zygomatic, infraorbital, buccal, and mandibular. The temporal and zygomatic branches laterally innervate the orbicularis oculi muscles. The infraorbital and buccal branches may also variably contribute to the inferior orbicularis.

Eyelids

The muscles of the eyelids are divided into an orbital (responsible for forced closure) and a palpebral component. The palpebral muscles are further separated into pretarsal (predominantly intermediate fast twitch fibers responsible for normal blinks) and preseptal muscles. This separation occurs at the upper lid crease, located approximately 6–7 mm

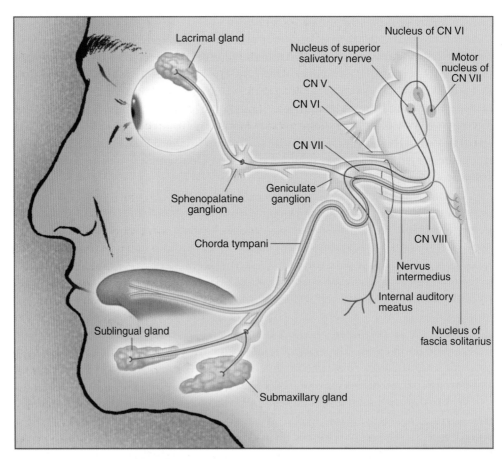

Figure 1-40 Functional anatomy of the facial nerve (CN VII) and diagnosis of peripheral facial weakness. Although CN VII has a long, circuitous path, the site of involvement can be deduced from the patient's clinical deficit. CN VII is predominantly motor in function. Its nucleus is in the caudal pons. CN VII courses dorsomedially and encircles the nucleus of the abducens nerve (CN VI). After bending around the abducens nucleus, CN VII lies close to CN VI. CN VII exits the pons in the cerebellopontine angle close to CNs V, VI, and VIII. CN VIII, the motor root of CN VII, and the nervus intermedius (the sensory and parasympathetic root of CN VII) enter the internal auditory meatus. Sensory cells located in the geniculate ganglion continue distally as the chorda tympani nerve, which carries taste fibers. Peripheral fibers of the nervus intermedius portion of CN VII initiate salivary, lacrimal, and mucous secretion. *(Reproduced with permission from Gilden DH. Clinical practice: Bell's palsy. N Engl J Med. 2004;351:1327.)*

above the lid margin. The superior lid crease is formed by collateral insertion of the levator aponeurosis to the skin of the eyelid. Closure of the lids is marked by an increase in activity of the orbicularis muscle and inhibition of the levator. The balance of tonic orbicularis and active levator activity determines the amount of lid opening. For discussion of eyelid abnormalities encountered in neuro-ophthalmic practice, see Chapter 11, The Patient With Eyelid or Facial Abnormalities. For further discussion, with illustrations, of eyelid anatomy, see BCSC Section 7, *Orbit, Eyelids, and Lacrimal System.*

Ocular Autonomic Pathways

The autonomic nervous system is also critical to normal functioning of the visual system. In particular, branches of the parasympathetic system play a role in lacrimal function, and pupil size is controlled by a balance between the innervation of the sympathetic fibers to the iris dilator muscles and the parasympathetic fibers to the sphincter muscles. The accessory retractor muscles, including the Müller muscle in the upper eyelid, receive sympathetic innervation.

Sympathetic Pathways

Sympathetic activity originates in the posterolateral region of the hypothalamus. Activity in the hypothalamus is influenced by signals in the frontal, sensorimotor, and occipital cortex and in the limbic system (cingulate gyrus). The course of sympathetic fibers destined for the orbit is divided into first-, second-, and third-order segments (Fig 1-41). Axons destined for the dilator muscles of the pupil and Müller muscle descend as the first-order segment, along with other sympathetic fibers, superficially in the anteromedial column through the brainstem to the spinal cord. Within the cervical cord, the sympathetic fibers continue in the intermediolateral column. From C8 to T2, the sympathetic fibers destined for the orbit synapse in the ciliospinal nucleus of Budge-Waller.

The postsynaptic second-order fibers leave the spinal cord through the ventral rami of the cervical (C8) and upper thoracic (T1 and T2) spinal cord before joining the paravertebral sympathetic plexus. Ascending rostrally, the sympathetic chain passes in the anterior loop of the ansa subclavia proximate to the innominate artery on the right and the subclavian artery on the left just above the lung apex. These fibers pass through the inferior and middle cervical ganglia to terminate in the superior cervical ganglion, at the level of the angle of the jaw (C2) and the carotid artery bifurcation.

The postganglionic third-order fibers continue in the wall of the bifurcated carotid. Sympathetic fibers innervating the sweat glands of the lower face follow the ECA.

The sympathetic fibers destined for the pupil continue along the ICA to enter the cranium through the carotid canal. Some sympathetic fibers leave the carotid artery as it exits the petrous bone and, along with the greater superficial petrosal nerve, form the *vidian nerve*. These sympathetic fibers parallel the parasympathetic fibers to the lacrimal gland. Within the cavernous sinus, sympathetic fibers destined for the dilator muscles leave the carotid in conjunction with CN VI for a few millimeters. Further anteriorly in the cavernous sinus, the sympathetic fibers join the nasociliary branch of the ophthalmic division of the trigeminal nerve. In the orbital apex, the fibers then pass through the ciliary ganglion (without synapsing). Along with the nasociliary branch, the sympathetic fibers reach the globe and travel with the long ciliary nerves to the dilator muscles of the pupil. The dilator muscle lies just superficial to the posterior pigment epithelium of the iris, which continues peripherally as the nonpigmented superficial layer of the ciliary body. The myoepithelial cells measure approximately 12.5 μm in thickness, with an apical epithelial portion and a basilar muscular portion that is oriented radially toward the pupillary opening. The muscular processes terminate peripheral to the sphincter muscle.

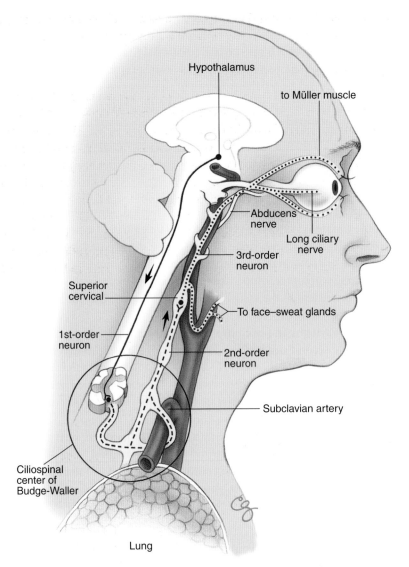

Figure 1-41 Anatomy of the sympathetic pathway showing first-order central neuron, second-order intermediate neuron, and third-order neuron pathways. Note the proximity of the pulmonary apex to the sympathetic chain. Note also the relationship of the intracavernous sympathetic fibers to CN VI. *(Illustration by Christine Gralapp.)*

Peripherally at the iris root, these cells are continuous with the pigmented epithelium of the ciliary body.

The fibers destined for the Müller muscle travel along the ophthalmic artery and its subsequent frontal and lacrimal branches. The Müller muscle originates near the origin of the levator aponeurosis and inserts 10–12 mm inferiorly on the superior border of the tarsus. It is very vascular and lies just deep to the superior cul-de-sac conjunctiva that extends superiorly from the tarsus. The superior orbital sympathetic fibers also innervate the sweat glands of the forehead. Thus, disruption of these sympathetic fibers is responsible for both the mild ptosis and the frontal anhidrosis seen with distal Horner syndrome.

Parasympathetic Pathways

Parasympathetic activity originates in various areas within the brainstem. Those fibers that control the pupil sphincter muscles originate in the Edinger-Westphal (EW) nuclei of the CN III nuclear complex within the midbrain. The main input to the EW nuclei is from the pretectal nuclei, both directly and via the posterior commissure. The pretectal nuclei, in turn, receive input directly from the afferent visual pathways via the pupillary tract, which leaves the optic tract in the brachium of the superior colliculus just anterior to the lateral geniculate (Fig 1-42). The cortex (especially the frontal lobes), the hypothalamus, and the reticular activating system provide tonic inhibitory signals to the EW nucleus. During sleep, the pupil becomes smaller due to loss of this inhibitory activity. In addition, the EW nucleus receives inputs from the more ventral and rostral midbrain, probably representing input related to bitemporal image disparity and serving as a stimulus for convergence and the near reflex.

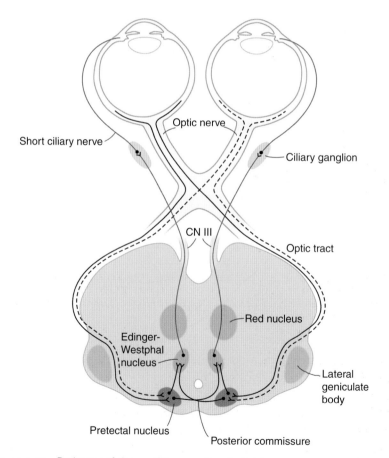

Figure 1-42 Pathway of the pupillary reaction to light. *(Illustration by Christine Gralapp.)*

The parasympathetic fibers and the CN III fascicles leave the CN III nucleus and exit in the interpeduncular fossa. Within the subarachnoid space, the parasympathetic fibers tend to run on the medial superficial surface of CN III. When CN III bifurcates in the anterior cavernous sinus, the parasympathetic fibers travel with the inferior division. In the orbital apex, these fibers enter the ciliary ganglion, where they synapse. The postsynaptic fibers then travel with the branch destined for the inferior oblique to join the posterior ciliary nerves to reach the anterior segment and the iris sphincter muscles. The sphincter muscle measures approximately 0.8 mm in diameter and 0.15 mm in thickness. It travels circumferentially around the pupillary margin just anterior to the posterior pigmented epithelium and central to the termination of the dilator muscle cells. The muscle itself is made of units composed of groups of 5–8 muscle cells.

Parasympathetic innervation to the lacrimal gland originates in the superior salivatory (salivary) nucleus located in the caudal pons posterolateral to the motor nucleus of CN VII. This nucleus receives sensory input from the trigeminal nerve and additional afferent fibers from the hypothalamus. Parasympathetic fibers leaving the nucleus join other parasympathetic efferents coming from the salivatory nucleus and run with gustatory afferents destined for the nucleus of the tractus solitarius parallel to the fascicles of the facial nerve in the nervus intermedius (see Fig 1-40; Fig 1-43). This nerve joins with

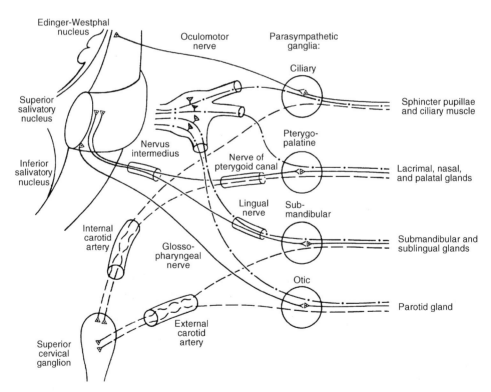

Figure 1-43 Connections of the 4 parasympathetic ganglia of the head and neck. *(Reproduced with permission from McMinn RMH. Last's Anatomy: Regional and Applied. 8th ed. Edinburgh: Churchill Livingstone; 1990.)*

CN VII to exit the brainstem on its ventral surface of the pontomedullary junction. With the other fascicles of CN VII, the parasympathetic fibers of the nervus intermedius run laterally to the internal auditory meatus. Within the petrous bone and fallopian canal, the parasympathetic fibers exit at the geniculate ganglion and then travel superficially over the petrous bone with the greater superficial petrosal nerve. This course parallels that of the carotid artery, and in the area where the carotid artery turns to rise into the cavernous sinus, the fibers join the vidian nerve. This travels through the sphenoid bone parallel and below the foramen rotundum to enter the pterygomaxillary space. The fibers synapse in the sphenopalatine ganglion. The postganglionic fibers travel superiorly through the inferior orbital fissure and then with the lacrimal nerve to reach the lacrimal gland. The parasympathetic fibers are responsible for reflex tearing.

Loewenfeld IE. *The Pupil: Anatomy, Physiology, and Clinical Applications.* 2nd ed. New York: Butterworth-Heinemann; 1999.

CHAPTER 2

Neuroimaging in Neuro-Ophthalmology

Glossary

BOLD (blood oxygenation level–dependent) MRI technique that allows functional imaging demarcating areas of high activity during a specific task.

CTA (computed tomographic angiography) CT technique used to image blood vessels.

DWI (diffusion-weighted imaging) MRI technique especially useful for acute and subacute stroke.

FLAIR (fluid-attenuated inversion recovery) MRI technique that highlights T2 hyperintense abnormalities adjacent to CSF (cerebrospinal fluid)-containing spaces, such as the ventricles, by suppressing CSF signal intensity.

fMRI (functional magnetic resonance imaging) MRI technique that allows visualization of more active brain areas during a specific task, such as reading.

Frequency-encoding analysis Gradient variation in the magnetic field results in a change in signal frequency; as the gradient is varied across the subject, the computer can localize the position of a particular signal.

Gadolinium Paramagnetic agent administered intravenously to enhance lesions.

Hounsfield unit 1/2000 of the x-ray density scale centered on water (at zero) and ranging from air (at -1000) to bone (approaching $+1000$).

IR (inversion recovery) Initial 180° pulses followed by a 90° pulse and immediate acquisition of the signal; in IR sequences, the interpulse time is given by TI.

MRA (magnetic resonance angiography) MRI technique for imaging blood vessels.

MRS (magnetic resonance spectroscopy) MRI technique that further characterizes the tissue composition of part of the brain, which helps differentiate tumor, demyelination, and necrosis.

Pixel Picture element; any of the small discrete elements that together constitute an image (as on a television screen); increasing pixels increases image resolution.

Relaxation Process by which an element gives up (reemits) energy after having absorbed it from the radiofrequency pulses.

SE (spin echo) In the most commonly employed spin-echo sequence, a 180° pulse follows a 90° pulse. For T2-weighted images, the 90° pulse is followed by two 180° pulses. The first 180° pulse is administered at one half the TE (time to echo), and the second 180° pulse is administered at one full TE later. The "first echo" image is referred to as *proton density*, and the "second echo" is T2-weighted.

SR (saturation recovery) With SR, the radiofrequency signal is recorded after a series of 90° pulses, with an interpulse interval less than or equal to an average tissue T1 (0.1–1.5 sec).

T1 Time required for 63% of protons to return to the longitudinal plane after cessation of a 90° radiofrequency pulse. This is also referred to as the *longitudinal*, or *spin-lattice*, relaxation time.

T2 Time required for 63% of the magnetic field in the transverse plane created by the radiofrequency pulse to dissipate. This dispersion of the magnetic vector corresponds to the exchange of spin among protons and is referred to as *spin-spin relaxation*; it is completed much more rapidly than is T1 relaxation.

TE (time to echo) Time following the pulse in which the signal is assessed.

Tesla Measure of magnetic field strength.

TI (interpulse time) See IR (inversion recovery).

TR Time to repetition of radiofrequency pulse.

Voxel Three-dimensional cube determined by the product of the pixel size and the slice thickness.

Jäger HR. Loss of vision: imaging the visual pathways. *Eur Radiol.* 2005;15(3):501–510.

Mafee MF, Karimi A, Shah JD, Rapoport M, Ansari SA. Anatomy and pathology of the eye: role of MR imaging and CT. *Magn Reson Imaging Clin N Am.* 2006;14(2):249–270.

Vaphiades MS. Imaging the neurovisual system. *Ophthalmol Clin North Am.* 2004;17(3): 465–480.

Computed Tomography

The orbit is particularly suited to x-ray–based imaging because fat provides excellent contrast to the globe (Fig 2-1), lacrimal gland, optic nerve, and extraocular muscles. Bone

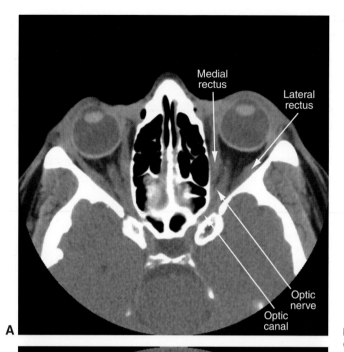

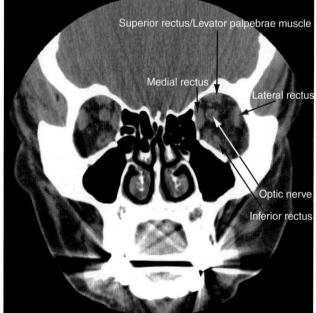

Figure 2-1 Normal orbital CT axial **(A)** and coronal **(B)** views. *(Courtesy of Rod Foroozan, MD.)*

and other calcium-containing processes can be easily visualized because of their marked x-ray attenuation. Soft-tissue details can be further enhanced by the injection of iodinated contrast material, which crosses a disturbed blood–brain barrier to accumulate within a local lesion and reveals inflammatory and neoplastic processes.

The advantages of *computed tomography (CT)* include rapid image acquisition, wide availability, and excellent spatial resolution. The speed and ability of CT to identify acute blood or bone abnormalities accurately make this technique especially useful in trauma, when a patient may be confused or combative, and identification of hemorrhage or bony abnormalities is critical. The disadvantages of CT include the use of ionizing radiation, contrast agent–related side effects, and poor soft-tissue resolution adjacent to bone or other radiodense objects. Iodinated contrast agents are associated with nephrotoxicity and relatively frequent allergic reactions. These drawbacks render CT less useful when a serial imaging technique is needed, when imaging brainstem or skull-based lesions, when a nonaxial plane (coronal or sagittal plane) is useful, or in patients with a history of iodinated contrast dye allergy or nephropathy.

Magnetic Resonance Imaging

Magnetic resonance imaging (MRI) is now the imaging study of choice for many disease processes. The technique depends on the physical properties of soft tissue for image generation. Atoms containing an odd number of nucleons (protons and neutrons) have a small magnetic moment. The most common element with these properties is hydrogen. When placed within a powerful magnet, these nuclei align with the magnetic field. Radiofrequency pulses can then transiently perturb the magnetic movements, knocking the protons out of alignment. Following a sequence of pulses, the rate of relaxation will correspond to the specific magnetic properties of the tissue, which results in tissue-specific signals. Varying the repeated radiofrequency pulses and the timing of signal recording yields different types of images. Modern MRI devices obtain a 3-dimensional data set that shows views in axial, coronal, sagittal, or even oblique planes without patient repositioning. MRI is sensitive to soft-tissue changes in water content, depending on how the water is bound and how it moves within tissue. Injection of gadolinium, a paramagnetic agent that also traverses a disrupted blood–brain barrier, alters the signal characteristics. This alteration may be critical in identifying certain tumors whose characteristics make them otherwise indistinguishable from normal cortical tissue. Although initially believed to be free of toxicity, gadolinium has been reported to cause a systemic fibrosis syndrome that often involves the skin (nephrogenic fibrosing dermopathy), especially in patients with preexisting renal disease. It is characterized by scleroderma-like thickening of the skin, subcutaneous edema, and ensuing joint contractures leading to profound disability. Involvement of other organs has also been described.

Magnetic resonance images are usually classified as being T1- or T2-weighted (Fig 2-2). Each tissue has its own characteristic T1 and T2 relaxation times resulting from a combination of the amount of water present and the tissue's bound state. In the most common spin-echo technique, a T1-weighted image is obtained by selecting appropriate pulse timing: a relatively short TR (time to repetition; approximately 200–700 msec) and a short TE (echo time; 20–35 msec) (Table 2-1). T1-weighted images are optimal for demonstrating anatomy. Resolution is also higher than in T2-weighted images, chiefly because of the increased intensity of the signal and thus the decreased acquisition times (minimizing motion artifact). However, T2-weighted images (long TR of 1500–3000 msec

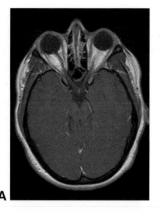 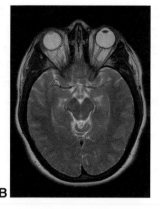 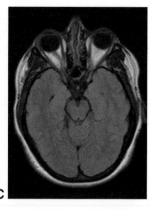

A   B   C

Figure 2-2 Normal axial MRI of the brain at the level of the orbits and midbrain. T1-weighted image with contrast **(A)** shows cerebrospinal fluid (CSF) and vitreous as hypointense (dark), orbital fat as hyperintense (bright), and gray matter as relatively hypointense compared to white matter. T2-weighted image **(B)** shows that CSF, vitreous, and orbital fat are hyperintense and gray matter is hyperintense compared to white matter. The FLAIR image **(C)** shows that orbital fat is hyperintense; however, vitreous and CSF appear hypointense, which facilitates detection of abnormalities in periventricular tissue. *(Courtesy of Rod Foroozan, MD.)*

Table 2-1 MRI Types and Parameters

Image	TR (time to repetition)	TE (time to echo)
T1	Short (200–700 msec)	Short (20–35 msec)
T2	Long (1500–3000 msec)	Long (75–250 msec)
Proton	Long (>1000 msec)	Short (<35 msec)
FLAIR	Very long (>6000 msec)	Long (>75 msec)

FLAIR = fluid-attenuated inversion recovery

and TE of 75–250 msec) maximize the differences in tissue water content and state. Thus, T2-weighted images are the most sensitive to inflammatory, ischemic, or neoplastic alterations in tissue (Figs 2-3, 2-4, 2-5). Proton density images, a third form (long TR and short TE), have intermediate properties between those of T1 and T2 weighting and are obtained simultaneously with the T2 image.

Very intense tissue signals (fat in T1-weighted images and cerebrospinal fluid [CSF]/vitreous in T2-weighted images) may obscure subtle signal abnormalities in neighboring tissues (Table 2-2). Special sequences have been designed to reduce these high signals. Fat-suppression techniques, such as *short tau inversion recovery (STIR),* are used to obtain relatively T1-weighted images without the confounding bright fat signal. This is particularly useful in studying the orbit (Figs 2-6, 2-7). *Fluid-attenuated inversion recovery (FLAIR)* provides T2-weighted images without the high-CSF signal, making FLAIR ideal for viewing the periventricular white matter changes in a demyelinating process such as multiple sclerosis (Fig 2-8). *Diffusion-weighted imaging (DWI)* is sensitive to recent vascular perfusion alterations and is thus ideal for identifying recent infarctions (Fig 2-9). An abnormal DWI signal develops within minutes of the onset of cerebral ischemia and persists for approximately 3 weeks, serving as a time marker for acute and subacute ischemic events.

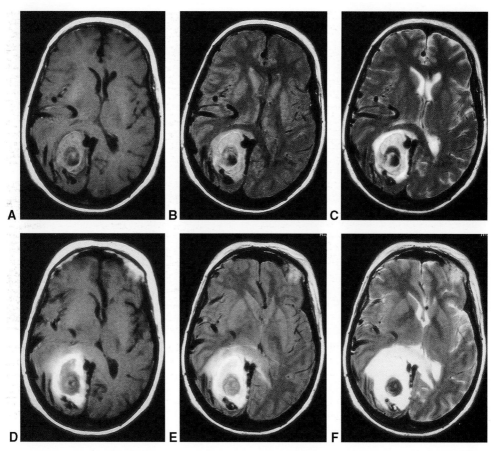

Figure 2-3 Comparison of T1 and T2 images can yield information about the characteristics of a lesion and can be particularly helpful in dating hemorrhages. A 61-year-old patient presented with acute onset of severe headache. A hemorrhage is apparent in the parieto-occipital region in the 3 scans originally taken: T1-weighted **(A)**, proton density **(B)**, and T2-weighted **(C)** images. The signal at the lesion periphery relates to the presence of oxyhemoglobin, whereas the core remains dark in all 3 images because of the presence of deoxyhemoglobin. When the MRI series was repeated 10 days later, the signal characteristics had changed as a result of the development of methemoglobin in the outer ring, which is bright on T1 **(D)**, proton density **(E)**, and T2 **(F)** sequences. The core remains dark. *(Courtesy of Steven A. Newman, MD.)*

Symms M, Jäger HR, Schmierer K, Yousry TA. A review of structural magnetic resonance neuroimaging. *J Neurol Neurosurg Psychiatry.* 2004;75(9):1235–1244.

Vascular Imaging

Several techniques are used to image blood vessels. These commonly used techniques are important because of the frequency with which ischemic processes affect the nervous system.

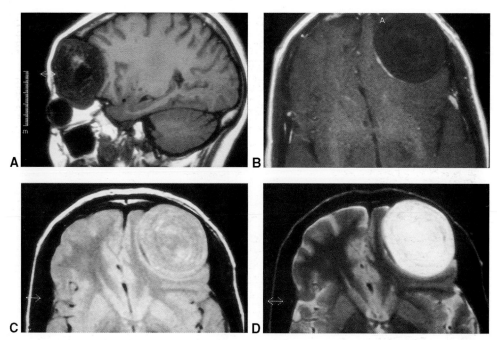

Figure 2-4 Various tumors may have specific sequence findings. This patient had a large frontal tumor invading the orbit. **A,** Sagittal T1 sequence shows the tumor to be heterogeneous but mostly hypointense to gray matter. **B,** Axial gadolinium-enhanced T1-weighted image demonstrates minimal rim enhancement. **C,** On the proton density image, the signal intensity becomes brighter, being isointense with gray matter and brighter than white matter. **D,** On T2 images, the lesion becomes extremely bright. These findings are characteristic of an epidermoid. *(Courtesy of Steven A. Newman, MD.)*

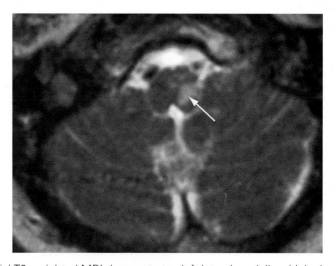

Figure 2-5 Axial T2-weighted MRI demonstrates left lateral medullary high signal *(arrow)* consistent with infarction in a patient with Wallenberg lateral medullary syndrome. The patient presented with left Horner syndrome, left facial numbness, skew deviation, right body numbness, and vertigo. *(Courtesy of Eric Eggenberger, DO.)*

Table 2-2 MRI Signal Intensity by Tissue

T1	Fat ≫ white matter > gray matter > CSF/vitreous > air
T2	CSF/vitreous ≫ gray matter > white matter > fat
Proton	CSF/vitreous > gray matter = white matter > fat > air
FLAIR	Fat > gray matter > white matter > CSF/vitreous > air
STIR	CSF/vitreous = gray matter > white matter > fat > air

FLAIR = fluid-attenuated inversion recovery; STIR = short tau inversion recovery

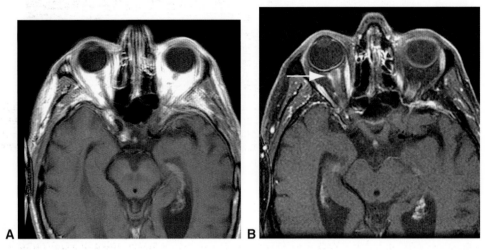

Figure 2-6 Axial T1-weighted orbital MRI with contrast **(A)** shows the normal hyperintense orbital fat. Suppression of the orbital fat **(B)** enables visualization of optic nerve sheath enhancement *(arrow)* consistent with a meningioma. *(Part A courtesy of Rod Foroozan, MD; part B reprinted with permission from Foroozan R, Hinckley L. Compression of the anterior visual pathways. In: Kline LB, Foroozan R, eds. Optic Nerve Disorders. 2nd ed. Ophthalmology Monograph 10. New York: Oxford University Press, in cooperation with the American Academy of Ophthalmology; 2007:109.)*

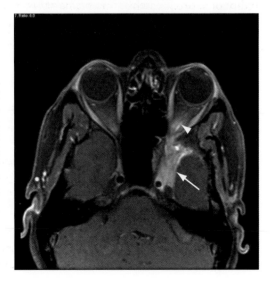

Figure 2-7 This 48-year-old female presented with slowly progressive decreased vision OS. This axial T1-weighted fat-suppressed postcontrast MRI shows a meningioma involving the middle cranial fossa of the skull base *(arrow)*, including the optic canal. Abnormal enhancement in the orbital apex indicates extension of the meningioma along the optic nerve sheath *(arrowhead)*. *(Courtesy of Eric Eggenberger, DO.)*

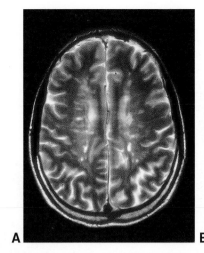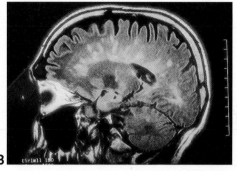

A   **B**

Figure 2-8 A 41-year-old patient presented with acute onset of decreased vision in his right eye. **A,** Axial T2-weighted image. **B,** Sagittal FLAIR technique demonstrates periventricular white matter spots characteristic of demyelinating disease. The FLAIR technique suppresses the high signal intensity of the CSF, thus allowing lesions around the ventricular system to be seen clearly. *(Courtesy of Steven A. Newman, MD.)*

Conventional/Catheter/Contrast Angiography

The "gold standard" for intracerebral vascular imaging remains catheter, or contrast, angiography (Fig 2-10). With this technique, a catheter is placed intra-arterially and iodinated radiodense contrast dye is injected. *Digital subtraction angiography (DSA)* is a technique that reduces artifacts by subtracting densities created by the overlying bony skull. The contrast dye outlines the column of flowing blood within the injected vessel and demonstrates stenosis, aneurysms, vascular malformations, flow dynamics, and vessel wall irregularities such as dissections or vasculitis. The procedure has an overall morbidity of approximately 2.5%, primarily related to ischemia from emboli or vasospasm, dye-related reactions, or complications at the arterial puncture site. The use of digital subtraction technology has enhanced the ability to visualize vascular structures with smaller amounts of contrast dye.

Magnetic Resonance Angiography

Because an MRI signal requires excitation and decay, moving tissue often passes out of the plane of assessment before the return signal can be detected. This is the basis of the black "flow void" characteristic of vascular channels with flow. Protons that are excited in 1 slice and then move to another slice may be specifically imaged. This 3-dimensional assessment underlies *magnetic resonance angiography (MRA)* and *magnetic resonance venography (MRV)*. Several techniques, such as 2- and 3-dimensional time-of-flight angiography, phase contrast angiography, and multiple overlapping thin-slab acquisition (MOTSA), have been used to obtain images. MRA signals may also be obtained from gadolinium-enhanced images. This technique is particularly useful for obtaining images of the proximal large vessels of the chest and neck. MRA with gadolinium has a very short acquisition

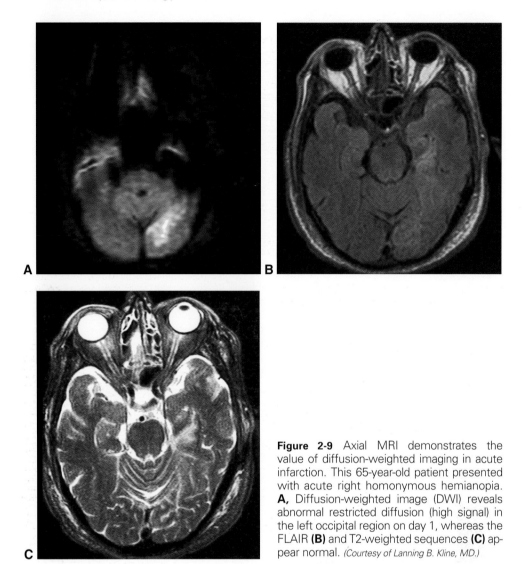

Figure 2-9 Axial MRI demonstrates the value of diffusion-weighted imaging in acute infarction. This 65-year-old patient presented with acute right homonymous hemianopia. **A,** Diffusion-weighted image (DWI) reveals abnormal restricted diffusion (high signal) in the left occipital region on day 1, whereas the FLAIR **(B)** and T2-weighted sequences **(C)** appear normal. *(Courtesy of Lanning B. Kline, MD.)*

time, making patient movement–related artifact less of an issue. MRA provides excellent noninvasive information about large and medium-size vessels. However, because MRA depends on flow physiology, it tends to overestimate vascular stenosis, and image resolution limits the ability to visualize smaller vessels or vasculitis. MRV may be helpful in excluding thrombosis within the dural venous sinuses (Fig 2-11), a condition that may cause papilledema (see also Chapter 14).

Computed Tomographic Angiography

Computed tomographic angiography (CTA), which uses a high-speed spiral scanner, provides excellent vessel resolution with 3-dimensional capability that is complementary to

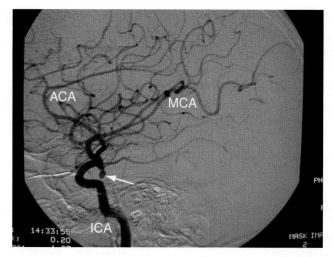

Figure 2-10 Contrast angiogram, lateral view, demonstrates aneurysm of the posterior communicating artery *(arrow)*. *ACA* = anterior cerebral artery, *ICA* = internal carotid artery, *MCA* = middle cerebral artery. *(Courtesy of Rod Foroozan, MD.)*

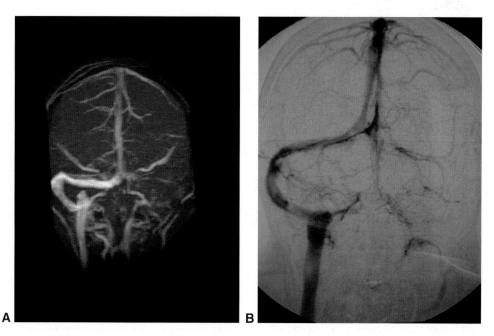

Figure 2-11 Venous sinus thrombosis. MRV **(A)** and cerebral angiography **(B)** in the venous phase showing absence of flow within the left transverse sinus, sigmoid sinus, and internal jugular vein. *(Reprinted with permission from Foroozan R, Kline LB. Papilledema. In: Kline LB, Foroozan R, eds.* Optic Nerve Disorders. *2nd ed. Ophthalmology Monograph 10. New York: Oxford University Press, in cooperation with the American Academy of Ophthalmology; 2007:55.)*

MRA. The technique requires iodinated contrast dye and ionizing radiation and takes approximately 15 minutes. Sensitivities in the detection of aneurysms >3 mm or stenosis >70% are approximately 95%. Some centers prefer the use of CTA over MRA in the detection of cerebral aneurysms, including those causing ocular motor cranial nerve palsies (see Chapter 8, Fig 8-10).

Osborn AG, Blaser S, Salzman KL. *Diagnostic Imaging: Brain.* Philadelphia: WB Saunders; 2004.

Metabolic and Functional Imaging

Magnetic resonance spectroscopy (MRS) provides information on tissue composition. This technique generally depends on hydrogen and phosphorus and produces 5 principal spectra: *N*-acetylaspartate (NAA), choline, creatinine, lipid, and lactate. NAA is associated with neuronal integrity; a decrease in NAA is associated with neuronal loss. Choline is a component of cell membranes. Creatinine is relatively stable within the brain and can serve as an internal control. Lactate is normally barely visible; it is a marker of anaerobic metabolism. Lipid is rarely used clinically. Differences in the pattern of these peaks are associated with different disease processes; nonnecrotic brain neoplasm typically produces an elevated choline peak and a reduced NAA peak. This technique can help characterize MRI abnormalities.

Functional MRI (fMRI) depends on changes in regional blood flow in the brain in accord with metabolic demand. With very fast MRI analysis, local differences in blood oxygenation (blood oxygenation level–dependent [BOLD]) can be evaluated. Based on this technique, areas of higher metabolic activity can be identified during specific tasks, such as reading, speaking, or moving a finger. Besides being less expensive than positron emission tomography (discussed next), fMRI has the additional advantages of faster imaging speed, higher spatial resolution, practical repeatability, and being less invasive. These advantages can be helpful not only in research but also in planning neurosurgical procedures to avoid eloquent areas of cerebral function such as those involved with language or vision.

Physiologic information is also available through the use of *positron emission tomography (PET)* or *single-photon emission computed tomography (SPECT)*. In the former, injection of a radioisotope with a short half-life is followed by imaging of the positrons produced during their decay. The uptake of short-lived radioactive isotopes such as fluorine (^{18}F), carbon (^{11}C), nitrogen (^{13}N), or oxygen (^{15}O) is related to metabolic activity. PET with [^{18}F]-fluoro-2-deoxyglucose has shown increased visual cortex metabolism during ictal visual hallucinations and has detected regions of hypoperfusion in cases associated with visual cortex ischemia. PET is usually combined with CT to enhance resolution. SPECT uses an iodinated radiotracer or technetium-99m agent as a cerebral perfusion and extraction agent. Because these agents depend on blood flow and cerebral metabolism, they can be used to study stroke, epilepsy, and dementia. SPECT is more widely available than PET, but it lacks sufficient resolution and specificity. Even after nondiagnostic or normal MRI results, functional imaging may reveal altered regional cerebral blood flow in patients with cerebral visual impairment from various causes.

Sonography

Sonography is an excellent noninvasive technique for imaging the orbit and the carotid. It does not require ionizing radiation and is relatively inexpensive, quick, and office-based; it does, however, require expertise in image acquisition and interpretation. Ultrasonography images are based on the reflection of 8–20 MHz ultrasound waves at acoustic interfaces. Carotid Doppler is generally accurate at detecting cervical carotid stenosis, but it does not provide information about more proximal or distal vessels. The major use of carotid Doppler imaging in neuro-ophthalmology is detecting cervical carotid stenosis following transient monocular blindness suggestive of retinal or optic nerve ischemia. Stenosis in this area of the carotid circulation may mitigate for carotid endarterectomy or carotid stenting, depending on the circumstances.

Orbital ultrasound provides useful data concerning the optic nerve and retrobulbar structures, including muscle, optic nerve, and vessels, but it does not provide accurate imaging of the orbital apex. Ultrasound is useful in the globe and may help distinguish disc edema from optic nerve head drusen, which are strongly echogenic (see Chapter 4, Fig 4-15).

Retinal and Nerve Fiber Layer Imaging

Several techniques for noninvasive imaging of the optic nerve head and retinal nerve fiber layer are in clinical use, including Heidelberg retinal tomography (HRT), GDx nerve fiber analysis, and optical coherence tomography (OCT). These techniques use laser or short coherence light to image the retina and optic nerve head rapidly and are increasingly being used to evaluate or follow certain optic nerve diseases such as glaucoma, in addition to being used in research in neuro-ophthalmic diseases. These techniques are discussed further in BCSC Section 10, *Glaucoma*.

Fundamental Concepts in Localization

The ultimate diagnostic goal is to determine the exact pathophysiology underlying a patient's symptoms. In neuro-ophthalmology, common symptoms include decreased vision, visual field defects, positive visual phenomena, double vision, oscillopsia, pain or numbness, ptosis, proptosis, or enophthalmos. The first goal of neuro-ophthalmic evaluation is clinical localization of the lesion. For an ophthalmologist, locations may be roughly divided into the orbit; the parasellar region, including the chiasm superiorly and cavernous sinuses laterally; the middle cranial fossa, which contains the retrochiasmal visual pathways, including the optic tract, geniculate and optic radiations, and occipital cortex; and the posterior fossa, containing the brainstem and cerebellum. Each of these areas is associated with unique neuroimaging challenges that influence the choice of imaging modality (Table 2-3). The pathophysiologic differential diagnosis is generated based on clinical localization, medical history, and imaging. Imaging results are maximized when the clinician and radiologist review images together, combining the clinical and radiographic features to rank-order the differential diagnosis and guide further evaluation (Table 2-4).

Osborn AG, Blaser S, Salzman KI. *Diagnostic Imaging Series: Brain*. Philadelphia: WB Saunders; 2004.

Table 2-3 Imaging Choice: Clinical Locations

Location	Imaging Study	Comments
Orbit	MRI, CT	Include fat suppression with MRI
Parasellar	MRI	CT: bony artifact
Chiasm	MRI	Poorly seen on CT
Middle cranial fossa	MRI, CT	
Posterior cranial fossa	MRI	CT: bony artifact
Cerebral vascular	MRA, CTA, angiography	
Cervical carotid	Doppler, MRA, CTA, angiography	Doppler often quickest
Bone	CT	
White matter	MRI	Poorly seen on CT
Meninges	MRI	Infection, inflammatory, or neoplastic process

Table 2-4 Imaging Choice: Clinical Situations

Clinical Situation	Imaging Study	Comments
Acute hemorrhage	CT, MRI	CT better for acute subarachnoid hemorrhage; MRI provides information on evolution of intraparenchymal hemorrhage
Aneurysm	MRA, CTA, angiography	May be missed by MRI and CT
Arteriovenous malformation (AVM)	Angiography	
Calcification	CT	Most forms poorly seen on MRI
Carotid cavernous fistula	Angiography	
Carotid dissection	MRI, MRA, angiography	
Carotid stenosis	Doppler, MRA, CTA, angiography	
Cerebral venous disease	MRI, MRA	
Demyelination/multiple sclerosis (MS)	MRI	
Foreign body	CT	MRI problematic with ferromagnetic objects, such as vascular clips
Infarct	MRI	DWI able to detect acute infarction
Infection	MRI	Abscess, meningitis
Neoplasm	MRI	MRI demonstrates edema and features better but is less useful with bony involvement
Optic neuritis	MRI	Include contrast and fat suppression; CT poor
Paranasal sinus disease	CT, MRI	CT shows bony details better than MRI
Pediatrics	CT (faster exam)	MRI may be preferable but may require sedation
Pituitary adenoma	MRI	CT in axial plane often misses pituitary abnormalities
Radiation damage	MRI	Include contrast with MRI; poorly seen on CT
Thyroid eye disease	MRI, CT, US	
Trauma	CT	CT: faster, shows acute blood and bony changes
White matter disease	MRI	FLAIR sequences best on MRI; poorly seen on CT

Critical Questions in Imaging

- *when* to order
- *what* to order
  - modality
  - location
- *how* to order
  - specify lesion and region of interest
  - discuss with radiologist before ordering
  - review with radiologist after imaging

When to Order

State-of-the-art imaging facilities are now widely available in the United States. Imaging, however, remains expensive, a potential drain on medical resources, and not without risks. The decision to order an imaging study should be based on clinical localization and the expectation of particular findings. Further, this information should have an effect on patient management or provide more accurate prognosis of the disease's natural history. Finally, the information should not be available by simpler or less expensive means. Transient visual phenomena without residual deficit are most frequently related to large-vessel disease and thereby require assessment of the vascular structures. Suspicion of a neoplastic mass lesion is one of the most common reasons for ordering an imaging study. Neoplasia, however, is not always the cause of optic neuropathy. For example, glaucoma is the most common cause of optic neuropathy, often manifested by increased optic disc cupping and classic arcuate visual field defects. Acuity in glaucoma, however, should be normal. When disc edema is present, the differential diagnosis should include anterior ischemic optic neuropathy (AION), papillitis, and intraorbital compression. Imaging is not required in the setting of classic AION. When central visual function is affected without disc edema, or field defects respect the vertical midline, parachiasmal pathology may be investigated with appropriate imaging studies.

Pisaneschi M, Kapoor G. Imaging the sella and parasellar region. *Neuroimaging Clin N Am.* 2005;15(1):203–219.

Weber AL, Caruso P, Sabates NR. The optic nerve: radiologic, clinical, and pathologic evaluation. *Neuroimaging Clin N Am.* 2005;15(1):175–201.

The workup of decreased vision should include imaging of the course of the optic nerve if there is evidence of optic neuropathy not explained by glaucomatous, ischemic, toxic, metabolic, infectious, or hereditary causes. Optic neuropathy should be confirmed by finding an afferent pupillary defect (if visual loss is asymmetric), along with some combination of acuity and visual field loss. Lack of these findings suggests consideration of anterior segment or macular pathology.

The Optic Neuritis Treatment Trial (ONTT) demonstrated that imaging was not required in the diagnosis of typical optic neuritis. The ONTT, however, also reported that a brain MRI obtained in this setting has critical prognostic significance with regard to recurrent episodes or progression to multiple sclerosis (MS). Thus, *in the setting of acute optic neuritis, a cerebral MRI scan should be ordered* to look for evidence of T2 hyperintensities within the white matter typical of MS; this evidence is best seen on T2-weighted or FLAIR images. A CT scan has no value in the setting of demyelinating disease. The publication of the Controlled High-Risk Subjects Avonex Multiple Sclerosis Prevention Study (CHAMPS) demonstrated the advantages of early treatment for patients with typical white matter lesions, which makes the initial scan even more important. (For further discussion of multiple sclerosis and these studies, see Chapter 14, Selected Systemic Considerations With Neuro-Ophthalmic Signs.)

Bitemporal visual field defects localize to the chiasm and should always lead to imaging. Some of the most frequent chiasmal compressive masses include pituitary adenoma with suprasellar extension, meningioma, craniopharyngioma, chiasmatic glioma, and aneurysm (Fig 2-12). Rarer lesions include metastases, chordomas, dysgerminomas, lymphoma, histiocytosis, epidermoids, Rathke cleft cysts, and granulomatous inflammatory disease.

Homonymous visual field defects imply retrochiasmal visual pathway pathology. These defects are most commonly vascular in origin but should be imaged unless clearly associated with an old stroke syndrome.

When a patient reports binocular double vision, anatomic localization is again critical, and the pattern of misalignment becomes all-important. Before a paretic syndrome is assumed, the clinician should exclude the possibility of a restrictive problem, most commonly related to trauma, inflammation, or thyroid eye disease. All restrictive phenomena (distinguished via forced duction testing) imply an orbital origin. Other signs of orbital involvement include proptosis, enophthalmos, or other globe position abnormalities, or orbital bruit. As with afferent system dysfunction involving the optic nerve, both CT and MRI may provide the necessary information regarding the extraocular muscles. MRI is somewhat more sensitive to the various changes associated with inflammation or infiltration, but CT well delineates the size of the extraocular muscles, particularly on direct (ie, not reformatted) coronal images (see Fig 2-1B).

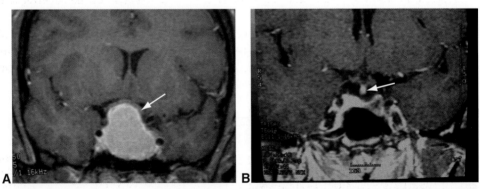

Figure 2-12 **A,** Coronal T1-weighted MRI postcontrast shows a large pituitary adenoma stretching and compressing the chiasm (visible as a gray ribbon superior to the adenoma [arrow]). This 45-year-old male presented with a bitemporal defect and impotence, and his prolactin level was elevated consistent with prolactinoma. **B,** MRI appearance several months after treatment with the dopamine agonist cabergoline shows near resolution of the prolactinoma; the enhancing structure in the suprasellar space is a normal-appearing infundibulum *(arrow),* with the chiasm above. *(Courtesy of Eric Eggenberger, DO.)*

When the pattern of deviation fits a cranial nerve palsy, the decision about imaging depends on the clinically suspected pathophysiology and whether the palsy is isolated. The acute onset of an isolated cranial nerve palsy in a patient in the vasculopathic age group (usually >50 years), especially when associated with a history of diabetes, hypertension, or vascular disease, is most likely microvascular, and imaging acutely may not be required. With multiple cranial nerve palsies, especially when the fifth nerve is involved, a cavernous sinus location is logical. Parasellar lesions are most effectively seen on MRI used in combination with gadolinium. The most common lesions affecting the parasellar region include meningioma (Fig 2-13), pituitary adenoma, aneurysm, neurilemoma, chordoma, chondrosarcoma, metastatic disease, and lymphoma.

Skew deviation is a supranuclear lesion producing vertical misalignment. That is, a vertical deviation without evidence of restrictive orbital involvement that does not fit the pattern of a fourth or third nerve palsy suggests a skew deviation. Imaging studies of the posterior fossa must be obtained. MRI is superior to CT at demonstrating posterior fossa pathology, including inflammatory, neoplastic, or ischemic processes.

Certain common clinical situations are associated with negative results on imaging. For example, in a patient older than 50 years, acute visual loss associated with evidence of optic neuropathy, ipsilateral disc edema, and lack of orbital signs or pain is almost always secondary to AION. Although giant cell arteritis may be considered in this setting, imaging is unlikely to be of benefit or change therapy. A second common clinical condition is the acute onset of an isolated cranial nerve palsy in a patient with a vasculopathic history. When the oculomotor nerve is involved, the status of the pupil becomes critical. Although microvascular disease can cause pupil dilation, the presence of a normally reactive pupil in the setting of an acute, otherwise complete, third nerve palsy essentially precludes a mass lesion, and scanning acutely in this setting may be unnecessary. Microvascular disease resulting in an acute cranial nerve palsy should be expected to clear completely. Failure to resolve over 3 months or evidence of aberrant regeneration (lid elevation on adduction or depression, miosis on adduction or elevation, or co-contraction of the superior and inferior recti) is a clear indication for scanning.

Pain unaccompanied by other findings (proptosis, motility disturbance, decreased vision, or, most important, numbness) is unlikely to be due to a pathology that can be imaged, particularly if the pain is episodic and brief. When the pain is associated with

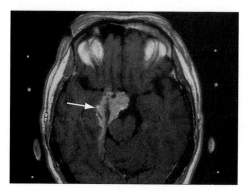

Figure 2-13 This 45-year-old patient presented with progressive third and sixth nerve palsies. An MRI scan reveals a cavernous sinus lesion on the right side, with an enhanced extension along the dural edge *(arrow)*. This so-called *dural tail* is characteristic of meningioma. *(Courtesy of Steven A. Newman, MD.)*

findings such as ptosis and miosis (Horner syndrome), carotid artery dissection should be suspected; MRI and MRA through the carotid artery and, rarely, contrast angiography may be needed for confirmation.

What to Order

With important exceptions (Table 2-5), MRI is usually more valuable than CT in both detecting a lesion and narrowing the differential diagnosis. The specific choice of imaging modality—including the sequence, orientation, and direction—depends on a combination of the suspected location and the expected pathology. In suspected large-vessel disease, MRA, CTA, and digital angiography may also be considered.

Table 2-5 Comparison of Magnetic Resonance and Computed Tomography Modalities

	Advantages	Disadvantages	Contraindications
MRI	Better for soft tissue Better resolution of optic nerve and orbital apex No ionizing radiation Better able to distinguish white from gray matter	Greater cost Contrast dye reactions and systemic nephrogenic fibrosis	Ferromagnetic implants/ foreign body Pacemakers Metallic cardiac valves Non–MRI compatible intracranial aneurysm clips Cochlear implants Technical considerations: Claustrophobia/too large for the bore
CT	Globe and orbital trauma (include high-resolution bone algorithms) Assessment of bony abnormalities Detection of calcification in lesions Assessment of orbital and hyperacute intracranial hemorrhage	Exposure to ionizing radiation dose Iodine-based dye contrast reactions Limited resolution in the posterior fossa Lack of direct sagittal imaging Poor resolution of the orbital apex	
MRA	Less invasive	Limited resolution (in aneurysms ≥3 mm) May overestimate carotid stenosis	Same as for MRI
CTA	Less invasive	Limited resolution (in aneurysms ≥3 mm) Artifacts from superimposed bone and adjacent vessels, especially where aneurysms lie within or close to bone	

Mafee MF, Rapoport M, Karimi A, Ansari SA, Shah J. Orbital and ocular imaging using 3- and 1.5-T MR imaging systems. *Neuroimaging Clin N Am.* 2005;15(1):1–21.

Neuroimaging should be done of both the brain and orbits. Orbital imaging provides details of the optic nerves and the surrounding tissues that are often not detected with brain imaging alone.

When pathology is localized to the orbit, either CT or MRI can provide useful information. Orbital fat produces excellent contrast with the other orbital components on both modalities, and both give excellent anatomical localization (see Figs 2-1, 2-4).

More important than the choice of the modality is the selection of orientation and specific sequences. Direct coronal images are useful in most orbital disorders (Fig 2-14). With MRI, direct coronal imaging is not a problem, but CT may require specific positioning (neck extension) that may be difficult to achieve with older patients. MRI of the orbit should be done with fat saturation techniques designed to eliminate the high T1 signal from fat (see Fig 2-6).

Each modality has advantages: CT provides information about the bony walls; MRI provides increased information about the optic nerve (eg, distinguishing meningioma from glioma and indicating the extent of the posterior tumor) and the state of the extraocular muscles, orbital apex, and optic canal in multiplanar views. MRI also avoids the artifact seen on CT related to dental fillings. When a calcified lesion is expected (eg, retinoblastoma, choroidal osteoma, optic nerve head drusen) or if there is a metallic intraorbital foreign body, CT should be used (see Table 2-5). MRI may have advantages in imaging melanomas due to their paramagnetic properties. MRI may also be preferred when attempting to distinguish inflammatory from lymphoproliferative changes. Resolution of the orbit may be further increased with special surface or orbital coils. Often,

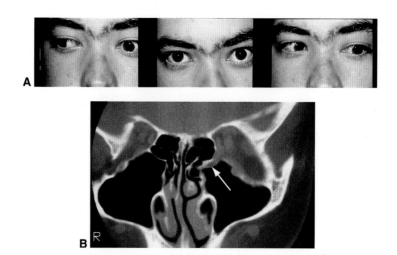

Figure 2-14 A 19-year-old man was referred for double vision following a motor vehicle accident. **A,** He had difficulty adducting the left eye, and attempted abduction caused palpebral fissure narrowing. **B,** A subsequent coronal CT scan demonstrates an entrapped medial rectus muscle *(arrow)* causing restriction. *(Courtesy of Steven A. Newman, MD.)*

however, the clinician loses the opportunity of comparing the 2 orbits when the sequences are coned down to 1 side.

For the parasellar region, MRI has marked advantages over CT (see Table 2-3), except in cases of trauma if small bone fragments or fractures are possible.

Intracranial soft tissue is generally better assessed with MRI than with CT, except with acute hemorrhage (including subarachnoid hemorrhage following rupture of an aneurysm or arteriovenous malformation), which does not show up well on T1- or T2-weighted MRI. (This is best seen on FLAIR sequences.) MRI does offer the advantage of establishing the evolution of intraparenchymal hemorrhage, and gradient echo MRI is sensitive to petechial hemorrhage from traumatic axonal shearing injury.

Because of the close proximity of bone, the posterior fossa is much better visualized with MRI than with CT. Suspicion of intra-axial or extra-axial brainstem or cerebellar pathology calls for MRI sequences of the posterior fossa.

If we look at most presumed pathology (see Table 2-4), MRI is again the choice in most clinical situations. Neoplasia, inflammation, demyelination, and ischemic changes, as well as cystic lesions, are better visualized on MRI than on CT. Computed tomography is better for acute hemorrhage (especially subarachnoid hemorrhage), bony lesions, and trauma.

How to Order

The ophthalmologist may have a role in the selection of the specific type of imaging procedure. The more pertinent information the radiologist is supplied, the more appropriately the imaging can be tailored to a particular patient. This information should at least include the expected location of the pathology and the suspected differential diagnosis (region and lesion of interest). Failure to supply such information often results in images that fail to show the area of interest or do so with insufficient detail. Inappropriate images (wrong location or orientation, lack of contrast administration, overly thick slices) are often worse than no images at all in that they may provide a false sense of security and may create third-party payer barriers to the required reimaging. By conveying as much specific clinical information to the radiologist as possible, the ophthalmologist will increase the usefulness of subsequent studies.

Negative Studies

The discipline of neuro-ophthalmology has been called "the reinterpretation of previously negative imaging studies." When an imaging study fails to demonstrate expected pathology or answer the clinical question, the first step is to reexamine the studies, ideally with a neuroradiologist. Were the appropriate studies performed, including required sequences and orientations? Was the area of interest adequately imaged (Fig 2-15)? Are the study results really negative (Figs 2-16, 2-17)? Even if the ophthalmologist cannot personally review the studies, speaking directly with the radiologist may prevent certain lesions from being overlooked and can provide the required clinical information to enhance the radiographic report's accuracy and usefulness.

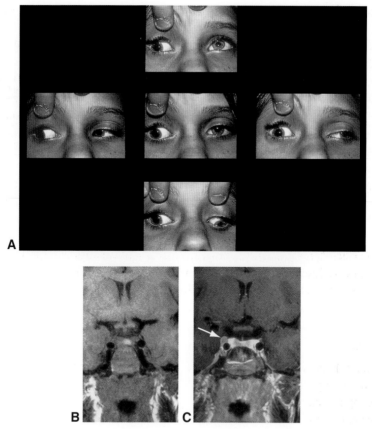

Figure 2-15 **A,** This 11-year-old patient was noted to have a third nerve palsy on the right side that began at age 5 and became complete by age 7. **B,** Initial studies were negative, but fine cuts through the cavernous sinus demonstrate asymmetry, with a slight nodule in the superior portion of the cavernous sinus on the right. **C,** This area became bright with administration of gadolinium, which indicated the presence of a right third nerve neurilemoma *(arrow)*. *(Courtesy of Steven A. Newman, MD.)*

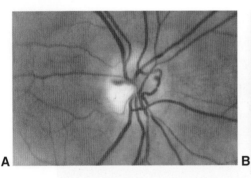
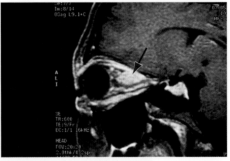

Figure 2-16 A 41-year-old woman was referred for progressive visual loss in the right eye. She had previously been told that she had a swollen optic nerve on the right and was diagnosed as having a "mild form of MS." Visual acuity was 2/200 OD and 20/20 OS, with a right afferent pupillary defect. She had reportedly had 2 previous MRI scans, which were negative. **A,** The right optic disc demonstrated temporal pallor with optociliary shunt vessels. The patient was referred for a third MRI scan, but this study was misdirected for workup of "microvascular brainstem disease" and revealed no abnormalities. **B,** Sagittal MRI through the orbit shows abnormal optic nerve sheath appearance consistent with optic nerve sheath meningioma *(arrow). (Part A courtesy of Steven A. Newman, MD; part B courtesy of Eric Eggenberger, DO.)*

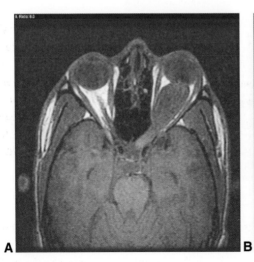
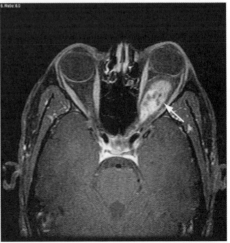

Figure 2-17 **A,** Axial T1-weighted precontrast and **(B)** fat-suppressed postcontrast MRIs reveal an enlarged enhancing intraorbital optic nerve OS *(arrow)* consistent with optic nerve glioma. Note the globular appearance of the mass containing cystic spaces (see Table 4-6). *(Courtesy of Eric Eggenberger, DO.)*

CHAPTER 3

The Patient With Decreased Vision: Evaluation

History

In addition to the age of the patient, 3 aspects of the history are critical in cases of impaired vision: (1) the type of involvement (unilateral vs bilateral), (2) the time course of visual loss, and (3) associated symptoms.

Unilateral vs Bilateral Involvement

Determining whether a lesion is unilateral or bilateral is crucial to localization: unilateral loss almost always indicates a lesion anterior to the chiasm, whereas bilateral loss may reflect bilateral optic nerve or retinal disease or a chiasmal or retrochiasmal process. A careful history is imperative to determine whether involvement is unilateral or bilateral. In *homonymous* visual field loss (involvement of the corresponding half-fields of each eye), patients often mistakenly attribute the loss to monocular involvement on the side of the affected temporal hemifield; such patients should be asked specifically if they have checked each eye individually. Often, binocular involvement is not appreciated until the patient is examined.

Time Course of Visual Loss

The speed of visual loss is important in determining etiology. Sudden onset (within minutes) usually indicates an ischemic (often embolic) retinal event, such as arterial occlusion. Rapid loss occurring over hours is also most often ischemic but is more characteristic of optic nerve involvement. A course evolving over days to weeks may also reflect ischemia but more frequently denotes inflammation. Gradual progression over months is typical of toxic lesions (although they may be more acute); progression over months or years is typical of compressive causes. Patients may become acutely aware of chronic processes when the uninvolved eye is covered or when the second eye becomes affected. The time course among causes overlaps significantly, so the history may be suggestive but not definitive.

Associated Symptoms

Pain associated with visual loss may aid in localization of affected areas. Periorbital pain ipsilateral to visual loss, increasing with eye movement, and possibly associated with globe tenderness, is common in optic neuritis. Additional symptoms related to demyelinating disease should be sought, including diplopia, ataxia, hemiparesis, and hemisensory changes. Nonspecific pain, facial numbness, or diplopia may indicate orbital or cavernous sinus lesions. Headache may suggest an intracranial mass or giant cell arteritis.

Examination

Examination of the patient with decreased vision is directed toward detecting, quantifying, and localizing the site of loss, with the goal of determining etiology. The process begins with assessment of visual acuity, the most common measure of central visual function.

Best-Corrected Visual Acuity

Best-corrected visual acuity, which measures the maximal foveal spatial discrimination, should be obtained with refraction. Pinhole visual acuity provides a rough approximation of best-corrected visual acuity but usually underestimates it. Occasionally, however, visual acuity measured with the pinhole is worse than visual acuity measured in other ways; this finding may direct the examiner to search for corneal or lenticular irregularities. For visual acuity levels worse than 20/200, the examiner should obtain a quantitative assessment by moving a standard 200 optotype E closer to the patient until its orientation is discerned. This distance is then recorded in standard Snellen notation (eg, "5/200"), providing a more accurate and reproducible measure than "finger counting @ 5 ft" for determining change in visual status over time.

Vision should be tested at distance and at near. With appropriate refractive correction, acuity for distance and near should be equivalent. Disparity of these 2 acuities may suggest a specific pathology. Vision that is better at near than at distance may be due to macular disease (in which near magnification may overcome small scotomata) or nuclear sclerotic cataract; vision that is better at distance—depending on ambient lighting and pupillary size—occasionally results from central posterior subcapsular or polar cataracts. The examiner should observe whether the patient requires eccentric fixation (possible central scotoma), tends to read only 1 side of the eye chart (possible hemianopic field defect), or reads single optotypes better than whole lines (possible amblyopia).

Pupillary Testing

Pupillary examination, as part of an evaluation of a patient with decreased vision, is aimed at detecting a *relative afferent pupillary defect (RAPD)*. This abnormality of pupillary reactivity, also known as a *Marcus Gunn pupil,* is a hallmark of impaired optic nerve conduction. In a person without this condition, the afferent pupillomotor signal carried along 1 optic nerve is transmitted to *both* pupils after synapse in the pretectal nuclei, producing a symmetric direct (ipsilateral) and consensual (contralateral) light pupillary constriction following light stimulation. Impaired conduction of the light stimulus along *1* optic nerve thus produces decreased pupillary constriction in *both* pupils when the light stimulus is presented to the affected eye. The RAPD is due to the asymmetric light response between the 2 eyes.

The RAPD is best elicited by means of the alternating light source in the swinging flashlight test (Practical Tips in Testing for a Relative Afferent Pupillary Defect). Using a bright focal light, the examiner shines the light into 1 pupil for 2–3 seconds and then rapidly swings the light into the other pupil for 2–3 seconds. This is repeated 4 or 5 times, and only the illuminated pupil (direct light response) is observed. The amplitude and velocity of pupillary constriction should be symmetric when stimulating either eye. In the patient with impaired optic nerve conduction in 1 eye, light stimulation of the affected eye will produce a sluggish pupil constriction of low amplitude. Often the pupil will redilate during the 3 seconds of light stimulation, a process called *pupillary escape* (Fig 3-1). When the light stimulus is then moved to the unaffected eye, the relative increase in pupillomotor input results in visibly greater pupil constriction, both in speed and amplitude.

PRACTICAL TIPS IN TESTING FOR A RELATIVE AFFERENT PUPILLARY DEFECT

1. Dim the ambient lighting; it is easier to evaluate pupillary movement when the pupil size is larger.
2. Ensure that the patient fixates at distance so that accommodation (and the accompanying miosis) is controlled.
3. Use a bright steady light source, such as a standard "muscle light," that is completely charged. Too dim a light source may produce false-positive results, whereas too bright a light source produces false-negative results if the pupil is driven into a state of sustained miosis.
4. Stimulate 1 eye for 2–3 seconds and quickly move across the bridge of the nose to stimulate the other eye for 2–3 seconds. Make several alternations and mentally average the pupil responses. Do not rely on a single observation.
5. Observe the initial pupillary constriction (velocity and amplitude) as well as the timing and amount of pupillary escape (or dilation) during the 2–3 seconds of light stimulation.
6. A dense RAPD is easily detected when the affected eye's pupil dilates in response to the swinging flashlight test.
7. A small to moderate RAPD is more difficult to detect as the affected eye's pupil may still constrict in response to the swinging flashlight test but is less vigorous than that of the unaffected side.
8. An RAPD may be detected even if the pupillary response in 1 eye may not be evaluated because of mechanical injury (iris trauma, synechiae) or pharmacologic blockade of reactivity (mydriasis or miosis). In such cases, evaluation of the direct and consensual response of the only working pupil may demonstrate asymmetry of responses and thus indicate the side of the RAPD.

9. Bilateral optic neuropathy, when fairly symmetric, may show sluggish pupillary responses but not a *relative* difference (and therefore no RAPD) between the 2 eyes when pupillary responses are compared.

10. The RAPD may be graded 1–4+ in increasing severity or may be quantified using neutral-density filters. These commercially available filters decrease the intensity of light reaching the retina and are placed in front of the good eye. Beginning with the lowest 0.3 log unit filter over the good eye, the swinging flashlight test is repeated. If an RAPD is still detectable, the 0.6 log unit filter is placed over the good eye and the test repeated in similar fashion until an RAPD is no longer observable. At this balance point, the light input from the good eye with filter now matches the light input from the bad eye. Increasing the strength of the filter in front of the good eye results in an RAPD in the good eye, a process known as "overshooting the balance point." The RAPD is quantified by the strength of the neutral-density filter needed over the good eye to reach the balance point.

11. The magnitude of the RAPD correlates with the overall degree of damage to retinal ganglion cells and their axons and to the amount of corresponding visual field. The magnitude will not necessarily parallel visual acuity if the papillomacular bundle is not significantly affected. Thus, it is possible to detect a prominent RAPD in the presence of normal visual acuity.

12. The presence of an RAPD does not result in anisocoria. Although the affected pupil is poorly reactive to light, it is not dilated at baseline. The consensual response from the normal input of the fellow eye maintains the pupil at equal size.

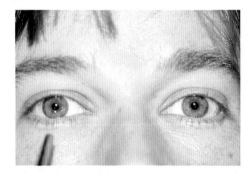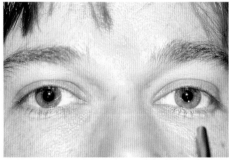

Figure 3-1 This 19-year-old patient was noted to have decreased vision in her left eye when she was evaluated for headaches. The swinging flashlight test demonstrated a left afferent pupillary defect. Funduscopy showed left optic atrophy, and MRI revealed an optic nerve glioma.

An RAPD is an extremely reliable and sensitive indicator of asymmetric optic nerve dysfunction. The absence of an RAPD should prompt reevaluation of the diagnosis of optic neuropathy or should cause consideration of bilateral optic nerve involvement. An RAPD may also result from any lesion that decreases the ganglion cell input to the optic nerve, such as severe macular disease or another retinal disorder such as detachment. The degree of the RAPD relates to the number of fibers affected; thus, a relatively small lesion of the optic nerve affects a large number of fibers and results in a large RAPD, whereas a retinal lesion must be substantially larger to produce a similar RAPD. Chiasmal lesions may produce an RAPD if fibers from the optic nerves are involved asymmetrically. Optic tract lesions may result in a mild RAPD in the contralateral eye (ie, the eye with the temporal visual field loss) because each tract contains more crossed than uncrossed pupillary fibers, and a lesion will damage more fibers crossing from that eye. With extremely rare exceptions, an RAPD does not result from media opacities such as cataract or vitreous hemorrhage. A mild RAPD may be detected in the setting of dense amblyopia, but the RAPD may also reflect superimposed optic nerve hypoplasia, optic neuropathy, or retinal pathology.

Fundus Examination

Two aspects of the fundus examination are important: the *clarity of the view* and the *appearance of the structures*. Both the retina (particularly the macula) and the optic nerve may show changes explaining a patient's decreased visual acuity.

The direct ophthalmoscope remains a valuable tool for assessing the fundus; it not only gives a highly magnified view of the fundus but also allows the examiner to evaluate the *visibility of the fundus,* which can be impaired by media opacities. (Unlike with indirect ophthalmoscopy and slit-lamp biomicroscopy, the optics and light source of direct ophthalmoscopy do not permit viewing through a media opacity.) The direct ophthalmoscope is first focused on the red reflex to screen for opacities or irregularities in the cornea, lens, or vitreous (such opacities appear black on the contrasting red background). As the lenses are focused on the posterior pole, the clarity of the view of the macular region suggests how much visual impairment the lesions might cause. Finally, the appearance of the optic disc and macular regions is assessed. The disc is examined for evidence of atrophy, edema, excavation, or other abnormality; the macula is examined for pigmentary disturbance, edema, scar, or other disruption of structural integrity. Used with the slit lamp, the 66, 78, or 90 D indirect lens improves viewing of the contour of both optic disc and macula by affording a stereoscopic view of the structures.

Optic atrophy is the hallmark of damage to the retinal ganglion cells. Although atrophy is visualized at the level of the optic nerve head, it may result from damage to any portion of the ganglion cells, from cell bodies to their synapses at the lateral geniculate nucleus. Optic atrophy does not occur immediately but takes 4–6 weeks from the time of axonal damage. Severe damage is usually easily identified by the chalky white appearance of the disc (Fig 3-2), with increased sharpness of the margins in contrast with the dull red appearance of the peripapillary retina, which is devoid of the normal softening effect of

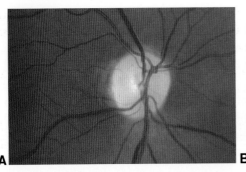 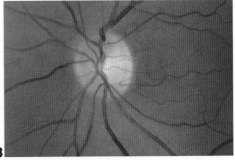

A   **B**

Figure 3-2 Fundus photographs demonstrating diffuse optic atrophy **(A)**, compared with normal optic disc appearance **(B)**. *(Courtesy of Steven A. Newman, MD.)*

the overlying nerve fiber layer (NFL). Milder forms of atrophy, with less whitening of the normally orange-pink disc color, are more difficult to detect but may become more apparent with close attention to the following aspects:

- *Comparison of the color of the 2 discs.* In some cases, subtle pallor is noticeable only in relation to the normal fellow eye. (Comparison may be difficult following unilateral cataract extraction.)
- *Evaluation of the surface vasculature of the disc.* Normally, this capillary net is easily visible with the high magnification of the direct ophthalmoscope, but the net becomes thin or is absent in early atrophy, even when pallor is still very mild.
- *Assessment of the peripapillary NFL.* Dropout of these fibers, an early sign of damage that may precede visible optic atrophy, may be seen as a loss of the normal translucent, glistening quality of the retina. Such loss produces a dull red appearance, which may be seen in broad or fine radial patches (Fig 3-3). The fine defects appear earliest in the superior and inferior arcades, where the NFL is normally thickest, as dark bands among the normal striations. These defects have been termed *rake defects* for their similarity to rake marks in soil. NFL dropout is also common in the papillomacular bundle as a broader region of damage.

Optic disc edema is a manifestation of swelling of the nonmyelinated nerve fibers. The edema results from impaired axoplasmic flow from any cause, including increased

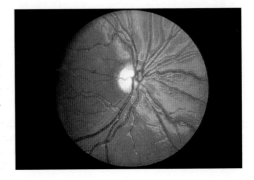

Figure 3-3 Optic disc showing temporal atrophy with a broad region of nerve fiber layer dropout *(left)*, contrasted with glistening intact nerve fiber layer *(right)*. *(Courtesy of Anthony C. Arnold, MD.)*

intracranial pressure, local mechanical compression, ischemia, and inflammation. Optic disc and retinal vascular changes are associated with the disc edema (Fig 3-4). Regardless of cause, the major clinical features are as follows:

- elevated appearance of the nerve head, with variable filling in of the physiologic cup; the retinal vessels may appear to drape over the elevated disc margin
- blurring of the disc margins
- peripapillary NFL edema (typically grayish white and opalescent, with feathered margins) obscures portions of the retinal vessels, which course within this level of the retina; the opacification of the NFL also blurs the border between the disc and the surrounding choroid
- hyperemia and dilation of the disc surface capillary net
- retinal venous dilation and tortuosity
- peripapillary hemorrhages and exudates

Additional findings may include retinal or choroidal folds, macular edema, and pre-retinal hemorrhage. True optic disc edema must be distinguished from other causes of elevation of the disc or blurring of its margins (pseudopapilledema). This distinction is discussed more fully in Chapter 4.

Visual Fields

Evaluation of the visual field is essential in all patients with visual loss. Visual field testing supplements visual acuity in establishing visual loss; helps localize the lesion along the afferent visual pathway; and quantifies the defect, enabling measurement of change over time. The choice of technique depends on the degree of detail required and the patient's

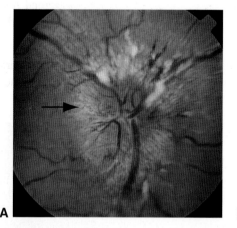
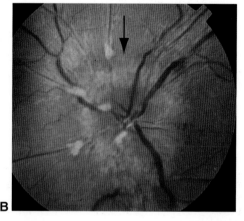

A **B**

Figure 3-4 Papilledema. **A,** Right eye. **B,** Left eye. The disc margins are blurred, with grayish white, opalescent thickening of the peripapillary nerve fiber layer *(arrows)*, cotton-wool spots, and flame hemorrhages. The retinal vessels are partially obscured at the disc margin and within the peripapillary retina. *(Courtesy of Sophia M. Chung, MD.)*

ability to cooperate. Testing may be considered qualitative (simply looking for the pattern of any visual field abnormality) or quantitative (measuring the degree of damage). Patterns of visual field loss are discussed in detail in Chapter 4.

Confrontation testing

Confrontation testing is a rapid, simple technique performed easily at the bedside or in the examination suite and should be a part of every ophthalmic examination. Confrontation testing, however, is only a screening test and must be followed with more sensitive perimetry whenever possible.

The examiner is seated approximately 1 m opposite the patient, who is directed to cover 1 eye and fixate on the examiner's nose. The patient is asked whether the examiner's entire face is visible or specific portions are missing; this often identifies central or altitudinal visual field defects. The examiner then asks the patient to identify a target of 1, 2, or 5 fingers presented at the midpoint of each of the 4 quadrants (3 or 4 fingers are more difficult to identify). Children and nonverbal patients may be asked to mimic the examiner's finger target. The patient is then asked to add the total number of fingers presented in opposing quadrants *(double simultaneous stimulation)*. By using an asymmetric number of fingers in the opposite quadrants, the examiner can identify the involved visual field. Consistently missed responses in a quadrant or hemifield may indicate a subtle visual field defect or extinction. ("Extinction" refers to the inability to see a target in an affected hemifield *only* when both hemifields are stimulated simultaneously; when a target is presented in this hemifield alone, it is seen. This finding is characteristic of parietal lobe lesions.) If the patient cannot identify fingers, the examiner presents progressively stronger stimuli (such as hand movement or light perception) in each quadrant. Accurate saccadic movement to an eccentric target is also evidence of at least relative preservation of the peripheral visual field.

Subjective comparisons may be helpful in detecting subtle sensitivity defects. With an eye occluded, the patient is asked to compare the clarity of the examiner's 2 hands presented in opposing hemifields, the less clear hand indicating a relative impairment. Color comparisons have long been used to identify the subtle red desaturation seen in anterior visual pathway disease, even without demonstrable defects that occur with stronger stimuli. The examiner presents identical small red targets (such as buttons or mydriatic bottle tops) in each hemifield, asking the patient if the stimuli appear equal. Color may appear altered, washed out, or absent in a damaged hemifield; with slow movement of the target, the examiner may be able to identify a change precisely as it crosses the vertical midline. This suggests damage to the chiasmal or retrochiasmal pathway. Alternatively, comparison of the central with the peripheral visual field in an eye may identify similar impairment centrally, suggesting optic neuropathy.

Amsler grid

Amsler grid testing is useful as a rapid screening suprathreshold test of the central 20° of the visual field (10° from fixation). The Amsler grid plate is held at ⅓ of a meter (13 inches) from the patient's face. The patient, optically corrected for near vision, covers 1 eye and looks at a fixation point in the center of the grid. The examiner asks the patient to describe any central areas of distortion *(metamorphopsia)*; any such areas suggest macular rather than optic nerve disease. Peripheral "bending" of the grid may represent optical aberration from spectacles and should be disregarded. The patient is also asked to identify any scotomata, which are less specific in terms of diagnosis but suggest visual pathway damage and the need for more detailed analysis. It is important to watch that the patient fixates on the central point rather than scans and to avoid suggesting a visual field defect during patient instruction. Amsler grid testing is rapid and simple, but sensitivity is relatively low. Perimetry should be performed whenever visual field defects are suspected, even in the face of negative results with the Amsler grid technique.

Schuchard RA. Validity and interpretation of Amsler grid reports. *Arch Ophthalmol.* 1993; 111(6):776–780.

Perimetry

More detailed evaluation of the visual field is obtained by perimetry. Both *static* and *kinetic* techniques are important. In static testing, stimuli of varying intensity (a combination of brightness and size) are presented at designated (static) points within the region of the visual field to be tested. The goal is to find the minimal stimulus that is consistently detected by the patient. In kinetic testing, a fixed-intensity stimulus is moved from a nonseeing to a seeing area of the visual field to determine the location at which it is consistently detected by the patient. Thus, the 2 techniques have the same goal but achieve it by different methods. In kinetic testing, all points of equal sensitivity for a specific stimulus are connected to form an *isopter,* which represents the outer limit of visibility for that stimulus. Analysis of several isopters (plotted with different stimuli) produces a "contour map" of the *island of vision.* In both static and kinetic techniques, the visual field is analyzed for areas of decreased sensitivity, in both location and degree.

Tangent screen   The tangent screen has been supplanted by automated perimetry but can be particularly helpful in the setting of nonorganic disease. The patient is seated 1 m from a black screen and, while fixating on a central white target, is asked to identify incoming targets from the peripheral, nonseeing field into the central field along each radial meridian. A black wand with various-sized targets attached to the tip is used to map 1 or 2 isopters kinetically. Static visual fields can be mapped by rotating the target to present the opposite black side. The field is repeated with the patient now seated farther from the screen. If the patient is now 2 m from the screen, for example, the target size should be doubled. The patient with nonorganic disease will fail to show appropriate doubling of the visual field. (See Chapter 13.)

Goldmann bowl perimetry   Goldmann bowl perimetry uses both kinetic and static techniques and has the advantage of evaluating the entire visual field.

Stimuli (usually white) of varying size and light intensity are presented in the same manner as in kinetic tangent screen testing, along each radial meridian from a peripheral to central location. Typically, 2 or 3 isopters are plotted, because relative defects that might not be detected using stronger stimuli may be found by using weaker ones. Static testing, using the on–off feature of the light stimulus, is performed within each isopter to identify scotomata. The borders of these defects may then be delineated by kinetic testing and their severity measured by varying stimulus size and intensity. Although near correction is used for the central 30° part of the testing, detailed visual fields of this area are best assessed by automated static perimetry.

The technician-dependent nature of both tangent screen and Goldmann bowl perimetry is both beneficial and disadvantageous. It confers the *advantage* of active interaction with patients to produce optimal cooperation, and it confers 2 *disadvantages:* the requirement for an experienced perimetrist who does not tire with repetitive examinations and technician bias.

Automated static perimetry In the 1990s, automated static perimetry became the standard for most clinicians in the United States. Although this technique is difficult for certain patients, particularly the elderly and those with a limited attention span, it has numerous advantages over manual kinetic techniques:

- standardized testing conditions, which allow better serial and interinstitutional comparisons of visual fields
- less technician dependence
- improved sensitivity
- numerical data that are amenable to statistical analysis for comparisons and clinical studies
- electronic data storage

With most automated perimeters, the presentation is static: stimuli (usually the Goldmann standard size III white) are randomly presented at predetermined locations within a specified region of the visual field. Visual field testing is typically restricted to the central 24° or 30° (Fig 3-5) for speed and patient compliance—but equally important, because of the overwhelming representation of the central visual field in the human striate cortex. The central 24° tests 80% of the visual cortex, whereas the central 30° tests 83% of the cortical area. More recent studies, however, reflect variations in total surface area of the occipital to be dedicated to macular function.

The brightness of the stimuli are varied, with patient responses determining the minimum visible stimulus at each location (sensitivity *threshold*). In automated perimetry, this threshold is defined as the dimmest target identified 50% of the time at a given location. Individual sensitivity values are printed on a topographic map of the region tested. Values are displayed in *decibels* (the unit of a logarithmic scale of power or intensity, measuring attenuation from the maximal stimulus of the perimeter); a higher value at a certain point indicates that the patient is able to see a stimulus with higher attenuation (less intensity), reflecting greater visual sensitivity at that point. These values are not absolute numbers and are not directly comparable among perimeters because there are differences in the maximal intensities, background, and other parameters (including duration of presentation).

For clinical interpretation, these values are compared with age-matched normal values at each point, and a statistical evaluation is made of the probability that each point value is abnormal. This information is plotted on topographic displays, along with a symbolic representation of the sensitivity values, the *grayscale map* (Fig 3-6). This map

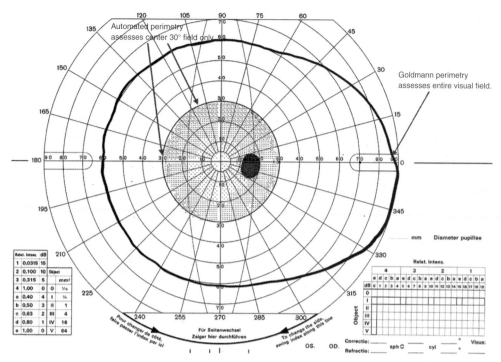

Figure 3-5 Diagrammatic representation of the extent of the visual field evaluated by Goldmann perimetry vs the 30° central program in automated static perimetry. The largest isopter in Goldmann testing extends 90° temporally and 60° in other quadrants; typical automated static perimetry evaluates only the central 30°. *(Courtesy of Anthony C. Arnold, MD.)*

depicts an overall topographic impression of the visual field data by using dark symbols for low-sensitivity points and lighter symbols for high-sensitivity points. The computer interpolates between tested points to provide a user-friendly picture (Fig 3-7). Additional statistical analysis may be selected to measure point-by-point visual field sensitivity depression compared with that of age-matched normal subjects (the total-deviation plot). Because sensitivity of the entire visual field may be depressed by ocular media abnormalities (eg, corneal surface problems, cataract), the pattern-deviation plot may be useful: the sensitivity values for all points are shifted (by the seventh-highest point) and reanalyzed based on age-expected values. This compensates for the overall depression and allows recognition of abnormal patterns (eg, scotomata, arcuate defects, homonymous defects) that might have been masked by the overall depression.

The original full-threshold perimetry proved to be long in duration and tiresome for patients, causing poor reliability and poor patient acceptance. A shorter version, known as the FASTPAC, was developed, but the test proved to be too short and therefore of questionable reliability. A compromise was achieved with the widely accepted Swedish interactive threshold algorithm (SITA), which shortens the time of the full-threshold test by 50% but maintains the accuracy necessary for reliability. (See BCSC Section 10, *Glaucoma.*)

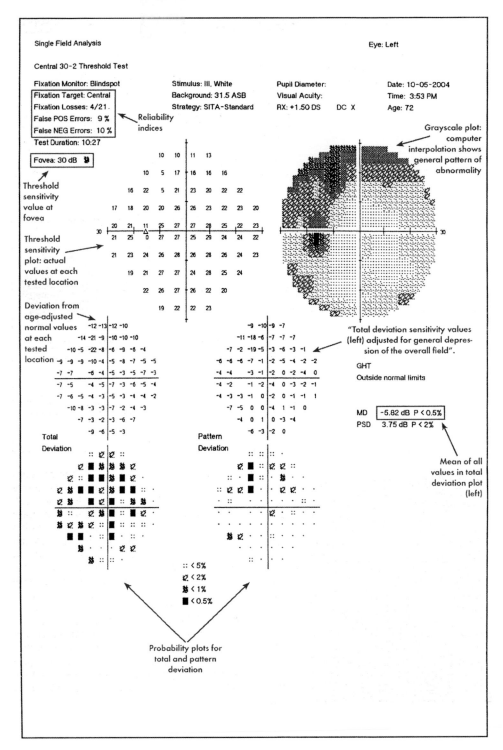

Figure 3-6 Printout from a Humphrey 30-2 automated static perimetry program, with explanations of statistical analysis, grayscale, and probability plots. *(Courtesy of Anthony C. Arnold, MD.)*

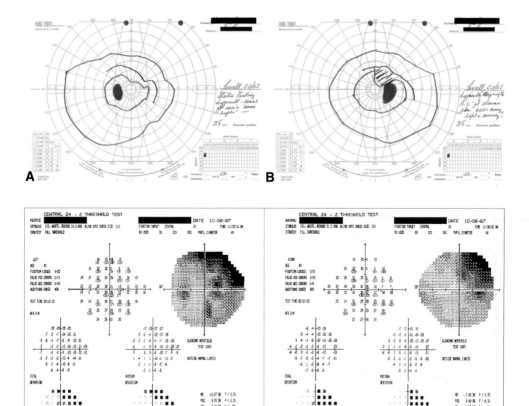

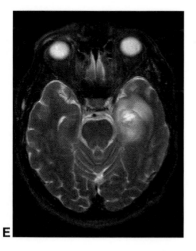

Figure 3-7 This 43-year-old woman presented with flashing lights seen off to the right side. Visual acuity was 20/30 bilaterally. **A, B,** Visual fields done by Goldmann perimetry suggest a possible superior arcuate defect on the left and superior temporal desaturation on the right. **C, D,** Automated static perimetry suggests possible superior and inferior arcuate defects on the left, but the total-deviation and pattern-deviation plots clearly demonstrate relative nasal depression OS, temporal desaturation OD, with respect to the vertical midline, indicating incomplete superior right homonymous hemianopia. **E,** MRI reveals a left temporal lobe mass, causing her visual symptoms. Both the total-deviation and pattern-deviation plots should be studied when determining visual field patterns; this combination provides the statistical significance to emphasize pathology. *(Parts A–D courtesy of Steven A. Newman, MD; part E courtesy of Joel Curé, MD.)*

Global indices are calculated to help determine change over time. These include a center-weighted mean of all point sensitivity depressions from normal (mean deviation) and various means of addressing localized defects (eg, pattern standard deviation, corrected pattern deviation, loss variance). These indices can be used to assess change in sensitivity over time (either overall or point by point).

Patient test reliability is assessed by identifying the following:

- *False-positive response rate:* how frequently the patient signals when no light is displayed (The acceptable rate is typically below 25%, but ideally these errors are reduced by technician–patient interaction during the testing.)
- *False-negative response rate:* how often the patient fails to signal when a target brighter than the previously determined threshold for that spot is displayed (The acceptable rate is typically below 25%, but the incidence increases in regions of true visual field loss, as the patient is unable to accurately reproduce responses.)
- *Fixation loss:* how often the patient signals when a target is displayed within the expected physiologic location of a blind spot (response not expected), indicating that the eye is not aligned with the fixation target
- *Short-term fluctuation measurement:* how consistent the patient responses are at specific points at which repeated testing is performed to evaluate consistency (double determinations)

Adams DL, Sincich LC, Horton JC. Complete pattern of ocular dominance columns in human primary visual cortex. *J Neurosci.* 2007;27(39):10391–10403.

Anderson DR, Patella VM. *Automated Static Perimetry.* 2nd ed. St Louis: Mosby; 1999.

Bengtsson B, Heiji A, Olsson J. Evaluation of a new threshold visual field strategy, SITA, in normal subjects. Swedish Interactive Thresholding Algorithm. *Acta Ophthalmol Scand.* 1998;76(2):165–169.

Horton JC, Hoyt WF. The representation of the visual field in human striate cortex: a revision of the classic Holmes map. *Arch Ophthalmol.* 1991;109(6):816–824.

Newman SA. Automated perimetry in neuro-ophthalmology. *Focal Points: Clinical Modules for Ophthalmologists.* San Francisco: American Academy of Ophthalmology; 1995, module 6.

Wong AM, Sharpe JA. Representation of the visual field in the human occipital contex: a magnetic resonance imaging and perimetric correlation. *Arch Ophthalmol.* 1999;117(2):208–217.

Adjunctive Testing

Color vision

Testing of color vision complements the assessment of visual acuity. In optic nerve disease, particularly demyelinating optic neuritis, the degree of dyschromatopsia may be proportionately greater than the degree of Snellen visual acuity loss; in macular disease, visual acuity and color vision tend to decline to corresponding degrees. Thus, in an eye with 20/30 visual acuity but severe color loss, optic neuropathy would be a more likely cause than macular disease. Persistent dyschromatopsia is common even after recovery of visual acuity in optic neuropathy.

Color vision testing is performed separately for each eye to detect unilateral disease. Pseudoisochromatic color plate testing was designed to screen for congenital red-green color deficiencies but may miss many mild cases of acquired dyschromatopsia. It is, however, commonly used clinically as a gross test of color vision, because optic neuropathies often manifest prominent red-green defects. Asymmetric defects between the 2 eyes are more significant than mild bilateral loss, which often represents a congenital defect, particularly in males. The AO HRR (American Optical Hardy-Rand-Rittler) plates are designed to screen for tritan defects as well as red-green defects. Blue-yellow color defects may accompany macular disease but also are common in dominant optic atrophy and may be an early sign in glaucoma. *Lanthony tritan plates* may be used to detect blue-yellow defects but are less commonly available than pseudoisochromatic plates.

More detailed color testing using arrangement tests comprehensively characterizes a color vision defect and may help distinguish acquired from congenital abnormalities. The *Farnsworth Panel D-15 test,* which requires the patient to arrange 15 colored discs in order of hue and intensity, is a good basic test if performed under standardized lighting conditions. This test can be made more sensitive by desaturation of the color chips *(Lanthony desaturated 15-hue test).* The *Farnsworth-Munsell 100-hue test* is far more detailed and provides better discrimination, using 85 discs, although the large amount of time required for testing and scoring limits its use for routine clinical testing. A shortened version, using only 21 of the color chips in the set, may be effective for discriminating among optic neuropathies.

Color vision testing is discussed further and illustrated in BCSC Section 12, *Retina and Vitreous.*

Melamud A, Hagstrom S, Traboulsi E. Color vision testing. *Ophthalmic Genet.* 2004;25(3): 159–187.

Nichols BE, Thompson HS, Stone EM. Evaluation of a significantly shorter version of the Farnsworth-Munsell 100-hue test in patients with 3 different optic neuropathies. *J Neuroophthalmol.* 1997;17(1):1–6.

Spatial contrast sensitivity

Visual acuity testing measures contrast discrimination by using targets that vary in size (and the resultant space between contrasting light and dark lines) but that are presented at a single (high) level of contrast. A more sensitive and comprehensive assessment may be made by varying contrast levels as well. Two types of contrast sensitivity tests are used today: grating and letter tests. The grating tests (Vistech [Vistech Consultants, Dayton, OH]; Sine Wave Contrast Test, or SWCT [Stereo Optical, Chicago]; Functional Acuity Contrast Test, or FACT [Stereo Optical, Chicago]) use rows of sine wave grating patches, each row reflecting a different spatial frequency. The minimum contrast seen at each spatial frequency level (the *contrast threshold*) is plotted, and the resulting graph of threshold versus frequency—the *contrast sensitivity function (CSF)*—represents the sensitivity of the central retinal region over a range of contrast levels rather than only the one seen with standard visual acuity testing. These grating tests, although arguably superior to letter tests, are difficult to administer and reliably reproduce. A simpler screening test using a single size of optotype with gradually diminishing contrast level (the Pelli-Robson chart) is more commonly used.

Because less severe damage to the visual system may manifest only as poor discrimination at lower contrast levels, contrast sensitivity testing may be useful for the detection and quantitation of visual loss in the presence of normal visual acuity measurements. The contrast sensitivity test is not specific for optic nerve dysfunction; media irregularities and macular lesions may also yield abnormal results. Interpreting contrast sensitivity test data is more complex than interpreting visual acuity data, particularly with regard to differentiating subtle abnormalities from normal; the test has not gained widespread acceptance in clinical practice.

Contrast sensitivity testing is discussed further in BCSC Section 3, *Clinical Optics*, and Section 12, *Retina and Vitreous*.

Owsley C. Contrast sensitivity. *Ophthalmol Clin North Am.* 2003;16(2):171–177.

Pelli DG, Robson JG, Wilkins AJ. The design of a new letter chart for measuring contrast sensitivity. *Clinical Vision Sciences.* 1988;2(3):187–199.

Photostress recovery test

The photostress recovery test is a simple clinical test that may help to differentiate central visual loss caused by a macular lesion or ocular ischemia from that derived from optic neuropathy. Each eye is tested separately. Best-corrected visual acuity is measured (the test is accurate only with visual acuity of 20/80 or better), after which the patient is instructed to gaze directly into a strong light (eg, a direct ophthalmoscope or slit-lamp beam) for 10 seconds held 2–3 cm from the affected eye. The patient is then directed to read the previously measured best visual acuity line as soon as possible. Normal recovery time is typically 45–60 seconds, but patients with maculopathy show prolonged recovery times, frequently 90–180 seconds or more. Patients with optic neuropathy maintain normal recovery times from photostress.

Glaser JS, Savino PJ, Sumers KD, McDonald SA, Knighton RW. The photostress recovery test in the clinical assessment of visual function. *Am J Ophthalmol.* 1977;83(2):255–260.

Potential acuity meter

Potential acuity meter (PAM) testing is useful when a media irregularity or opacity is suspected to be the cause of decreased vision. Optotypes are projected onto the retina through very small apertures in the cornea, lens, or vitreous, allowing for an estimate of best visual acuity as if the media abnormality were absent. The test may under- or overestimate true potential visual acuity and therefore is not universally accepted as a predictor of postoperative visual acuity following cataract extraction. However, it can be useful as an approximation, particularly in cases of visual loss from multiple factors. Thus, for a patient with 20/200 visual acuity and a potential visual acuity of only 20/60, a search should be made for a cause other than media opacity, such as optic neuropathy or maculopathy. Conversely, a patient with diffuse visual field loss and 20/100 visual acuity who improves to 20/20 on PAM testing probably does not require further testing. PAM testing may also be useful in cases of functional visual loss, when testing reveals a substantially better potential visual acuity than is measured by standard Snellen testing.

Minkowski JS, Palese M, Guyton DL. Potential acuity meter using a minute aerial pinhole aperture. *Ophthalmology.* 1983;90(11):1360–1368.

Reid O, Maberley DA, Hollands H. Comparison of the potential acuity meter and the visometer in cataract patients. *Eye.* 2007;21(2):195–199.

Fluorescein angiography

Fluorescein angiography may help differentiate macular from optic nerve–related visual loss. Although most cases of maculopathy show an obvious retinal abnormality, certain disorders—such as retinal capillary dropout due to diabetes or other vasculopathies, mild cystoid macular edema, minor collections of submacular fluid (eg, central serous retinopathy), toxic maculopathies (eg, chloroquine), and early cone dystrophies—may demonstrate only subtle clinical signs. These may be more obvious on angiography as avascular zones, dye leakage, or irregularities of the retinal pigment epithelium (RPE). The angiographic filling pattern of the edematous optic nerve head may provide additional diagnostic information. Significant filling delay suggests ischemic optic neuropathy and helps rule out papillitis and other nonischemic causes of optic disc edema.

Angiography may also demonstrate delayed or absent choroidal filling, either with or without disc edema. This finding may explain visual loss due to choroidal ischemia and may suggest or help to confirm a diagnosis of giant cell arteritis (Fig 3-8). Indocyanine green (ICG) angiography may better assess choroidal blood flow; it may be useful as a supplement to fluorescein angiography in suspected choroidal ischemia.

For further discussion of fluorescein angiography, see BCSC Section 12, *Retina and Vitreous*.

Arnold AC, Badr M, Hepler RS. Fluorescein angiography in nonischemic optic disc edema. *Arch Ophthalmol.* 1996;114(3):293–298.

Arnold AC, Hepler RS. Fluorescein angiography in acute nonarteritic anterior ischemic optic neuropathy. *Am J Ophthalmol.* 1994;117(2):222–230.

Berkow JW, Flower RW, Orth DH, Kelley JS. *Fluorescein and Indocyanine Green Angiography: Technique and Interpretation.* 2nd ed. Ophthalmology Monograph 5. San Francisco: American Academy of Ophthalmology; 1997.

Galor A, Lee MS. Slowly progressive vision loss in giant cell arteritis. *Arch Ophthalmol.* 2006;124(3):416–418.

Siatkowski RM, Gass JD, Glaser JS, Smith JL, Schatz NJ, Schiffman J. Fluorescein angiography in the diagnosis of giant cell arteritis. *Am J Ophthalmol.* 1993;115(1):57–63.

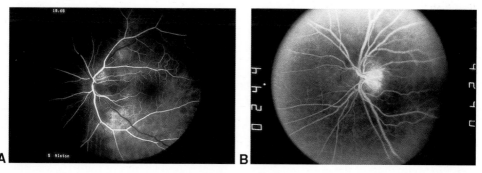

Figure 3-8 Fluorescein angiography in anterior ischemic optic neuropathy (AION). **A,** In *arteritic* AION, the optic disc shows segmental filling delay associated with marked choroidal perfusion defect. **B,** In contrast, the disc in *nonarteritic* AION shows segmental filling delay with normal choroidal filling. *(Reprinted from Arnold AC, Hepler RS. Fluorescein angiography in acute nonarteritic anterior ischemic optic neuropathy. Am J Ophthalmol. 1994;117(12):222–230.)*

Optical coherence tomography

Optical coherence tomography (OCT) provides noninvasive, high-resolution, rapid real-time acquisition, and in situ visualization of the retinal layers and optic nerve. The images are achieved by measuring light waves reflected back from the retina and optic nerves and creating 2- and 3-dimensional tomographic images. OCT has become instrumental in evaluating and managing a variety of retinal disease, intraocular tumors, and glaucoma. Its use in neuro-ophthalmology is still in its infancy. (See BCSC Section 10, *Glaucoma*, and Section 12, *Retina and Vitreous*, for more discussion.)

Electrophysiologic testing

With central and/or peripheral visual loss but no obvious fundus abnormality, ancillary electrophysiologic testing may help to confirm or rule out occult abnormalities of the optic nerve or retinal function. Electrophysiologic testing is discussed at length in BCSC Section 12, *Retina and Vitreous*.

Visual evoked potential   The *visual evoked potential (VEP)*, or *visual evoked response (VER)*, is a measurement of the electrical signal recorded at the scalp over the occipital cortex in response to light stimulus. The light-evoked signal, small in amplitude and hidden within the normal electroencephalographic (EEG) signal, is amplified by repetitive stimulation and time-locked, signal-averaging techniques, separating it from the background EEG readings. The precise origin of the VEP signal remains unclear, but it reveals the integrity of the afferent visual pathway; damage anywhere along the path may reduce the signal. The VEP is primarily a function of central visual function, because such a large region of occipital cortex is devoted to macular projections. Thus, peripheral visual loss might be overlooked by VEP testing.

Flash stimulus is useful for patients with very poor vision, in whom the response to pattern-reversal stimulus, which is more subtle, may be limited or absent. If measurable, however, the pattern response provides a more quantifiable and reliable waveform. The pattern may be studied by the number of cycles per second as well as the size of the checkerboard pattern. Smaller sizes allow detection of smaller changes in function. The most commonly studied VEP waveform typically contains an initial negative peak (N1), followed by a positive peak (P1, also known as P100 for its usual location at 100 msec); second negative (N2) and second positive (P2) peaks follow. The *latency* of onset of a peak after light stimulus and (to a lesser degree) the *amplitude* of the peak are the most useful features analyzed.

The examiner can compare readings from each eye with standardized normal values, readings from the 2 eyes, and readings from the 2 hemispheres. Peak latencies are relatively consistent, and accurate normative data are available; amplitude data are less consistent and thus less useful. Abnormalities in the waveform result from impairment anywhere along the visual pathways, but unilateral abnormalities may reflect optic neuropathy and thus may help to reveal lesions in the absence of clear-cut fundus abnormalities. Demyelination of the optic nerve results in increased latency of the P100 waveform, without significant effect on amplitude; ischemic, compressive, and toxic damage reduce amplitude primarily, with less effect on latency.

For most clinical situations, the VEP is of limited usefulness. It is subject to numerous factors that may produce abnormal waveforms in the absence of visual pathway damage, including uncorrected refractive error, media opacity, amblyopia, fatigue, and inattention (either intentional or unintentional). In most cases, the VEP is unnecessary for the diagnosis of optic neuropathy and is less accurate for its quantification than perimetry. The 2 scenarios in which VEPs remain clinically useful are (1) evaluation of the visual pathway in infants or inarticulate adults and (2) confirmation of intact visual pathways in patients suspected of nonorganic disease. A consistently abnormal flash response in the infant or inarticulate adult reflects gross impairment. An abnormal pattern response, however, is less useful, as it may indicate damage or may be a false-negative result from inattention or the reasons just cited. Normal responses confirm intact visual pathways.

A new technique being developed is the *multifocal VEP (mfVEP)*; it is designed to detect small abnormalities in optic nerve transmission and provide topographic correlation along the visual pathway. Limited studies to date of the anterior visual pathways correlate visual field abnormalities to the abnormalities confirmed by mfVEP.

Fishman GA, Birch DG, Holder GE, Brigell MG. *Electrophysiologic Testing in Disorders of the Retina, Optic Nerve, and Visual Pathway.* 2nd ed. Ophthalmology Monograph 2. San Francisco: American Academy of Ophthalmology; 2001.

Hood DC, Odel JC, Winn BJ. The multifocal visual evoked potential. *J Neuroophthalmol.* 2003; 23(4):279–289.

Electroretinogram   The *electroretinogram (ERG)* is a measure of electrical activity of the retina in response to light stimulus. Electrical activity is measured at the corneal surface by electrodes embedded in a corneal contact lens that is worn for testing.

The *full-field* response is generated by stimulating the entire retina with a flashlight source under varying conditions of retinal adaptation. Major components of the electrical waveform generated and measured include the *a-wave,* primarily derived from the photoreceptor layer; the *b-wave,* derived from the inner retina, probably Müller and ON-bipolar cells; and the *c-wave,* derived from the RPE and photoreceptors. Rod and cone photoreceptor responses can be separated by varying stimuli and the state of retinal adaptation during testing.

This form of testing is useful in detecting diffuse retinal disease in the setting of generalized or peripheral visual loss. Disorders such as retinitis pigmentosa (including the forms without pigmentation), cone–rod dystrophy, toxic retinopathies, and the retinal paraneoplastic syndromes—cancer-associated retinopathy (CAR) and melanoma-associated retinopathy (MAR)—may present with variably severe visual loss and minimal visible ocular abnormality. The ERG is invariably severely depressed by the time visual loss is significant, and thus testing is extremely useful. The full-field test, however, measures only a mass response of the entire retina; minor or localized retinal disease, particularly maculopathy—even with severe visual acuity loss—may not produce an abnormal response.

Fishman GA, Birch DG, Holder GE, Brigell MG. *Electrophysiologic Testing in Disorders of the Retina, Optic Nerve, and Visual Pathway.* 2nd ed. Ophthalmology Monograph 2. San Francisco: American Academy of Ophthalmology; 2001.

A special technique using a handheld direct ophthalmoscope–stimulator to produce localized flicker stimulation and recordings from the macular region has been termed the *focal* or *macular ERG.* This method reliably detects subtle macular dysfunction in cases of central visual loss with a normal-appearing macula on fundus and fluorescein evaluations; however, it is being supplanted by the *multifocal ERG* (discussed later in this section).

Fish GE, Birch DG. The focal electroretinogram in the clinical assessment of macular disease. *Ophthalmology.* 1989;96(1):109–114.

The ERG response generated by a pattern-reversal stimulus similar to VEP testing has been studied and is termed the *pattern ERG,* or *PERG.* It is thought that ganglion cell activity is reflected in the N95 component of the waveform, and thus the technique may detect subtle optic neuropathies. Reports have suggested the usefulness of PERG in distinguishing between ischemic and demyelinating optic neuropathy: the N95 component remains relatively normal in demyelination (if not atrophic) and appears abnormal in ischemia. The test has not gained wide clinical use.

Holder GE. Pattern electroretinography (PERG) and an integrated approach to visual pathway diagnosis. *Prog Retin Eye Res.* 2001;20(4):531–561.

A newer technique, by which simultaneously recorded ERG signals from up to 250 focal retinal locations within the central 30° are mapped topographically, is termed *multifocal ERG* (Fig 3-9). Because it does not rely on a massed retinal response, as does full-field ERG, it has demonstrated great value in detecting occult focal retinal abnormalities within the macula or more peripherally. The technique is useful in distinguishing between optic nerve and macular disease in occult central visual loss, as the signal generally remains normal in optic nerve disease. Also, it may detect regions of peripheral retinal dysfunction too small to measure by the full-field technique.

Hood DC, Bach M, Brigell M, et al. ISCEV guidelines for clinical multifocal electroretinography (2007 edition). *Doc Ophthalmol.* 2008;116(1):1–11.

Hood DC, Odel JG, Chen CS, Winn BJ. The multifocal electroretinogram. *J Neuroophthalmol.* 2003;23(3):225–235.

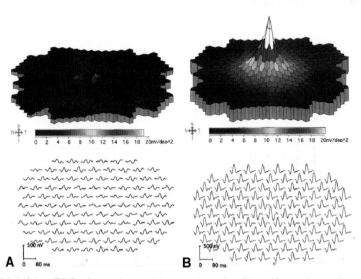

Figure 3-9 Multifocal ERG of a patient with maculopathy. The affected eye shows flattening of the foveal peak in the graphic display **(A),** compared with normal **(B).** A detailed topographic display of waveforms at each retinal location shows diffusely decreased amplitudes that are worse at the fovea. *(Courtesy of Anthony C. Arnold, MD.)*

CHAPTER 4

The Patient With Decreased Vision: Classification and Management

Decreased vision may arise from abnormalities in the ocular media, retina, optic nerve, optic tracts, visual radiations, and occipital cortex. Evaluation of the patient with visual loss requires consideration of the clinical history, examination, and ancillary testing, as outlined in Chapter 3. To further localize the source of visual loss, specific attention should be directed to the following points in the examination:

- *evidence of ocular media abnormality:* clarity of the view of the fundus
- *evidence of retinopathy*: appearance of the macula and peripheral retina
- *pattern of visual loss:* central (visual acuity loss); peripheral (visual field loss)
- *evidence of optic neuropathy:* presence of afferent pupillary defect; appearance of the optic disc
- *evidence of chiasmal lesion*
- *evidence of retrochiasmal lesion*

Ocular Media Abnormality

Irregularities or opacities of the ocular media may degrade the quality of the image presented to the anterior visual pathway and may result in decreased vision. Such conditions should be sought on slit-lamp examination and by direct ophthalmoscopic examination. These conditions include

- *corneal lesions,* both obvious (scars and severe conic distortion from keratoconus) and subtle (irregular or oblique astigmatism, early cone formation in keratoconus); keratometry or corneal topographic mapping may be required to detect these abnormalities. Subtle tear-film abnormalities (as in keratitis sicca and exposure keratopathy), subepithelial dystrophies, and corneal thickening with stromal edema may also degrade vision.
- *lenticular irregularities,* also either obvious (cortical, nuclear, subcapsular, or polar opacities) or subtle (central nuclear darkening, irregularity of lenticular tissue, "oil droplet" formation, posterior lenticonus)

- *vitreous abnormalities,* such as cellular infiltrate with haze, blood, inflammatory membranes, and asteroid hyalosis

Maculopathy

Diseases of the macula produce central visual loss, including decreased visual acuity and color vision and central visual field loss, and can sometimes mimic an optic neuropathy. However, unless there is severe macular disease, a relative afferent pupillary defect (RAPD) is absent. Furthermore, maculopathy tends to cause parallel losses in color discrimination and visual acuity, unlike optic nerve disease, which often causes color vision loss that is disproportionately greater than that of visual acuity. Visual field deficits in maculopathy tend to be focal and centered on the fixation point; deficits in optic neuropathies are larger, often cecocentral, and part of a generalized depression of visual field sensitivity. In addition, patients with macular lesions may complain of metamorphopsia, not typically a feature of optic neuropathy. In general, maculopathies produce visible fundus abnormalities that allow correct diagnosis, but these findings can be subtle, evanescent, or absent. Optical coherence tomography (OCT), fluorescein angiography, and, occasionally, multifocal electroretinography (mfERG) may help detect an abnormality of retinal structure or function. (See Chapter 3 and BCSC Section 12, *Retina and Vitreous,* for further discussion of these tests.)

The most common maculopathies and retinopathies often confused with optic nerve disease include acute idiopathic blind-spot enlargement syndrome, which overlaps with multiple evanescent white dot syndrome; vitamin A deficiency; and cone dystrophy. Patients with these entities may present with normal funduscopic examinations. Rarer entities are the paraneoplastic retinopathies: cancer-associated retinopathy (CAR) and melanoma-associated retinopathy (MAR). Patients with these entities present with significant visual symptoms but may also have a fundus that is, on examination, normal or that shows minimal changes later in the disease. Other retinal disorders sometimes confused with optic neuropathies such as central serous retinopathy, cystoid macular edema, and acute zonal occult outer retinopathy (AZOOR) are discussed in detail in BCSC Section 12, *Retina and Vitreous.*

Acute Idiopathic Blind-Spot Enlargement

Traditionally, enlargement of the blind spot on visual field testing is associated with changes of the optic disc such as edema or drusen. However, the term *acute idiopathic blind-spot enlargement (AIBSE)* has been used to describe a number of clinical entities that present with enlargement of the normal blind spot on perimetry but may show a variety of funduscopic appearances. (See BCSC Section 9, *Intraocular Inflammation and Uveitis,* and Section 12, *Retina and Vitreous,* for further discussion.) Some patients have a normal fundus appearance without optic disc edema and retinal lesions, whereas others demonstrate disc edema, peripapillary abnormalities, choroiditis, retinal pigment epithelium (RPE) changes, and uveitis. This variability has led to controversy as to whether these entities are separate or a spectrum of 1 disorder. In addition to the common feature of blind-spot enlargement, photopsias are a prominent symptom thought to reflect disease of the outer retina. Electroretinography (ERG), both full field and multifocal, can detect abnormalities. Thus, this clinical syndrome is a reflection of outer retina, RPE, and choroidal dysfunction and not primarily an optic neuropathy. In general, patients with AIBSE have a good visual prognosis.

Fletcher WA, Imes RK, Goodman D, Hoyt WF. Acute idiopathic blind spot enlargement: a big blind spot syndrome without optic disc edema. *Arch Ophthalmol.* 1988;106(1):44–49.

Volpe NJ, Rizzo JF III, Lessell S. Acute idiopathic blind spot enlargement syndrome: a review of 27 new cases. *Arch Ophthalmol.* 2001;119(1):59–63.

Multiple Evanescent White Dot Syndrome

In *multiple evanescent white dot syndrome (MEWDS)*, which most frequently affects women under 30 years of age, presenting features include photopsias, decreased visual acuity, and visual field defects ranging from an enlarged blind spot to a cecocentral/central scotoma to a diffuse depression of visual field sensitivity (Fig 4-1). An RAPD is present in some cases but is generally mild. The characteristic small, deep retinal white spots in the posterior retina are transient, usually lasting weeks and resolving spontaneously; the retina may appear normal at first examination. The optic disc is normal or shows mild edema. On fluorescein angiography, the retinal lesions, if demonstrable, show early wreathlike hyperfluorescence and late staining. Indocyanine green angiography produces a very striking pattern of small hypofluorescent lesions overlying larger hypofluorescent

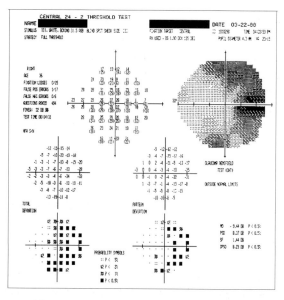

Figure 4-1 This 32-year-old woman presented with a 6-month history of continuously flashing lights to the right side in the right eye. Visual acuity was 20/15 bilaterally with a less than 0.3 log unit right afferent pupillary defect. Automated quantitative perimetry shows a broad region of temporal visual field depression arising from blind spot and not respecting the vertical midline. *(Courtesy of Steven A. Newman, MD.)*

lesions that are concentrated in a peripapillary distribution corresponding to the enlargement of the physiologic blind spot. An ERG typically demonstrates depressed a-wave responses. Multifocal ERG often demonstrates focal areas of retinal dysfunction. (See Section 9, *Intraocular Inflammation and Uveitis,* and Section 12, *Retina and Vitreous,* for further discussion.)

Gross NE, Yannuzzi LA, Freund KB, Spaide RF, Amato GP, Sigal R. Multiple evanescent white dot syndrome. *Arch Ophthalmol.* 2006;124(4):493–500.

Quillen DA, Davis JB, Gottlieb JL, et al. The white dot syndromes. *Am J Ophthalmol.* 2004;137(3): 538–550.

Vitamin A Deficiency

Vitamin A is a fat-soluble vitamin essential in the photoreceptor visual pigment rhodopsin, as well as in the differentiation of basal cells into mucous epithelium, which includes the conjunctiva. It is absorbed by the small intestine, transported to the liver, where it is stored, then redistributed to target organs, including the RPE. Malnutrition, malabsorption, liver disease, and zinc deficiency (zinc is a cofactor in the conversion of retinol to 11-*cis*-retinal) contribute to vitamin A deficiency. Manifestations of deficiency include xerosis, conjunctival Bitôt spots, keratomalacia, nyctalopia, peripheral visual field loss, and sometimes central visual loss. Ancillary testing reveals marked rod dysfunction (on ERG) and elevated thresholds of rods and cones (on dark adaptation). Patients often show dramatic recovery with treatment, which includes vitamin A supplementation and treatment of any underlying systemic disorder.

Purvin V. Through a shade darkly. *Surv Ophthalmol.* 1999;43(4):335–340.

Cone Dystrophy

Cone dystrophy is a rare disorder characterized by unexplained visual loss that may be confused with an optic neuropathy. Patients typically present in the first or second decade of life with a gradually progressive bilateral decline in visual acuity and color vision. Photophobia and hemeralopia ("day blindness") are common. In the early stages, mild to moderate visual loss may be accompanied by a normal fundus appearance or a slight decrease in foveal reflex and granular macular pigmentation. As the disease progresses, the macular RPE becomes atrophic in a central oval region. A "bull's-eye" pattern of depigmentation may be present, similar to that seen in chloroquine maculopathy. Fluorescein angiography may highlight these abnormalities before they become clinically apparent. ERG results may be normal initially but eventually show markedly depressed photopic (cone) response and less prominently affected scotopic (rod) response. Multifocal ERG is helpful in early cone dystrophy.

Paraneoplastic Syndromes

Cancer-associated retinopathy

Cancer-associated retinopathy (CAR) presents with photopsias, nyctalopia, impaired dark adaptation, dimming, ring scotoma, and peripheral and/or central visual field loss. In contrast to the episodic positive visual phenomena of migraine, the symptoms of CAR tend to be continuous. Symptoms develop over weeks to months, often (in 50% of cases) before the underlying malignancy is identified (usually small cell carcinoma of the lung, although other lung tumors and breast, uterine, and cervical malignancies have been implicated). Deterioration is progressive, with eventual bilateral involvement and severe visual loss. The fundus may initially appear normal, although the ERG is typically markedly reduced in amplitude, even in the early stages. As the disease course progresses, the retinal arterioles become attenuated, the RPE thinned and mottled, and the optic discs atrophic.

Investigators believe that in most patients, the underlying tumor expresses an antigen that is homologous to a 23-kd retinal photoreceptor protein; originally termed the *CAR antigen,* this protein has now been identified as the calcium-binding protein *recoverin.* Circulating autoantibodies against the tumor-associated antigen presumably cross-react with retinal recoverin to produce immune-mediated photoreceptor degeneration of both rods and cones. On the basis of this presumed mechanism, several modes of therapy have been attempted. Keltner and colleagues described a patient whose antibody levels diminished and visual function improved and stabilized on systemic corticosteroid therapy. Treatment benefit has also been attributed to various combinations of corticosteroids, plasmapheresis, and intravenous immunoglobulin. In general, however, the prognosis for vision is poor. Treatment of the inciting tumor has an unclear effect on retinal function.

Melanoma-associated retinopathy

Melanoma-associated retinopathy (MAR) is an extremely rare syndrome that primarily involves rods, with corresponding symptoms of photopsia, nyctalopia, and bilateral peripheral visual loss. MAR usually develops rapidly over weeks to months but may have a sudden onset. Visual symptoms typically develop in the setting of previously diagnosed melanoma, and investigation of visual loss often reveals metastasis. Visual acuity, color vision, and the central visual field are often initially normal, with peripheral visual field abnormalities predominant. The fundus may be normal or may show RPE irregularity, retinal arteriolar attenuation, and optic disc pallor in cases that have been symptomatic for months. ERG abnormalities in patients with MAR syndrome suggest rod dysfunction. Visual function may remain stable and nonprogressive in MAR (which is not the case in CAR). No treatment has been proven effective.

Chan JW. Paraneoplastic retinopathies and optic neuropathies. *Surv Ophthalmol.* 2003;48(1): 12–38.

Goldstein SM, Syed NA, Milam AH, Maguire AM, Lawton TJ, Nichols CW. Cancer-associated retinopathy. *Arch Ophthalmol.* 1999;117(12):1641–1645.

Guy J, Aptsiauri N. Treatment of paraneoplastic visual loss with intravenous immunoglobulin: report of 3 cases. *Arch Ophthalmol.* 1999;117(4):471–477.

Keltner JL, Thirkill CE, Tyler NK, Roth AM. Management and monitoring of cancer-associated retinopathy. *Arch Ophthalmol.* 1992;110(11):48–53.

Kim RY, Retsas S, Fitzke FW, Arden GB, Bird AC. Cutaneous melanoma-associated retinopathy. *Ophthalmology.* 1994;101(11):1837–1843.

Sawyer RA, Selhorst JB, Zimmerman LE, Hoyt WF. Blindness caused by photoreceptor degeneration as a remote effect of cancer. *Am J Ophthalmol.* 1976;81(5):606–613.

Amblyopia

In cases of unexplained monocular visual loss, previously existing amblyopia must be considered. Causes such as anisometropia, astigmatism, or small-angle heterotropia should be sought. Improvement of visual acuity with the testing of isolated letters rather than entire lines suggests the crowding phenomenon noted in amblyopia. Occasionally, severe amblyopia results in an RAPD, but the degree is small (rarely more than 0.6 log unit). Visual fields are generally normal or show mild generalized depression rather than the focal scotoma or more severe depression seen with visual pathway damage. Records from previous ophthalmic examinations may be extremely helpful.

Optic Neuropathy

Optic neuropathies typically are associated with visual field loss, as described in the following sections. Most demonstrate an afferent pupillary defect, although in cases with very mild optic nerve dysfunction or with bilateral symmetric dysfunction, the defect may not be detectable. The optic disc may be abnormal or normal in appearance; abnormal discs may be edematous or may show other abnormalities, such as drusen, excavation, or atrophy. Certain causes of optic neuropathy may present in more than one way; for example, orbital compressive or infiltrative lesions may initially demonstrate either normal, edematous, or atrophic optic discs. In this chapter, we have classified optic neuropathies by their most common presentations, but it must be remembered that there is considerable overlap in these categories.

Visual Field Patterns

Retinal ganglion cell nerve fibers enter the optic nerve head in 3 major groups (Fig 4-2), and lesions of the optic nerve thus result in 3 categories of visual field loss. In general, defects may be classified as noted in Table 4-1.

- *papillomacular fibers:* cecocentral scotoma (Fig 4-3A, left), paracentral scotoma (Fig 4-3A, right), and central scotoma (Fig 4-3B)
- *arcuate fibers:* arcuate scotoma (nerve fiber bundle defect) (Fig 4-3C), broad (altitudinal) defect (broader region of arcuate fibers) (Fig 4-3D), and nasal (step) defect (nasal portion of arcuate fibers) (Fig 4-3E). These fibers align along a temporal horizontal retinal raphe, so that damage to them produces defects that align along the corresponding nasal horizontal meridian.
- *nasal radiating fibers:* temporal wedge defect

Blind-spot enlargement results from optic disc edema of any cause, because of displacement of surrounding retina (Fig 4-3F).

Anterior Optic Neuropathies With Optic Disc Edema

Acute papilledema

The term *papilledema* refers to edema of the optic nerve head that results from increased intracranial pressure (ICP). The appearance of the disc in papilledema is indistinguishable

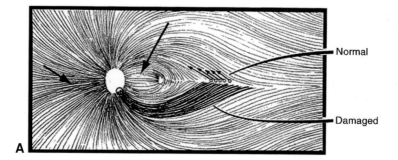

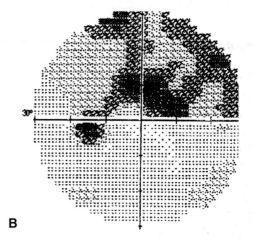

Figure 4-2 **A,** Diagram of retinal nerve fiber layer entering the optic disc. The fibers are classified as arcuate *(inferior bundle highlighted)*, papillomacular *(long arrow)*, and nasal radiating *(short arrow)*. **B,** Humphrey perimetry grayscale diagram, showing superior arcuate visual field defect corresponding to the inferior arcuate nerve fiber bundle damage highlighted. *(Part B courtesy of Anthony C. Arnold, MD.)*

from that in other causes of edema (eg, papillitis). Acute papilledema produces hyperemia of the optic disc, with dilation of the existing disc surface capillary net, telangiectasia of the surface and radial peripapillary vessels, and often flame hemorrhages. The edematous peripapillary retinal nerve fiber layer (NFL) is grayish white and opalescent, with feathered, striated margins that obscure the disc edge and retinal vessels coursing through it. In early papilledema, NFL involvement may be incomplete, with only partial obscuration of vessels. Absence of the physiologic cup is a late finding in papilledema; such absence more frequently reflects a congenitally full optic disc, as seen in pseudopapilledema (see the discussion later in this section). Absence of spontaneous venous pulsations may reflect increased ICP, but absence at initial examination is of limited value: 20% of the normal population does not show spontaneous venous pulsations. Their disappearance after prior documented presence, however, is suggestive of ICP elevation. Other ophthalmoscopic findings with more severe papilledema may include disc and retinal cotton-wool spots, exudates, and hemorrhage.

Most patients with elevated ICP have symptoms, including headache, nausea, and vomiting. Patients may also note transient visual obscurations, episodes of unilateral or bilateral visual loss lasting seconds. These are described as "grayouts," "whiteouts," "smokiness or fogginess," or "blackouts" of vision, and often occur with orthostatic changes. In acute papilledema, optic nerve function, including visual acuity and color vision, is usually normal. Pupillary responses are also normal; visual fields demonstrate only enlargement of the blind spot.

Table 4-1 Perimetric Terms

Term	Characteristics
Characteristics of the visual field defect	
Absolute	No stimulus perceived in the affected area
Relative	Bigger and brighter stimuli may be perceived in the affected field, but smaller, dimmer targets are not seen. The size and shape of the field defect, therefore, change inversely with changes in size and/or intensity of the presented stimulus. Defects may be described as shallow when only the smallest or dimmest targets fail to be identified or deep if bright objects are not detected in the central portion of the defect.
Terms describing visual field defects	
Scotoma	Area of depressed visual function surrounded by normal visual function (eg, the blind spot)
Central	Involves fixation only
Cecocentral	Extends from fixation temporally to the blind spot
Paracentral	Involves a region next to, but not including, fixation
Pericentral	Involves a region symmetrically surrounding, but not involving, fixation
Arcuate	Corresponds to and represents nerve fiber bundle loss
Altitudinal	A more extensive arcuate defect involving 2 quadrants in either the superior or inferior field
Quadrantanopia	One quadrant of visual field involved
Hemianopia	One half of visual field involved, either nasal or temporal
Description of bilateral visual field defects with respect to spatial localization and extent	
Homonymous	Same side of visual space affected in each eye
Bitemporal	Opposite temporal sides of visual field space affected in each eye
Complete	Entire field affected
Incomplete	A portion of the field spared
Congruity	Tendency for homonymous field defect to be symmetric (ie, to have a similar size, location, and shape in each eye's field)

The clinician's first step in managing suspected papilledema is to rule out pseudo-papilledema. To make this distinction, 3 questions should be answered:

1. *Is the optic disc hyperemic?* Disc edema—except for the pallid form of ischemic optic neuropathy (giant cell arteritis) or advanced chronic papilledema with atrophy (in which there is significant optic nerve dysfunction as well)—is usually associated with congestion of the disc microvasculature, which increases the disc's reddish hue.

2. *Are there microvascular abnormalities on the surface of the disc?* Edema of the disc usually demonstrates dilation and telangiectasia of the surface disc capillaries and may be associated with flame hemorrhages on or adjacent to the disc. These findings are absent in pseudopapilledema. They differ from the peripapillary telangiectatic vessels seen with Leber hereditary optic neuropathy, which are primarily peripapillary and do not leak fluorescein.

3. *At what depth in the retina does the blurring of the disc margin originate?* The margin of the disc is blurred in disc edema because the thickened and opacified disc

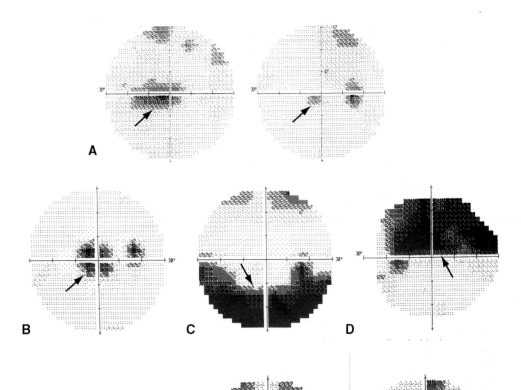

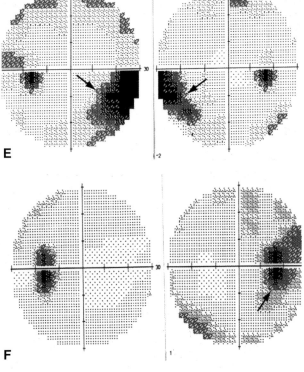

Figure 4-3 Patterns of visual field loss in optic neuropathies. **A,** Cecocentral scotoma *(left; arrow);* paracentral scotoma *(right; arrow).* **B,** Central scotoma *(arrow).* **C,** Arcuate scotoma *(arrow).* **D,** Broad arcuate (altitudinal) defect *(arrow).* **E,** Nasal arcuate (step) defects *(arrows).* **F,** Enlarged blind spot *(arrow).* *(Parts E, F courtesy of Anthony C. Arnold, MD.)*

and peripapillary NFL obscure both the retinal vessels and the disc margin. In most cases of pseudopapilledema, the optic disc borders appear indistinct and the disc is elevated, but the retinal blood vessels are clearly visible as they cross the disc margin.

Most cases of pseudopapilledema are due to the presence of optic disc drusen (ODD). However, with ODD the disc is not hyperemic and typically shows no dilation of the surface microvasculature. Blurring of the disc margin arises from axoplasmic stasis in the axons deep within the optic disc, which creates a yellowish, hazy appearance that obscures the border between disc and retina but leaves the view of the retinal vessels intact. This contrasts with the whitish, fluffy, striated appearance of NFL edema in true papilledema. Buried drusen are frequently accompanied by other features, including anomalous branching of the retinal vessels (loops, trifurcations, and generally increased branching); a disc margin with a scalloped appearance; and peripapillary RPE dispersion, with a gray or black region adjacent to the disc (Fig 4-4). Ancillary diagnostic testing may aid in the detection or confirmation of ODD (see Fig 4-15).

Other causes of an elevated disc appearance mimicking papilledema are hyaloid remnants and glial tissue on the disc surface, congenital "fullness" of the disc associated with entry of the optic nerve into the eye through a relatively small scleral canal, and disc fullness associated with hyperopia. Optic disc margins may also be blurred without elevation of the disc by NFL opacities other than edema, including myelination of the NFL (Fig 4-5). Myelination typically occurs at the disc margin, where it obscures the disc–retina border; myelination in the NFL also obscures the retinal vessels and results in a feathered edge that resembles true edema. Myelination may be readily differentiated from

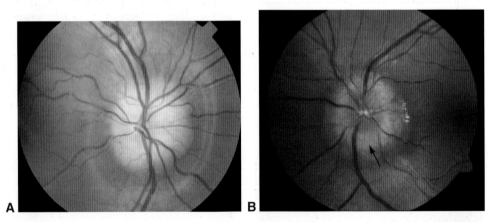

A   **B**

Figure 4-4 **A,** Fundus photograph of the optic disc with buried drusen. The disc margin is blurred, with yellowish opacity of the deep peripapillary tissue. The retinal vessels are clearly seen overlying the disc. **B,** Fundus photograph of the optic disc with papilledema. The disc margin is blurred, with grayish white, opalescent thickening of the peripapillary nerve fiber layer *(arrow)*. The retinal vessels are partially obscured at the disc margin and within the peripapillary retina. There are exudates just temporal to the disc from chronic edema. *(Courtesy of Sophia M. Chung, MD.)*

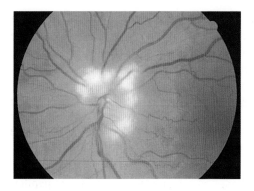

Figure 4-5 Myelinated nerve patches are often seen within the arcuate bundles, occasionally abutting the disc. When they are contiguous, these nerve patches may be confused with disc edema or cotton-wool spots. *(Courtesy of Anthony C. Arnold, MD.)*

edema, however, by its dense, white opacity, as compared with the partially translucent, grayish white appearance of true edema.

Papilledema may result from a variety of conditions, including an intracranial mass, hydrocephalus, central nervous system (CNS) infection (meningitis or meningoencephalitis), infiltration by a granulomatous or neoplastic process, or pseudotumor cerebri (see "Idiopathic intracranial hypertension" later in the chapter). Suspicion of papilledema warrants *urgent* neuroimaging to rule out an intracranial mass lesion. Normal imaging results should prompt neurologic consultation with evaluation of the cerebrospinal fluid (CSF) opening pressure and composition.

Chronic papilledema

In patients with chronically elevated ICP (months to years) and long-standing papilledema, optic nerve function may deteriorate. The disc may no longer be hyperemic but becomes pale from chronic axonal loss (Fig 4-6). Additional features may include

- *Gliosis of the peripapillary NFL.* The opacification appears grayish, less fluffy, and more membranous than with edema. Gliosis tends to follow retinal vessels, producing vascular sheathing.
- *Optociliary shunt vessels (retinochoroidal collaterals), preexisting venous channels on the disc surface that dilate in response to chronic central retinal vein obstruction from elevated ICP.* Unlike the retinal vascular anomalies often accompanying drusen and congenital disc anomalies, these collateral vessels follow an evolving course of

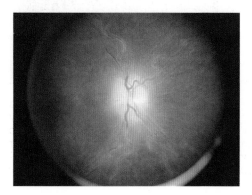

Figure 4-6 Chronic atrophic papilledema with gliosis and retinal vascular sheathing. *(Courtesy of Anthony C. Arnold, MD.)*

enlargement over time and characteristically dive deep into the choroid immediately adjacent to the disc.

- *Refractile bodies of the disc, the result of chronic lipid-rich exudation* (Fig 4-7). They differ from drusen in that they tend to be smaller and noncalcified, remaining on the disc surface rather than within its substance, with frequent clustering at the disc margin; they disappear as papilledema resolves.

With chronic papilledema, visual field defects may include nasal field loss, arcuate scotomata, and generalized peripheral depression; central visual field involvement with decreased visual acuity is a typically late finding. The process is usually bilateral, and if asymmetric, there may be an RAPD.

Arnold AC. Differential diagnosis of optic disc edema. *Focal Points: Clinical Modules for Ophthalmologists.* San Francisco: American Academy of Ophthalmology; 1999, module 2.

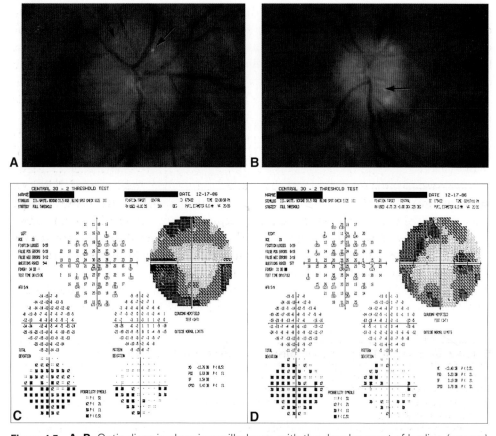

Figure 4-7 A, B, Optic discs in chronic papilledema, with the development of bodies *(arrows)*, representing lipid exudates from chronic microvascular leakage. **C, D,** Visual fields confirm the presence of mild diffuse depression in sensitivity and superior and inferior arcuate defects.
(Parts A, B courtesy of Anthony C. Arnold, MD; parts C, D courtesy of Steven A. Newman, MD.)

Idiopathic intracranial hypertension

Patients with *idiopathic intracranial hypertension (IIH)*, also known as *pseudotumor cerebri*, present with symptoms and signs of elevated ICP. Headache, nausea, and vomiting are common; additional complaints may include transient visual obscurations (secondary to papilledema), diplopia (secondary to abducens nerve paresis), visual field loss, pulsatile tinnitus, and dizziness. Most patients (>90%) with IIH have papilledema. Typically, other neurologic abnormalities are absent (other than abducens palsy related to increased ICP). As is typical with acute papilledema, visual acuity is most often normal; visual fields may show enlarged blind spots but usually no additional defects. In long-standing, untreated, or severe cases, optic nerve function may deteriorate, with the development of visual field defects of chronic papilledema, as described in the previous section. Table 4-2 gives the diagnostic criteria of IIH.

The incidence of IIH peaks in the third decade of life, and there is a strong female preponderance; most patients are obese. The disease occurs less commonly in children (with obesity less a factor) and infrequently in lean adults. IIH is associated with the use of exogenous substances such as vitamin A (>100,000 U/day), tetracycline, nalidixic acid, cyclosporine, and oral contraceptives, as well as the use of or withdrawal from corticosteroids. Although hormonal changes such as pregnancy and hormonal abnormalities have been implicated, IIH has not been definitely associated with any specific endocrinologic dysfunction. The mechanism for the increase in ICP in idiopathic IIH remains obscure. Absorption of CSF across the arachnoid granulations into the dural venous sinuses is probably impaired, but the specific cause is unknown.

An associated condition such as cerebral venous obstruction (eg, due to trauma, childbirth, a hypercoagulable state, or middle ear infection), systemic or localized extracranial venous obstruction (eg, radical neck dissection), a dural arteriovenous malformation, or systemic vasculitis may lead to decreased venous outflow and thus increased ICP. Such conditions may resemble IIH, and therefore patients with suspected IIH should undergo neuroimaging (MRI) to rule out tumor, hydrocephalus, and meningeal lesion. In addition, *magnetic resonance venography (MRV)* should be considered to assess for venous sinus occlusion (see Chapter 2, Fig 2-11). Lumbar puncture should always be performed to confirm elevated ICP and to rule out a meningeal process.

The ophthalmologist plays a critical role in the management of IIH. Careful long-term follow-up is essential to ensure that papilledema resolves. Regular examinations,

---

Table 4-2 Criteria for Diagnosis of Idiopathic Intracranial Hypertension

Symptoms, if present, representing increased ICP or papilledema
Signs representing increased ICP or papilledema
Documented elevated ICP during lumbar puncture measured in the lateral decubitus position
Normal CSF composition
No evidence of ventriculomegaly, mass, structural, or vascular lesion on MRI scan or contrast-
    enhanced CT scan for typical patients, and MRI scan and magnetic resonance venography for
    all others
No other cause (including medication) of intracranial hypertension identified

including visual acuity testing, color vision testing, and quantitative perimetry, document the level of optic nerve function. Stereophotographs of the optic nerve are essential during patient follow-up. The frequency of visual field testing depends on the severity of papilledema, the level of optic nerve dysfunction, and the response to treatment.

Treatment for IIH depends on symptomatology and visual status. The disease may be self-limited; if headache is controlled with minor analgesics and there is no optic nerve dysfunction, no therapy may be required. However, the natural history of IIH may be one of severe visual loss: 26% of patients in a long-term study developed visual acuity of less than 20/200 in the worse eye. For obese patients, weight loss is an effective treatment and is always recommended. In patients requiring medical therapy, acetazolamide (Diamox) is usually the first choice. Topiramate (Topamax) has also been used with success; it has multiple beneficial effects—control of headache, appetite suppression, and carbonic anhydrase inhibition—and therefore lowers ICP. Furosemide (Lasix) is frequently used in patients intolerant of acetazolamide or topiramate. The use of corticosteroids is controversial. Although elevated ICP is frequently decreased with corticosteroids, recurrence is common when the corticosteroids are tapered; indeed, corticosteroid withdrawal is a documented cause of IIH. However, a short course of high-dose intravenous corticosteroids may be useful in the acute phase of fulminant papilledema with very high ICP and severe visual loss. Repeated lumbar punctures are not recommended therapy.

Intractable headache or progressive visual loss on maximally tolerated medical therapy mandates surgical therapy. In some cases of severe visual loss and papilledema from markedly elevated ICP, surgical intervention may be considered without waiting for definite evidence of progression. The primary surgical options are optic nerve sheath decompression (fenestration) or CSF diversion procedure (lumboperitoneal or ventriculoperitoneal shunt).

When headache is a lesser component and progressive visual loss occurs, optic nerve sheath fenestration is typically preferred because it directly protects the optic nerve and has lower morbidity than shunting. However, optic nerve surgery carries a 1%–2% risk of blindness from optic nerve injury, central retinal artery occlusion (CRAO), or central retinal vein occlusion (CRVO). It does not lower ICP and thus does not treat headache. Although a reduction of papilledema in the contralateral eye occasionally is reported, bilateral surgery is generally required. The long-term success rate is low, estimated at 16% with 6-year follow-up. Optic nerve sheath fenestration may be repeated but is technically more difficult because of scarring.

Lumboperitoneal or ventriculoperitoneal shunting procedures effectively lower ICP, with improvement of headache, abducens palsy (if present), and papilledema; moreover, shunting entails no direct risk to the optic nerve. A shunt, however, may become occluded, infected, or altered in position, requiring reoperation in more than 50% of cases. In cases of severe morbid obesity, gastric bypass surgery has been shown to effectively reduce both weight and ICP.

Idiopathic intracranial hypertension also occurs in the pediatric population, but controversy exists as to the criteria for pediatric IIH. The word *pediatric* typically refers to children under the age of 18 years. However, some authors believe the term should be reserved for children who are prepubescent, or without any physical changes of sexual maturation. IIH appears to be a different disorder in prepubescent children, with more boys and nonobese children affected. Unlike with adult IIH, a variety of cranial neuropathies have been associated with pediatric IIH, including those of CNs III, IV, VI, VII, IX, and XII, which reverse with lowering of the ICP. Furthermore, papilledema without headache or visual symptoms is more common in younger patients. Finally, the CSF opening pressures in children are different from those in adults, and both CSF content and pressure are different in neonates. The treatment for pediatric IIH is similar to that for adult IIH.

Celebisoy N, Gökcay F, Sirin H, Akyürekli O. Treatment of idiopathic intracranial hypertension: topiramate versus acetazolamide, an open label study. *Acta Neurol Scand.* 2007;116(5): 322–327.

Feldon SE. Visual outcomes comparing surgical techniques for management of severe idiopathic intracranial hypertension. *Neurosurg Focus.* 2007;23(5):E6.

Friedman DI, Jacobson DM. Idiopathic intracranial hypertension. *J Neuroophthalmol.* 2004; 24(2):138–145.

Rangwala LM, Liu GT. Pediatric idiopathic intracranial hypertension. *Surv Ophthalmol.* 2007; 52(6):597–617.

Shah VA, Kardon RH, Lee AG, Corbett JJ, Wall M. Long-term follow-up of idiopathic intracranial hypertension: the Iowa experience. *Neurology.* 2008;70(8):634–640.

Anterior ischemic optic neuropathy

Anterior ischemic optic neuropathy (AION) is the most common acute optic neuropathy in patients over 50 years of age, reflecting ischemic damage to the optic nerve head. Patients present with painless monocular visual loss developing over hours to days. Visual acuity may be diminished. Visual field loss is always present: altitudinal and other variants of arcuate defects are the most common, although central and cecocentral scotomata and generalized (especially nasal) depression may also occur. An RAPD is present unless the optic neuropathy is bilateral. Optic disc edema is visible at onset and may precede the visual loss. Diffuse hyperemia is the most common presentation, although the disc edema may be pale and segmental. Peripapillary flame hemorrhages and retinal arteriolar narrowing are often seen.

AION is classified as either *arteritic (AAION),* in which case it is associated with giant cell arteritis (GCA), or *nonarteritic (NAION)* (Table 4-3). The most important initial step in the management of AION is the search for evidence of GCA.

Arteritic anterior ischemic optic neuropathy AAION is less frequent (5%–10% of AION cases) than NAION and usually occurs in older patients (mean age 70 years). It is caused by inflammatory and thrombotic occlusion of the short posterior ciliary arteries. Systemic symptoms of GCA are usually present, especially headache and tenderness of the temporal arteries or scalp. Jaw claudication is the symptom most specific for the disorder, but other symptoms include malaise, anorexia and weight loss, fever, joint and muscle pain, and ear pain. Occult GCA, without overt systemic symptoms, may occur in up to 20% of patients with AAION. Transient dimming and visual loss may precede AAION by several weeks.

Visual loss is typically severe (visual acuity is <20/200 in over 60% of patients). Optic disc edema is typically pale in AAION compared with NAION (Fig 4-8). Cotton-wool

Table 4-3 **Arteritic vs Nonarteritic Ischemic Optic Neuropathy**

Characteristic	Arteritic	Nonarteritic
Age	Mean, 70 years	Mean, 60 years
Sex	F > M	F = M
Associated symptoms	Headache, scalp tenderness, jaw claudication, transient visual loss	Usually none
Visual acuity	<20/200 in >60% of cases	>20/200 in >60% of cases
Disc/fundus	Pallid disc edema common	Hyperemic disc edema
	Cup normal	Cup small
	Cotton-wool spots	
Erythrocyte sedimentation rate	Mean, 70 mm/hr	Mean, 20–40 mm/hr
C-reactive protein	Elevated	Normal
Fluorescein angiography	Disc delay and choroid delay	Disc delay
Natural history	Rarely improve	31% improve
	Fellow eye, 54%–95%	Fellow eye, 12%–19%
Treatment	Systemic steroids	None proven

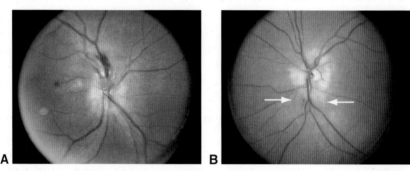

Figure 4-8 **A,** Optic disc appearance in nonarteritic AION. Edema is segmental, with mild superimposed pallor and flame hemorrhages. **B,** Optic disc appearance in arteritic AION. Pallor is more pronounced, and in this case, peripapillary choroidal ischemia creates pale swelling of the peripapillary deep retina and choroid *(arrows),* further obscuring the disc–retinal border. *(Reprinted from Arnold AC. Differential diagnosis of optic disc edema. Focal Points: Clinical Modules for Ophthalmologists. San Francisco: American Academy of Ophthalmology; 1999, module 2.)*

spots indicative of concurrent retinal ischemia may be present. Accompanying choroidal ischemia may produce peripapillary pallor and edema deep to the retina, exacerbating the visual loss. Fluorescein angiography reveals delayed choroidal filling, helping to differentiate AAION from NAION (see Fig 3-8). The optic disc diameter of the fellow eye is usually normal, as is the physiologic cup.

When AAION is suspected, immediate therapy is critical. Confirmational temporal artery biopsy may be delayed without compromising test results. Intravenous methylprednisolone (1 g/day for the first 3–5 days) is most often recommended, after which oral prednisone may be used (up to 100 mg/day, tapered slowly over 3–12 months or more, depending on response). Alternate-day corticosteroid therapy is inadequate for AAION.

The major goal of therapy (apart from avoiding systemic vascular complications) is to prevent contralateral visual loss. Untreated, the fellow eye becomes involved in up to 95% of cases, within days to weeks. Although the initially affected eye may improve somewhat, recovery is not generally anticipated. The risk of recurrent or contralateral optic nerve involvement on corticosteroid withdrawal has been reported at 7%; thus, tapering must be slow and careful. Recurrent symptoms should prompt reevaluation for disease activity.

For a discussion of systemic involvement, diagnostic evaluation, and therapy for GCA, see Chapter 14.

Aiello PD, Trautmann JC, McPhee TJ, Kunselman AR, Hunder GG. Visual prognosis in giant cell arteritis. *Ophthalmology.* 1993;100(4):550–555.

Hayreh SS, Podhajsky PA, Raman R, Zimmerman B. Giant cell arteritis: validity and reliability of various diagnostic criteria. *Am J Ophthalmol.* 1997;123(3):285–296.

Liu GT, Glaser JS, Schatz NJ, Smith JL. Visual morbidity in giant cell arteritis. Clinical characteristics and prognosis for vision. *Ophthalmology.* 1994;101(11):1779–1785.

Nonarteritic anterior ischemic optic neuropathy   The nonarteritic form of AION is more common (accounting for 90%–95% of AION cases) and occurs in a relatively younger age group (mean age 60 years). NAION is presumed to be related to compromise of the optic disc microcirculation in the setting of structural "crowding" of the disc. Histopathologic confirmation of the site of vascular occlusive disease is not available. Patients frequently report visual impairment on awakening, possibly related to nocturnal systemic hypotension. The initial course may be *static,* with visual loss stable from onset, or *progressive,* with either episodic, stepwise decrements or a steady decline of vision over weeks to months prior to eventual stabilization. The progressive form has been reported in 22%–37% of nonarteritic cases. Associated systemic symptoms are generally absent.

Visual loss is usually less severe than in AAION (visual acuity >20/200 in over 60% of cases). The optic disc edema in NAION may be diffuse or segmental and hyperemic or pale, but pallor is less common than in the arteritic form (see Fig 4-8). Focal telangiectasia of the edematous disc surface vasculature occasionally resembles a vascular mass. The retinal arterioles are focally narrowed in the peripapillary region in up to 68% of cases. The optic disc in the contralateral eye is typically small in diameter and demonstrates a small or absent physiologic cup ("disc at risk").

The optic disc usually becomes visibly atrophic within 4–8 weeks; persistence of edema past this point suggests an alternative diagnosis. The 5-year risk of contralateral involvement is 14.7%. Occurrence in the second eye produces the clinical appearance of "pseudo–Foster Kennedy syndrome," in which the previously affected disc is atrophic and the currently involved nerve head is edematous. Both eyes show visual field loss characteristic of AION. This is in contrast to the true Foster Kennedy syndrome (Fig 4-9), secondary to intracranial mass, in which 1 optic disc is atrophic because of chronic compression by the mass, whereas the other disc is edematous because of elevated ICP. In this true syndrome, the eye with optic disc edema typically has no visual field loss other than an enlarged blind spot.

Risk factors for NAION include structural crowding of the disc ("disc at risk"), systemic hypertension, diabetes (particularly in young patients), smoking, and hyperlipidemia. Neither carotid occlusive disease nor prothrombotic disorders have been shown to be significant risk factors. Hyperhomocysteinemia, platelet polymorphisms, sleep apnea, and nocturnal hypotension have been proposed as risk factors but are currently unproven. NAION has been reported in association with the use of phosphodiesterase inhibitors

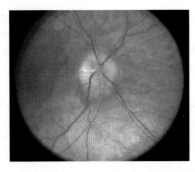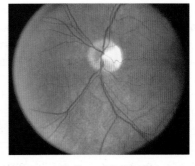

Figure 4-9 Optic discs in true Foster Kennedy syndrome. Unlike with NAION, the edematous disc is usually hyperemic with normal visual function, and the contralateral disc does not show an altitudinal pattern of atrophy. *(Courtesy of Steven A. Newman, MD.)*

(eg, sildenafil or Viagra), presumably because of its hypotensive effect, although causation has not been proven.

NAION must be differentiated from optic neuritis; infiltrative optic neuropathies; anterior orbital lesions producing optic nerve compression; and other forms of optic disc edema, including diabetic papillopathy. Optic neuritis may resemble NAION with regard to rate of onset, pattern of visual field loss, and optic disc appearance. NAION, however, usually occurs in patients over age 50, typically without pain on eye movement; moreover, altitudinal visual field loss and diffuse hyperemic disc edema (with associated retinal flame hemorrhages) are more common in NAION (Table 4-4). In unclear cases, fluorescein angiography of the optic disc may help. Delayed optic disc filling is present in 75% of NAION cases, whereas filling is normal in nonischemic disc edema, including optic neuritis. Contrast-enhanced MRI may also aid in distinction; the affected optic nerve is most commonly normal in NAION, with enhancement present early in the course of optic neuritis.

Untreated NAION generally remains stable after reaching the low point of visual function, but recovery of at least 3 Snellen visual acuity lines has been reported in 31% of patients after 2 years in the Ischemic Optic Neuropathy Decompression Trial (IONDT). Recurrent episodes of visual loss in the same eye after 3 months are unusual in NAION (up to 6.4%), occurring most often in young patients.

There is no proven therapy for NAION. The IONDT showed no benefit of surgery for NAION, and it has therefore been abandoned as a treatment modality. Neuroprotective

Table 4-4 NAION vs Optic Neuritis: Typical Features

	NAION	Optic Neuritis
Age	>50	<40
Pain	Unusual	With eye movement 92%
Pupil	+ RAPD	+ RAPD
Visual field defect	Altitudinal	Central
Optic disc	Edema 100%; may be pale	Edema 33%; hyperemic
Retinal hemorrhage	Common	Unusual
Fluorescein angiography	Delayed disc filling	No delayed disc filling
MRI scan	No optic nerve enhancement	Optic nerve enhancement

agents have demonstrated beneficial effects against secondary neuronal degeneration in animal models of ischemic retinal ganglion cell damage and optic nerve crush injury; however, clinical studies have been unsuccessful in recruiting sufficient patients in a timely manner. For example, a European study of 36 patients demonstrated a nonstatistical trend toward improved visual field, but not visual acuity, in a brimonidine-treated-group, but the study was terminated because of the difficulty in enrolling patients within 7 days after onset of NAION.

There is also no proven prophylaxis for NAION. Although aspirin has a proven effect in reducing the incidence of stroke in patients at risk, its role in reducing the incidence of fellow eye involvement after the initial episode is unclear.

Arnold AC. Pathogenesis of nonarteritic anterior ischemic optic neuropathy. *J Neuroophthalmol.* 2003;23(2):157–163.

Hayreh SS, Podhajsky PA, Zimmerman B. Ipsilateral recurrence of nonarteritic anterior ischemic optic neuropathy. *Am J Ophthalmol.* 2001;132(5):734–742.

Ischemic Optic Neuropathy Decompression Trial: twenty-four month update. Ischemic Optic Neuropathy Decompression Trial Research Group. *Arch Ophthalmol.* 2000;118(6):793–798.

Newman NJ, Scherer R, Lagenberg P, et al; Ischemic Optic Neuropathy Decompression Trial Research Group. The fellow eye in NAION: report from the ischemic optic neuropathy decompression trial follow-up study. *Am J Ophthalmol.* 2002;134(3):317–328.

Optic nerve decompression surgery for nonarteritic anterior ischemic optic neuropathy (NAION) is not effective and may be harmful. The Ischemic Optic Neuropathy Decompression Trial Research Group. *JAMA.* 1995;273(8):625–632.

Tesser RA, Niendorf ER, Levin LA. The morphology of an infarct in nonarteritic anterior ischemic optic neuropathy. *Ophthalmology.* 2003;110(10):2031–2035.

Wilhelm B, Lüdtke H, Wilhelm H; BRAION Study Group. Efficacy and tolerability of 0.2% brimonidine tartrate for the treatment of acute non-arteritic anterior ischemic optic neuropathy (NAION): a 3-month, double-masked, randomised placebo-controlled trial. *Graefes Arch Clin Exp Ophthalmol.* 2006;244(5):551–558.

Papillitis

In approximately 35% of cases of optic neuritis, the inflammation is located anteriorly in the nerve, the optic disc is edematous, and the term *papillitis* is applied. The disc edema is usually hyperemic and diffuse. Papillitis is more common in postviral and infectious neuritis than in demyelinating neuritis, but overlap is considerable. Children in particular manifest postviral optic neuritis, which is bilateral and associated with profound visual loss. But papillitis in adults is, in all other aspects, managed in the same manner as retrobulbar neuritis (see the discussion later in the chapter).

In the 15-year follow-up to the Optic Neuritis Treatment Trial (ONTT), patients with normal MRIs but severe papillitis, peripapillary hemorrhages, or retinal exudates did not develop multiple sclerosis (MS).

Beck RW, Trobe JD, Moke PS, et al; Optic Neuritis Study Group. High and low-risk profiles for the development of multiple sclerosis within 10 years after optic neuritis: experience of the optic neuritis treatment trial. *Arch Ophthalmol.* 2003;121(7):944–949.

Optic Neuritis Study Group. Multiple sclerosis risk after optic neuritis: final optic neuritis treatment trial follow-up. *Arch Neurol.* 2008;65(6):727–732.

Neuroretinitis

Neuroretinitis is a clinical syndrome characterized by acute loss of vision, typically without pain, in association with disc edema and a star pattern of exudates in the macula (Fig 4-10). The disc edema is diffuse and spreads through the outer plexiform layer along the papillomacular bundle and around the fovea. As the fluid is resorbed, the lipid precipitates in a characteristic radial pattern in the Henle layer. Although the macular star may be present at the time of initial presentation, it may be delayed by days. Recognition of fluid in the papillomacular bundle or the lipid exudates is critical in establishing the correct diagnosis. In addition, patients with neuroretinitis do not have an increased risk of demyelinating disease. Two thirds of patients with neuroretinitis have been shown to have cat-scratch disease caused by the *Bartonella henselae* or *B quintana* organisms. Other potential infectious causes include syphilis, Lyme disease, viruses, and diffuse unilateral subacute neuroretinitis (DUSN). Serologic testing for specific infections should be considered in cases of neuroretinitis, particularly if additional clinical findings such as skin rash or uveitis are present. See BCSC Section 9, *Intraocular Inflammation and Uveitis,* for a complete discussion of ocular bartonellosis and neuroretinitis.

Cunningham ET, Koehler JE. Ocular bartonellosis. *Am J Ophthalmol.* 2000;130(3):340–349.

Suhler EB, Lauer AK, Rosenbaum JT. Prevalence of serologic evidence of cat scratch disease in patients with neuroretinitis. *Ophthalmology.* 2000;107(5):871–876.

Diabetic papillopathy

Diabetic papillopathy was originally described in young patients with type 1 diabetes but is now understood to occur more frequently in older adults with type 2 disease. Patients often have no visual complaints or may have nonspecific complaints of "blurred vision" or "distortion" without pain. Vision may be normal or decreased, the finding of an RAPD is variable, and the visual field may demonstrate an enlarged blind spot or a pattern of optic nerve dysfunction. The optic nerve reveals hyperemic edema, but 50% of patients show marked dilation of the disc surface microvasculature (Fig 4-11) that is often mistaken for neovascularization of the disc (NVD). A characteristic radial pattern of the dilated vessels

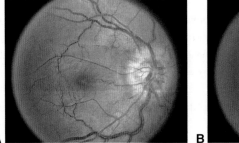 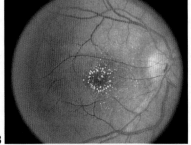

A **B**

Figure 4-10 A 23-year-old man with a 2-day history of blurred vision on the right (visual acuity: 20/40 OD, 20/20 OS). **A,** The optic disc on the right side is elevated and hyperemic, with obscuration of the nerve fiber layer. **B,** 5 weeks after onset, funduscopic examination shows a macular star, characteristic of neuroretinitis. Optic disc edema is now less prominent. *(Courtesy of Steven A. Newman, MD.)*

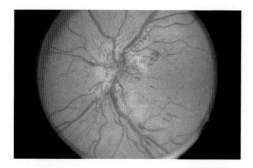

Figure 4-11 Optic disc in diabetic papillopathy shows disc edema with prominent surface telangiectasia. *(Reprinted from Arnold AC. Differential diagnosis of optic disc edema.* Focal Points: Clinical Modules for Ophthalmologists. *San Francisco: American Academy of Ophthalmology; 1999, module 2.)*

may help distinguish diabetic papillopathy from NVD; in the latter, the vessels proliferate into the vitreous cavity and leak into the vitreous on fluorescein angiography. Diabetic retinopathy is present in 63%–80% of patients with diabetic papillopathy and is a contributing factor to diminished visual acuity.

Bilateral diabetic papillopathy warrants investigation to rule out papilledema associated with raised ICP. Untreated, the radial vessels and disc edema resolve slowly over 2–10 months. Optic atrophy occurs in 20% of cases, but the visual prognosis is often related to the degree of accompanying diabetic retinopathy. In rare cases, diabetic papillopathy progresses to AION, with residual pallor and arcuate visual field defects. The pathophysiology is unproven but suspected to be mild, reversible ischemia. Therefore, the distinction of diabetic papillopathy as an entity unique from AION remains controversial. There is no proven therapy for this disorder. Diabetes is discussed in BCSC Section 1, *Update on General Medicine*; associated ocular disorders are discussed in BCSC Section 12, *Retina and Vitreous*.

Arnold AC. Ischemic optic neuropathies. *Ophthalmol Clin North Am.* 2001;14(1):83–98.

Bayraktar Z, Alacali N, Bayraktar S. Diabetic papillopathy in type II diabetic patients. *Retina.* 2002;22(6):752–758.

Regillo CD, Brown GC, Savino PJ, et al. Diabetic papillopathy. Patient characteristics and fundus findings. *Arch Ophthalmol.* 1995;113(7):889–895.

Papillophlebitis

The syndrome of unilateral retinal venous congestion and optic disc edema in healthy young patients was originally termed *papillophlebitis* by Lonn and Hoyt in 1966; it has also been known as *optic disc vasculitis* and *benign retinal vasculitis*. It is a subset of CRVO in the young, in which the disc edema is unusually prominent.

The disorder typically presents with vague visual complaints of blurring, occasionally with transient visual obscurations. Visual acuity is typically normal or is mildly diminished because of macular hemorrhage or edema. An RAPD is absent, color vision is normal, and visual field testing shows enlargement of the blind spot. Fundus examination shows marked retinal venous engorgement associated with hyperemic optic disc edema (Fig 4-12). Retinal hemorrhages extending to the equatorial region are common. Fluorescein angiography typically shows marked retinal venous dilation, staining, and leakage associated with circulatory slowing; regions of capillary occlusion (usually seen

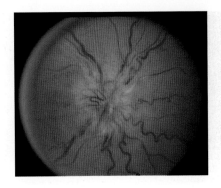

Figure 4-12 Papillophlebitis. Optic disc edema in a 28-year-old woman with engorgement and tortuosity of retinal venous system. Visual acuity is 20/30. *(Reprinted from Kline LB, Foroozan R, eds.* Optic Nerve Disorders. *2nd ed. Ophthalmology Monograph 10. New York: Oxford University Press, in cooperation with the American Academy of Ophthalmology; 2007:218.)*

with ischemic CRVO) are rare. Systemic vasculitis has occasionally been reported, and rheumatologic consultation may be considered. The condition usually resolves spontaneously over 6–12 months, with either no visual loss or only mild impairment related to incompletely resolved maculopathy. For further discussion of CRVO, see BCSC Section 12, *Retina and Vitreous.*

Fong ACO, Schatz H. Central retinal vein occlusion in young adults. *Surv Ophthalmol.* 1993; 37(6):393–417.

Lonn LI, Hoyt WF. Papillophlebitis: a cause of protracted yet benign optic disc edema. *Eye Ear Nose Throat Mon.* 1966;45(10):62–68.

Anterior orbital compressive or infiltrative lesions

Most orbital compressive lesions do not produce optic disc edema, but anterior orbital masses may compress the anterior intraorbital optic nerve and its venous drainage, producing disc edema, sometimes associated with optociliary shunt vessels (retinochoroidal collaterals) and occasionally with full-blown CRVO. Compressive lesions or enlarged extraocular muscles (in thyroid eye disease) at the orbital apex that spare the exiting retinal venous system may or may not result in disc edema but do produce optic nerve dysfunction and eventual atrophy. In all other respects, the clinical syndrome is the same as for other intraorbital and intracanalicular compressive lesions.

Similarly, infiltration of the optic nerve (eg, inflammatory, infectious, neoplastic) most often is a retrobulbar process, but anterior involvement may present with optic disc edema. The optic disc may simply be edematous or display features of superimposed cellular infiltration. Visible prelaminar cellular infiltrate (diffuse or focal) tends to be more opaque, with a grayish or yellowish discoloration (Fig 4-13); the infiltrate may be denser and more opaque than in nonspecific edema. Focal granulomatous infiltration may consist of a focal nodule on the disc surface. When edema and visual loss persist or progress in a way that is atypical for the common causes of optic neuropathy or when prelaminar infiltrate is visible, ancillary testing for an infiltrative lesion should be performed.

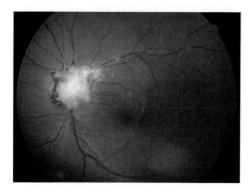

Figure 4-13 Sarcoid optic neuropathy. Left fundus of a 25-year-old man with a 1-month history of blurred vision. Visual acuity was 20/50 and he had a 1.2 log left afferent pupillary defect. The dense white elevation on the disc represents granulomatous inflammation. A chest x-ray showed hilar adenopathy, and bronchoscopy confirmed sarcoidosis. *(Courtesy of Steven A. Newman, MD.)*

Anterior Optic Neuropathies Without Optic Disc Edema

Optic disc drusen

Optic disc drusen (ODD), also known as *hyaline* or *colloid bodies,* are refractile, often calcified nodules located within the optic nerve head (Fig 4-14). Their reported prevalence has ranged from 0.34% (clinical) to 2% (autopsy) of population studies. ODD occur with equal frequency in males and females but rarely affect non-Caucasian people. They are bilateral in 75%–86% of cases but are often asymmetric. Although an irregular dominant inheritance pattern has been described, a significant number of cases are isolated. The pathophysiology of ODD is unproven. Most theories invoke impaired ganglion cell axonal transport, probably related to a small scleral canal and mechanical obstruction. Metabolic abnormalities associated with impaired transport may result in intra-axonal mitochondrial damage, the drusen being products of deteriorating axons. ODD may be associated with retinitis pigmentosa and with pseudoxanthoma elasticum.

Most patients with ODD are asymptomatic, but transient visual obscurations have been reported, with an incidence as high as 8.6%; such obscurations are probably secondary to transient disc ischemia. Visual acuity typically remains normal; decreased visual acuity, especially if progressive, should arouse suspicion of another lesion (eg, an intracranial mass). Visual field loss is present in 75%–87% of cases, most frequently manifested as an enlarged blind spot (60%), arcuate defects (59%), and peripheral depression. Visual field defects either remain stable or very slowly worsen. The location of visible drusen does not necessarily correlate with the location of visual field loss. An RAPD is present in cases with asymmetric visual field loss.

The optic discs of patients with ODD appear elevated and small in diameter, with indistinct or irregular margins and associated anomalous vascular branching patterns. In childhood, ODD tend to be buried, but they become more visible over the years. When visible, ODD appear as round, whitish yellow refractile bodies. They are frequently present at the nasal disc margin, where they may produce a scalloped appearance. Occasionally, they are located within the NFL just adjacent to the disc. These so-called *extruded drusen* may be more common in patients with retinitis pigmentosa. Although disc color

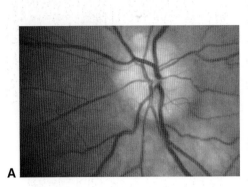

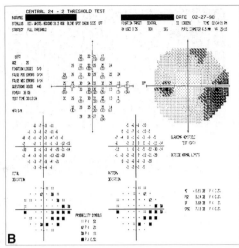

Figure 4-14 **A,** Fundus photograph of optic disc drusen, showing blurred disc margin with scalloped edge, refractile bodies on the disc surface and at the superior pole, mild pallor, and no obscuration or retinal blood vessels. **B,** Visual fields confirmed the presence of an inferior greater than superior arcuate defect on the left produced by drusen involving the left disc. *(Courtesy of Steven A. Newman, MD.)*

tends to be normal with buried drusen, the disc may appear relatively pale with surface drusen. Moreover, ODD may cause optic atrophy or NFL defects (54% of cases).

No treatment is proven to alter the clinical course, but visual impairment is usually mild. In rare cases, vascular complications (eg, flame hemorrhage, nonarteritic anterior ischemic optic neuropathy, or peripapillary subretinal neovascularization) occur.

Optic disc drusen vs papilledema   Buried ODD produce elevation of the disc and blurring of its margins, simulating optic nerve head edema. Major features differentiating ODD include

- lack of hyperemia
- lack of disc surface microvascular abnormalities (capillary dilation, telangiectasia, flame hemorrhage)
- normal or atrophic peripapillary retinal NFL; the retinal vessels at the disc margin are clearly visible (not obscured by NFL edema)
- blurring of the disc margins due to abnormalities at the level of the RPE, such as obscuration by buried drusen, pigment atrophy, and clumping
- anomalous retinal vascular patterns, including loops, increased branchings, and tortuosity

Ancillary testing may be useful in differentiating drusen from papilledema (Fig 4-15):

- *B-scan ultrasonography* may differentiate calcified drusen from papilledema in 2 ways. First, the optic nerve head with ODD is elevated and highly reflective; with a decrease in the sensitivity of the display, calcified drusen maintain this high signal

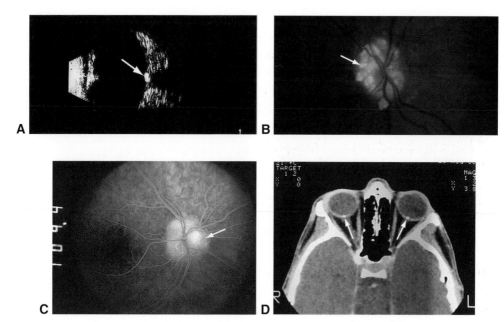

Figure 4-15 Diagnostic testing for optic disc drusen. **A,** B-scan ultrasonography, demonstrating focal, highly reflective (due to calcification) elevation within the optic disc *(arrow)*, which persists when the gain is decreased. **B,** Preinjection fundus photograph demonstrating autofluorescence *(arrow)*. **C,** Late-phase fluorescein angiogram of patient with optic disc drusen shows nodular staining pattern *(arrow)* without dye leakage. **D,** CT scan of the orbits. Calcified optic disc drusen are visible bilaterally at the posterior globe–optic nerve junction *(arrows)*. *(Parts A, C, and D courtesy of Anthony C. Arnold, MD; part B courtesy of Hal Shaw, MD.)*

intensity within the nerve head (Fig 4-15A), whereas with papilledema, the signal intensity decreases along with the remainder of the ocular signal. Ultrasonography may identify drusen in 48%–58% of suspected cases, although the ability of this technique to detect noncalcified buried ODD is unclear. Second, with papilledema, the intraorbital portion of the optic nerve is typically widened and will decrease in width with prolonged lateral gaze (the so-called *30° test*); drusen do not produce widening of the intraorbital nerve.

• *Fluorescein angiography* is also an effective method for distinction. First, certain drusen, if near enough to the disc surface, demonstrate *autofluorescence,* in which refractile bodies are brightly visible on preinjection frames of the angiogram (Fig 4-15B). Second, drusen, even in buried form, typically block fluorescence focally in early frames, with gradual dye uptake producing a nodular late staining without leakage from the disc surface capillaries (Fig 4-15C). Papilledema, in contrast, results in early diffuse hyperfluorescence, with late leakage overlying and adjacent to the disc.

- *Neuroimaging* may be indicated in rare cases to rule out an intracranial or optic nerve tumor and to attempt direct confirmation of calcified drusen. A CT scan remains superior to an MRI scan for detection of drusen; calcium is poorly imaged on an MRI scan but does produce a bright, easily detected signal at the junction of the posterior globe and optic nerve on a CT scan (Fig 4-15D).

With chronic papilledema, refractile bodies occasionally develop on the nerve head surface, simulating ODD (see Fig 4-7). These lesions (probably residual exudate) typically form near the temporal margin of the disc rather than within its substance, are usually smaller than ODD, and disappear with resolution of the papilledema.

Optic disc drusen vs astrocytic hamartomas   Astrocytic hamartomas of the retina, most common in tuberous sclerosis and neurofibromatosis, may take the form of so-called *mulberry lesions*. When located adjacent to the disc, they may closely resemble ODD, and in early reports they were termed *giant drusen of the optic disc* (Fig 4-16). In contrast to true ODD, disc hamartomas

- originate at the disc margin, with extension to the peripapillary retina
- arise in the inner retinal layers and typically obscure retinal vessels
- may have a fleshy, pinkish component
- do not autofluoresce and may show tumorlike vascularity on fluorescein angiography

Auw-Haedrich C, Staubach F, Witschel H. Optic disk drusen. *Surv Ophthalmol.* 2002;47(6): 515–532.

Davis PL, Jay WM. Optic nerve head drusen. *Semin Ophthalmol.* 2003;18(4):222–242.

Giarelli L, Ravalico G, Saviano S, Grandi A. Optic nerve head drusen: histopathological considerations—clinical features. *Metab Pediatr Syst Ophthalmol.* 1990;13(2–4):88–91.

Purvin V, King R, Kawasaki A, Yee R. Anterior ischemic optic neuropathy in eyes with optic disc drusen. *Arch Ophthalmol.* 2004;122(1):48–53.

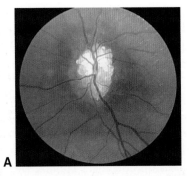 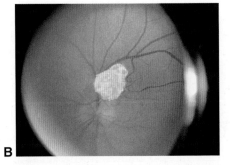

Figure 4-16   Optic disc drusen must be distinguished from astrocytic hamartoma. **A,** Drusen demonstrate prominent refractile nodules on the disc surface, which do not obscure retinal vessels. **B,** Astrocytic hamartomas are nodular masses arising from peripapillary retina and obscure the retinal vessels. *(Reprinted from Arnold AC. Optic disc drusen. Ophthalmol Clin North Am. 1991;4:505–517.)*

Leber hereditary optic neuropathy

Leber hereditary optic neuropathy (LHON) typically affects males age 10–30 years but may occur much later in life; women may account for 10%–20% of cases. The syndrome presents with acute, severe (<20/200), painless, initially monocular visual loss associated with an RAPD and central or cecocentral visual field impairment (Fig 4-17). The classic fundus appearance includes

- hyperemia and elevation of the optic disc and thickening of the peripapillary retina, giving rise to so-called pseudoedema of the disc ("pseudoedema" in this context refers to an optic disc that appears swollen but without leakage on fluorescein angiography)
- peripapillary telangiectasia
- tortuosity of the medium-sized retinal arterioles

These findings may also be present before visual loss begins. However, the fundus may be entirely normal (over 40% in one referral series). Fluorescein angiography demonstrates

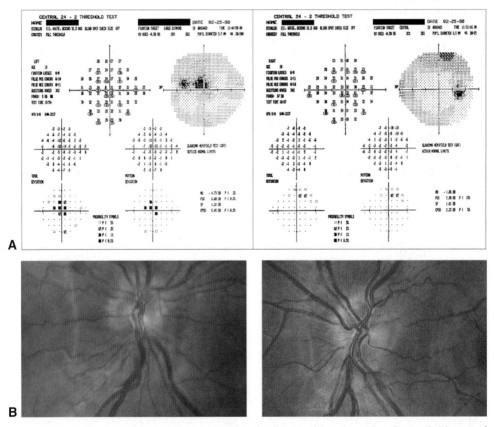

Figure 4-17 Leber hereditary optic neuropathy. A 17-year-old male with a 2-month history of decreased visual acuity in the left eye. **A,** Visual fields show cecocentral scotoma OS. **B,** Fundus photos demonstrate small optic discs with hyperemia and blurred margins. There was no leakage on fluorescein angiography.

no leakage or staining of the disc, in contrast to the appearance of inflammatory optic neuropathies with edema.

The asymptomatic second eye often has subclinical visual field abnormalities that progress rapidly over weeks to months to cecocentral scotomata. The initially involved optic disc becomes atrophic, with loss of peripapillary telangiectasia. In rare cases, the interval between involvement of the 2 eyes is longer (up to 8 years). Although visual loss is usually permanent, partial recovery of vision, up to years after the initial loss, has been reported in 10%–20% of cases.

LHON is related to a mitochondrial DNA mutation, most frequently at the 11778 position, less commonly at the 3460 or 14484 location. The corresponding single base-pair nucleotide substitution results in impaired mitochondrial adenosine triphosphate production, which tends to affect highly energy-dependent tissues (such as the optic nerve). Blood testing for these mutations may confirm the diagnosis, may permit genetic counseling, and may provide information about prognosis; patients with the 14484 mutation have a higher chance (up to 65%) of late spontaneous improvement in central visual function, whereas those with the 11778 mutation have a lower chance (estimated at 4%).

The mutation is transmitted by mitochondrial DNA, which is inherited from the mother, rather than from nuclear DNA. Thus only women transmit the disease. Not all men with affected mitochondria experience visual loss, and affected women only infrequently develop visual symptoms. The reasons for this selective male susceptibility are unclear, as is the precipitating event. At any one time, a variable percentage of DNA is affected (heteroplasmy); only when this fraction becomes high does the disease become clinically evident. Family history may be difficult to elicit, and in a significant number of cases there is a negative family history (suggesting a de novo mutation).

Differential diagnosis includes optic neuritis, compressive optic neuropathy, and infiltrative optic neuropathy. In patients without a positive family history, neuroimaging is advisable to rule out a treatable cause of visual loss. Occasionally, patients demonstrate cardiac conduction abnormalities or other mild neurologic deficits that warrant further evaluation. No treatment has been shown to be effective. Corticosteroids are not beneficial. Coenzyme Q_{10}, succinate, and other antioxidants and agents that may increase mitochondrial energy production have been used, but no definite benefit has been shown. Avoidance of agents such as tobacco or excess ethanol, which might stress such energy production, is recommended, although definitive studies of benefit are lacking.

Newman NJ. Leber's hereditary optic neuropathy: new genetic considerations. *Arch Neurol.* 1993;50(5):540–548.

Newman NJ, Biousse V, Newman SA, et al. Progression of visual field defects in Leber hereditary optic neuropathy: experience of the LHON treatment trial. *Amer J Ophthalmol.* 2006;141(6):1061–1067.

Nikoskelainen E, Hoyt WF, Nummelin K, Schatz H. Fundus findings in Leber's hereditary optic neuroretinopathy. III. Fluorescein angiographic studies. *Arch Ophthalmol.* 1984;102(7): 981–989.

Nikoskelainen EK, Huoponen K, Juvonen V, Lamminen T, Nummelin K, Savontaus ML. Ophthalmologic findings in Leber hereditary optic neuropathy, with special reference to mtDNA mutations. *Ophthalmology.* 1996;103(3):504–514.

Riordan-Eva P, Sanders MD, Govan GG, Sweeney MG, Da Costa J, Harding AE. The clinical features of Leber's hereditary optic neuropathy defined by the presence of a pathogenetic mitochondrial DNA mutation. *Brain.* 1995;118(Pt 2):319–337.

Autosomal dominant optic atrophy

The most common hereditary optic neuropathy (estimated prevalence is 1:50,000), *autosomal dominant optic atrophy (ADOA)* has an autosomal dominant inheritance pattern, but variable penetrance and expression make positive family history inconsistent. Genetic linkage studies have localized an ADOA gene *(OPA1)* to a region on chromosome 3. The OPA1 protein is widely expressed and most abundant in the retina. It encodes dynamin-related GTPase, which is anchored to mitochondrial membranes; thus mutations result in loss of mitochondrial membrane integrity and function, with subsequent retinal ganglion cell degeneration and optic atrophy.

Presentation is usually in the first decade of life, with insidious onset of visual loss, often first detected on routine school vision screenings. Involvement is usually bilateral but may be asymmetric. At detection, visual acuity loss is usually moderate, in the range of 20/50–20/70, although it may decline progressively. The majority of patients preserve vision >20/200. Color vision deficits are invariably present. In this clinical situation, tritanopia is highly suggestive of ADOA; detection of tritanopia usually requires testing by the Farnsworth 100-hue method. However, red-green or generalized defects are common in ADOA as well. Visual field testing demonstrates central or cecocentral loss in most cases, but enlargement of the blind spot with extension to the superotemporal periphery is occasionally mistaken for chiasmal syndromes (Fig 4-18). The defects typically do not respect the vertical midline. Affected optic discs usually show focal temporal optic atrophy but may be diffusely pale. A wedge-shaped temporal excavation may be present and is highly suggestive of ADOA, but its absence does not rule out the diagnosis.

Diagnosis is based on clinical findings and negative results on neuroimaging, which should be performed in all suspected cases. The clinical course is generally one of stability or of very slowly progressive worsening over the patient's lifetime. No treatment is available.

Alexander C, Votruba M, Pesch UE, et al. OPA1, encoding a dynamin-related GTPase, is mutated in autosomal dominant optic atrophy linked to chromosome 3q28. *Nature Genetics.* 2000;26(2):211–215.

Olichon A, Baricault L, Gas N, et al. Loss of OPA1 perturbates the mitochondrial inner membrane structure and integrity, leading to cytochrome c release and apoptosis. *J Biol Chem.* 2003;278(10):7743–7746.

Votruba M, Fitzke FW, Holder GE, Carter A, Bhattacharya SS, Moore AT. Clinical features in affected individuals from 21 pedigrees with dominant optic atrophy. *Arch Ophthalmol.* 1998;116(3):351–358.

Glaucoma

Patients with glaucoma may be completely unaware of impaired vision. Chronic open-angle glaucoma typically produces slowly progressive visual field loss in the arcuate and peripheral regions, sparing fixation until late in the course. The optic disc characteristically appears excavated (increased diameter and depth of the physiologic cup, often with

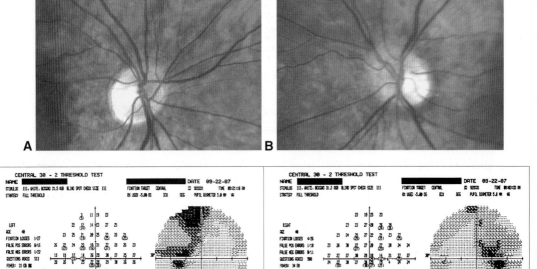

Figure 4-18 Autosomal dominant optic atrophy. 34-year-old man who had been aware of difficulty reading the blackboard in fourth grade, with mild gradual decrease in visual acuity OU since that time. **A, B,** Optic discs show temporal atrophy and papillomacular nerve fiber layer dropout. **C, D,** Visual fields demonstrate bilateral cecocentral scotomata, which extend superotemporally. *(Courtesy of Steven A. Newman, MD.)*

focal notching at the inferior or superior pole). Cup pallor develops only with relatively advanced damage. Intraocular pressure is often (but not invariably) elevated; so-called *normal-tension glaucoma* may be more likely to produce paracentral scotomata closer to fixation, but even this condition usually spares visual acuity. All aspects of glaucoma are discussed at length in BCSC Section 10, *Glaucoma*.

Excavation of the optic nerve head may also be seen in compressive, hereditary (LHON) and severe ischemic (AAION) processes. Compressive lesions are more likely to produce temporal rather than nasal or arcuate visual field loss; LHON usually produces central or cecocentral loss; ischemic damage may result in either pattern. In all of these forms, the optic disc often demonstrates earlier and more prominent pallor, with less severe excavation and notching than in glaucoma (Fig 4-19). Central visual acuity, as well as color vision, is preserved in glaucoma until late in the course, whereas both are usually reduced early in the other optic neuropathies.

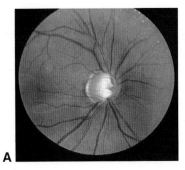 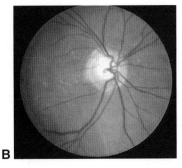

A **B**

Figure 4-19 Optic nerve excavation. **A,** With *glaucomatous* damage, the remaining temporal rim of neuroretinal tissue generally remains a relatively normal pink color despite severe excavation. **B,** With *nonglaucomatous* damage, the rim is pale relative to the degree of excavation. *(Courtesy of Anthony C. Arnold, MD.)*

Congenital optic disc anomalies

Optic nerve hypoplasia The severity of hypoplasia in optic nerve hypoplasia varies widely; patients may be asymptomatic with minimal visual field defect, or they may present with severe visual loss of uncertain duration. Visual field defects are typical for optic nerve damage, with peripheral and arcuate defects common. The prevalence of bilaterality is 56%–92%. The optic disc is small in diameter, usually one half to one third of normal; subtle cases may require a comparison of the 2 eyes. Comparison of horizontal disc diameter to the disc–macula distance may help in detection. Retinal vessel diameter may seem large relative to the disc size, and the vessels may be tortuous. The disc may be pale, gray, or (less commonly) hyperemic and may be surrounded by a yellow peripapillary halo, which in turn is bordered by a ring of increased or decreased pigmentation (the double-ring sign) (Fig 4-20).

Either unilateral or bilateral optic nerve hypoplasia may be associated with midline or hemispheric brain defects, endocrinologic abnormalities (deficiency of growth hormone and other pituitary hormones), and congenital suprasellar tumors. Skull-base defects may be associated with basal encephaloceles. The syndrome of optic nerve hypoplasia, absent septum pellucidum, and pituitary dwarfism (septo-optic dysplasia, de Morsier syndrome) is most common. The corpus callosum may be thinned or absent. An MRI scan is recommended in all cases of optic nerve hypoplasia, and endocrinologic consultation should be

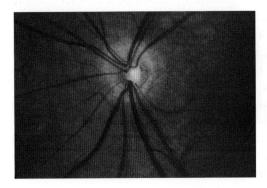

Figure 4-20 Optic disc hypoplasia. The small optic disc is surrounded by a relatively hypopigmented ring of tissue (double-ring sign). The retinal vessels are normal in appearance. *(Reprinted from Kline LB, Foroozan R, eds. Optic Nerve Disorders. 2nd ed. Ophthalmology Monograph 10. New York: Oxford University Press, in cooperation with the American Academy of Ophthalmology; 2007:158.)*

considered, because hypoglycemic seizures or growth retardation may develop without treatment. Recognized teratogens, including quinine, ethanol, and anticonvulsants, have also been associated with optic nerve hypoplasia. A variant of optic nerve hypoplasia, superior segmental hypoplasia, has a corresponding inferior visual field defect; it occurs most often in children of mothers with insulin-dependent diabetes. (For additional discussion, see BCSC Section 6, *Pediatric Ophthalmology and Strabismus*.)

Congenital tilted disc syndrome *Congenital tilted disc syndrome*, a usually bilateral condition (80% of cases), must be differentiated from simple myopic tilted optic discs with temporal crescent. The congenital syndrome also occurs in myopic patients, in whom it also produces an inferonasal crescent (actually a colobomatous excavation of the nerve tissue). The crescent leaves the remaining superotemporal oval portion of the disc relatively intact such that the disc appears tilted off the usual vertical axis and sometimes elevated, simulating mild edema (Fig 4-21). The retinal vessels are often nasalized. The maldeveloped inferior portion is ectatic and is associated with thinning of the inferonasal choroid and RPE, producing a visual field defect that is partially refractive (because the ectasia produces focal change in axial length) and partially neurogenic (because of focally diminished density of the optic nerve axon). The superotemporal visual field defects may mimic those of chiasmal compression but are differentiated by their failure to respect the vertical midline and by their partial improvement with myopic refractive correction. An MRI scan occasionally is indicated to rule out chiasmal

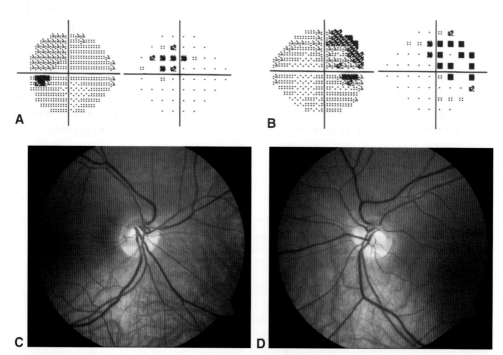

Figure 4-21 Visual fields **(A)** left and **(B)** right show bilateral relative superotemporal defects not respecting the vertical midline. Fundus photos show bilateral tilted discs OD **(C)** and OS **(D)**. *(Parts A, B courtesy of Anthony C. Arnold, MD; parts C, D courtesy of Sophia M. Chung, MD.)*

lesions, even in cases of visible tilted disc syndrome, if visual field defects respect the vertical midline.

Excavated optic disc anomalies   Excavated optic disc anomalies cover a spectrum of severity, ranging from optic pits through colobomas and dysplastic nerves to the morning glory disc anomaly (for additional discussion, see BCSC Section 6, *Pediatric Ophthalmology and Strabismus*):

- An *optic pit* is a depression of the optic disc surface that is often gray or white, located temporally, and associated with a mild visual field defect (usually paracentral or arcuate). Serous detachment of the macula develops in 25%–75% of cases, possibly related to liquid vitreous reaching the subretinal space through communication between the optic pit and the macula.
- *Colobomas* of the nerve result from incomplete closure of the embryonic fissure and usually occur inferiorly, with deep excavation of the optic nerve substance, possibly extending to the adjacent choroid and retina. Visual field defects and RAPD are associated and reflect the degree of abnormality. Colobomas of other structures, such as iris and choroid, may be present.
- The *dysplastic nerve* of papillorenal syndrome or renal coloboma syndrome is characterized by an excavated disc with absence or attenuation of the central retinal vessels and multiple cilioretinal vessels emanating and exiting from the disc edge. Vision is often normal, but visual fields may reflect superonasal visual field defects. Controversy exists as to whether the nerves are colobomatous from incomplete embryonic fissure closure or from a primary dysplasia of the optic nerve. This characteristic optic nerve appearance may reflect renal failure secondary to renal hypoplasia and is linked to mutations in the *PAX2* gene, which is inherited in an autosomal dominant fashion.
- The *morning glory disc anomaly* is a funnel-shaped staphylomatous excavation of the optic nerve and peripapillary retina. It is more common in females and most often unilateral. The disc is enlarged, pink or orange, and either elevated or recessed within the staphyloma. Chorioretinal pigmentation surrounds the excavation, and white glial tissue is present on the central disc surface. The characteristic feature is the emanation of retinal vessels from the periphery of the disc. Visual acuity is often 20/200 or worse, and an RAPD and a visual field defect are present. Nonrhegmatogenous serous retinal detachments occur in 26%–38% of cases. Occult transsphenoidal basal encephaloceles may be present and may be mistaken for nasal polyps; V-shaped infrapapillary depigmentation may be a marker for an encephalocele.

Brodsky MC. Congenital optic disk anomalies. *Surv Ophthalmol.* 1994;39(2):89–112.

Brodsky MC, Hoyt WF, Hoyt CS, Miller NR, Lam BL. Atypical retinochoroidal coloboma in patients with dysplastic optic discs and transsphenoidal encephalocele. *Arch Ophthalmol.* 1995;113(5):624–628.

Parsa CF, Silva ED, Sundin OH, et al. Redefining papillorenal syndrome: an underdiagnosed cause of ocular and renal morbidity. *Ophthalmology.* 2001;108(4):738–749.

Siatkowski RM, Sanchez JC, Andrade R, Alvarez A. The clinical, neuroradiographic, and endocrinologic profile of patients with bilateral optic nerve hypoplasia. *Ophthalmology.* 1997; 104(3):493–496.

Posterior Optic Neuropathies

Retrobulbar optic neuritis

Optic neuritis occurs in young patients (mean age 32), most often female (77%), and presents as subacute monocular visual loss developing over days to weeks. Periorbital pain, particularly with eye movement, occurs in 92% of cases and often precedes visual loss. The retrobulbar form occurs in 65% of cases and is associated with a normal optic disc appearance at onset. An RAPD is present unless the optic neuropathy is bilateral and symmetric. The central visual field is usually affected, with a decrease in visual acuity. However, visual field loss takes the form of an isolated central scotoma less commonly (8% in the ONTT) than it does diffuse loss within the central 30° visual field (48%) or altitudinal visual field loss (15%) (Fig 4-22). Dyschromatopsia is common, particularly for red, and is often more severe than is loss of visual acuity.

Retrobulbar neuritis may be isolated or associated with demyelinating, viral, vasculitic, or granulomatous diseases. Viral infections may involve the optic nerve meninges or parenchyma directly or by delayed immune response (postviral optic neuritis). Such involvement is common in children and is typically bilateral and simultaneous in onset. Demyelinating optic neuritis may be isolated or may be associated with MS (see Chapter 14). Systemic lupus erythematosus and other vasculitides may be associated with optic nerve inflammation, usually without optic disc edema. Finally, granulomatous processes such as syphilis and sarcoidosis (see Fig 4-13) may affect the optic nerves. Although the neuritis in these disorders tends to be associated with other ocular signs of the disease (eg, uveitis, chorioretinitis, retinal periphlebitis), it may occur in isolation.

The differential diagnosis of retrobulbar neuritis includes compressive, infiltrative, or toxic optic neuropathies. Typical optic neuritis begins to show improvement within 1 month; if patients recover most of their vision within 1–3 months, ancillary testing is generally unnecessary for diagnosis. In selected cases—particularly when associated ocular signs (such as retinal vasculitis, chorioretinitis, or uveitis), protracted pain or visual loss, or disc swelling raises the question of specific disease processes requiring treatment—additional hematologic, serologic, and other testing may be of value. In the setting of atypical optic neuritis, such studies may include serum and CSF VDRL and FTA-ABS tests, to rule out syphilis; chest x-ray, gallium scan, serum angiotensin-converting enzyme levels, and skin testing, to exclude sarcoidosis; and ESR, antinuclear antibody testing, and anti-DNA antibody testing, to assess for lupus and other vasculitic diseases.

MRI of the brain is recommended in every case of retrobulbar neuritis. The evaluation for periventricular white matter lesions consistent with demyelination is the single best test for assessing the risk of future MS and to guide subsequent decisions on the use of immunomodulation therapy (see the following section). The 15-year data from the ONTT demonstrate a risk for MS of 25% in patients with zero lesions on MRI versus 72% with at least 1 lesion, with the highest rate of conversion within the first 5 years. Patients with normal MRIs who had not developed MS by year 10 had only a 2% risk of developing the disease by year 15. The overall rate of conversion of all patients to MS is 50% at 15 years (see Chapter 14). Among patients with normal baseline MRIs, male gender, optic disc swelling, and atypical features of optic neuritis (absence of pain, no light perception vision, peripapillary hemorrhages, and retinal exudates) were all associated with a lower risk of future MS.

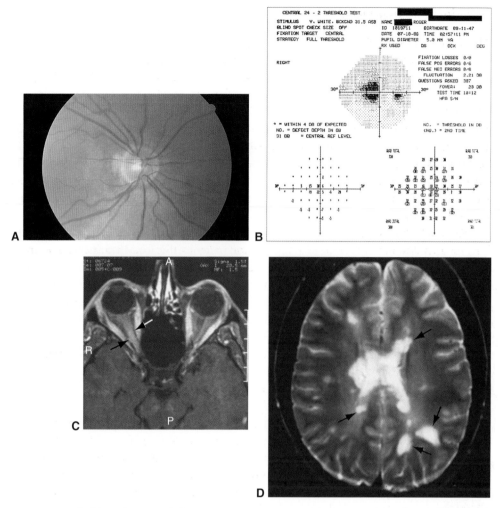

Figure 4-22 **A,** Disc photograph in retrobulbar optic neuritis, showing normal appearance. **B,** A central scotoma is present on automated perimetry. **C,** T1-weighted axial MRI scan of the orbits with fat-suppression and gadolinium administration, showing enhancement of the right intraorbital optic nerve *(arrows)*. **D,** T2-weighted axial MRI scan of the brain, demonstrating multiple white matter hyperintensities *(arrows)* consistent with demyelination. *(Parts A, B courtesy of Steven A. Newman, MD; parts C, D courtesy of Anthony C. Arnold, MD.)*

Visual recovery to a level of 20/40 or better occurs in 92% of patients with optic neuritis. Recovery is unrelated to the presence of pain, the occurrence of optic disc swelling, or the severity of visual loss. After 15 years of follow-up in the ONTT, overall visual acuity was 20/20 or better in 72% of affected eyes, 20/25 to 20/40 in 20% of affected eyes, and worse than 20/200 in 3%. Severe visual loss at onset led to a worse visual prognosis. The 10-year follow-up study reported that optic neuritis recurred in the affected or fellow eye in 35% of cases overall and in 48% of those developing MS. Most eyes with a recurrence regained normal or almost-normal vision. Despite the seemingly excellent prognosis of optic neuritis, patients usually remain aware of visual deficits in the affected eye after recovery. Studies using measures of visual function other than Snellen visual acuity (such as contrast sensitivity, sense of light brightness, stereopsis, visual fields, or color vision) show residual abnormalities in up to 90% of patients with at least 20/30 vision. Patients with MS had statistically significant lower contrast sensitivity and visual field function when compared to those without MS at the 15-year follow-up.

Treatment   The ONTT demonstrated that corticosteroid therapy had no long-term beneficial effect for vision, although the use of intravenous methylprednisolone 250 mg every 6 hours for 3 days, followed by oral prednisone 1 mg/kg/day for 11 days, sped recovery by 1 to 2 weeks. Oral prednisone alone showed no benefit and was associated with an increased recurrence rate double that of the other groups; its use is not recommended. Intravenous therapy also demonstrated a reduction in the rate of development of clinical MS after the initial optic neuritis only in the subgroup of patients with MRI scans showing 2 or more white matter lesions: at 2 years, these patients' risk for MS was 36% untreated, 16% treated. By follow-up year 3 and thereafter, however, this protective effect was lost. With benefits not clear, the value of both therapy and additional diagnostic evaluation for MS must be assessed on an individual basis. In cases in which a rapid return of vision is essential (eg, a monocular patient or an occupational need), intravenous methylprednisolone on an outpatient basis may be considered; otherwise, treatment for visual recovery is not indicated. An MRI scan is generally performed to assess MS risk, but additional evaluation, including CSF analysis and evoked potentials, is probably best deferred to a consulting neurologist. The value of intravenous corticosteroids alone to reduce the long-term risk of MS is unproven.

Immunomodulatory therapy is of proven benefit for reducing morbidity in the relapsing-remitting form of MS, and studies have shown that such agents delay the conversion of patients with acute optic neuritis or other clinical isolated syndrome with high-risk MRI characteristics to definite MS. (See Chapter 14 for a discussion of the treatment of MS.)

Beck RW, Cleary PA, Anderson MM Jr, et al. A randomized, controlled trial of corticosteroids in the treatment of acute optic neuritis. The Optic Neuritis Study Group. *N Engl J Med.* 1992;326(9):581–588.

Beck RW, Cleary PA, Trobe JD, et al. The effect of corticosteroids for acute optic neuritis on the subsequent development of multiple sclerosis. The Optic Neuritis Study Group. *N Engl J Med.* 1993;329(24):1764–1769.

Beck RW, Gal RL, Bhatti MT, et al. Visual function more than 10 years after optic neuritis: experience of the optic neuritis treatment trial. *Am J Ophthalmol.* 2004;137(1):77–83.

The 5-year risk of MS after optic neuritis. Experience of the Optic Neuritis Treatment Trial. Optic Neuritis Study Group. *Neurology.* 1997;49(5):1404–1413.

Ghezzi A, Martinelli V, Torri V, et al. Long-term follow-up of isolated optic neuritis: the risk of developing multiple sclerosis, its outcome, and the prognostic role of paraclinical tests. *J Neurol.* 1999;246(9):770–775.

Optic Neuritis Study Group. Multiple sclerosis risk after optic neuritis: final optic neuritis treatment trial follow-up. *Arch Neurol.* 2008;65(6):727–732.

Optic Neuritis Study Group. Visual function 15 years after optic neuritis: a final follow-up report from the optic neuritis treatment trial. *Ophthalmology.* 2008;115(6):1079–1082.

Neuromyelitis optica

Neuromyelitis optica (NMO), also known as *Devic syndrome,* has been characterized by optic neuritis in association with acute myelitis. However, diverse clinical presentations and conflicting diagnostic criteria have led to confusion about the accuracy of diagnosis. Therefore, the diagnostic criteria have been redefined as the following:

- optic neuritis (unilateral or bilateral)
- myelitis
- plus at least 2 of the following:
  - a contiguous spinal cord lesion on MRI involving 3 vertebral segments or more
  - a brain MRI nondiagnostic for MS
  - a positive NMO-IgG serologic test

Patients may present with neurologic symptoms outside the visual pathways and spinal cords. These criteria provide 99% sensitivity and 90% specificity. The NMO-IgG autoantibody alone has 76% sensitivity and 94% specificity; it binds to aquaporin-4, the principal water channel protein expressed in astroglial foot processes that are involved in fluid homeostasis in the CNS. Both the visual and neurologic prognosis in NMO are poorer than in MS; episodes of visual loss are recurrent, with severe visual impairment (<20/200) common in at least 1 eye in NMO. The treatment of NMO has not been well studied, although immunosuppressive agents such as corticosteroids remain the mainstay of therapy for acute episodes.

Papais-Alvarenga RM, Carellos C, Alvarenga MP, Holander C, Bichara RP, Thuler LC. Clinical course of optic neuritis in patients with relapsing neuromyelitis optica. *Arch Ophthalmol.* 2008;126(1):12–16.

Wingerchuk DM, Lennon VA, Pittock SJ, Lucchinetti CF, Weinshenker BG. Revised diagnostic criteria for neuromyelitis optica. *Neurology.* 2006;66(10):1485–1489.

Optic perineuritis

Distinct from optic neuritis is *optic perineuritis,* or *perioptic neuritis.* Clinically, optic perineuritis may present, as it does in optic neuritis, with acute painful loss of vision, more commonly in women; however, patients are often older (36% >50 yrs), central vision is spared in over 50% of patients, and visual loss can progress over several weeks. With neuroimaging, enhancement involves the dural sheath rather than the optic nerve itself; sometimes the condition may be confused with an optic nerve sheath meningioma. Distinguishing optic perineuritis from optic neuritis is important with respect not only to treatment but also to prognosis as to the development of MS. Patients with optic perineuritis respond immediately and dramatically to corticosteroids, but relapses are common with short courses. Without treatment, patients show progressive visual loss. Optic perineuritis is not associated with an increased risk of demyelinating disease.

Purvin V, Kawasaki A, Jacobson DM. Optic perineuritis: clinical and radiographic features. *Arch Ophthalmol.* 2001;119(9):1299–1306.

Thyroid eye disease

Enlargement of the extraocular muscles in thyroid eye disease (TED) may compress the optic nerve at the orbital apex (Fig 4-23). Patients usually present with associated signs

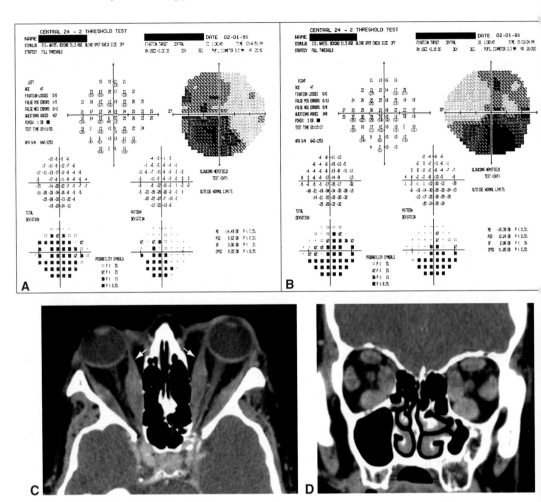

Figure 4-23 Thyroid eye disease in a 48-year-old man with a 6-month history of weakness; gradual swelling around the eyes; and, over the last month, progressively decreased visual acuity. Visual acuity was 20/200 OD, 20/80 OS, with a 0.3 log unit right afferent pupillary defect. **A, B,** Automated perimetry shows bilateral central and inferior visual field loss. Axial **(C)** and coronal **(D)** CT scans show the optic nerve becoming encroached upon by enlarged extraocular muscles. Enlargement of extraocular muscle in thyroid eye disease typically spares the muscle tendon *(arrows). (Parts A, B courtesy of Steven A. Newman, MD; parts C, D courtesy of Sophia M. Chung, MD.)*

(eg, eyelid retraction and lag) and may show signs of orbital congestion (eg, eyelid and conjunctival edema) in addition to proptosis. However, some patients have few of the typical findings.

The visual loss associated with TED is usually slowly progressive, insidious, and most often bilateral. Visual fields show central or diffuse depression, and an RAPD is present when the optic neuropathy is asymmetric. The optic disc is commonly normal but may be edematous. Optic atrophy may be present in more chronic cases.

Management of this optic neuropathy involves decompression of the increased orbital tissue volume. Systemic corticosteroids may be used in the acute phase but are not recommended for long-term use. If symptoms recur on tapering doses, surgical decompression of the orbit is generally performed. Thyroid eye disease is discussed at greater length in Chapter 14 of this volume and in BCSC Section 7, *Orbit, Eyelids, and Lacrimal System.*

Intraorbital/intracanalicular compressive optic neuropathy

Patients with intraorbital or intracanalicular compressive lesions typically present with slowly progressive visual loss, an RAPD, and monocular visual field loss (usually central or diffuse). There may be subtle associated signs of orbital disease such as eyelid edema, retraction, or lag; ptosis; proptosis; or extraocular muscle abnormality. The optic disc may be normal or mildly atrophic at presentation, although anterior orbital lesions may produce optic disc edema. Optociliary shunt vessels (retinochoroidal collaterals) or choroidal folds may also be present. The lesions that most commonly produce optic neuropathy include optic nerve sheath meningioma and glioma. Cavernous hemangioma, although common in the orbit, produces compressive optic neuropathy only occasionally.

If an orbital compressive lesion is suspected, neuroimaging is indicated. Although MRI is best for evaluating soft-tissue abnormalities in the orbit, particularly in differentiating meningioma from glioma, a thin-section CT scan remains a highly satisfactory option and is preferred for evaluation of calcification and bony abnormalities.

Optic nerve sheath meningioma Optic nerve sheath meningioma (ONSM) arises from proliferations of the meningoepithelial cells lining the sheath of the intraorbital or intracanalicular optic nerve (Fig 4-24; see also Chapter 2, Fig 2-7). Although these tumors are uncommon (1%–2% of all meningiomas), they account for one third of primary optic nerve tumors, second only to optic nerve glioma. They are usually detected in adults age 40–50 and affect women 3 times as often as men; 4%–7% of optic nerve sheath meningiomas occur in children. The incidence of neurofibromatosis type 1 in these patients is increased. Patients may present with the classic diagnostic triad:

- painless, slowly progressive monocular visual loss (see Chapter 2, Fig 2-16)
- optic atrophy
- optociliary shunt vessels

Optociliary shunt vessels are distinctive vascular structures, preexisting channels that dilate in response to chronic obstruction of outflow through the central retinal vein. These vessels shunt retinal venous outflow to the choroidal circulation and may be more correctly termed *retinochoroidal collaterals*. They occur in approximately 30% of patients with ONSM but are nonspecific; they are also present in sphenoid wing meningioma, optic glioma, CRVO, and chronic papilledema. Patients also demonstrate an RAPD and an optic nerve–related visual field defect. Minimal to mild proptosis and mild ocular motility defects may also be present. Disc edema may be present, especially if the tumor extends anteriorly. Diagnosis is confirmed by neuroimaging findings (Table 4-5).

Current literature suggests that 3-dimensional, stereotactic, conformal (fractionated) radiation is the treatment of choice for ONSM and has been reported to produce stability or visual improvement in up to 94.3% of patients. However, it remains unclear whether radiation should be administered immediately upon diagnosis or when tumor growth or

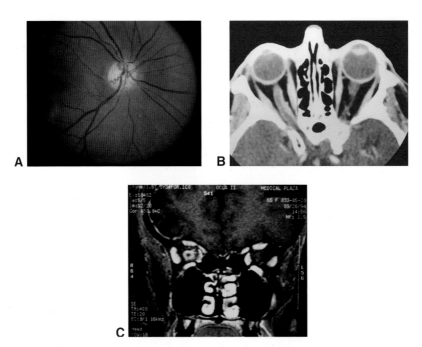

Figure 4-24 A, Fundus photograph shows optic disc atrophy, with optociliary shunt vessels (retinochoroidal collaterals) visible at the 8 and 12 o'clock positions. **B,** CT scan reveals "tram track sign"; diffuse enlargement of the right intraorbital optic nerve extending anteriorly to the globe, with enhancement of the optic nerve sheath. **C,** "Ring sign" in meningioma. Coronal orbital MRI scan shows similar sheath enhancement surrounding relatively normal, darker optic nerve on the right. *(Parts A, C reprinted from Arnold AC. Optic nerve meningioma. Focal Points: Clinical Modules for Ophthalmologists. San Francisco: American Academy of Ophthalmology; 2004, module 7. Part B courtesy of Steven A. Newman, MD.)*

Table 4-5 Neuroradiologic Features of Optic Nerve Sheath Meningioma

Diffuse, tubular enlargement of the optic nerve
Sheath thickening and enhancement, with relative sparing of optic nerve substance ("tram track" or "railroad track" signs)
Apical expansion of the tumor
Extradural tumor extension
Calcification of the nerve sheath on CT scan
Adjacent bony hyperostosis on CT scan
Isointense or mildly hyperintense to brain on T1- and T2-weighted MRI scan
Prominent contrast enhancement on CT and MRI scan

progressive visual loss is documented. Radiation retinopathy and pituitary dysfunction are reported as late radiation complications.

Surgery for biopsy or excision is typically ill-advised because the potential for significant visual loss is considerable. However, if the tumor extends intracranially or, very rarely, across the planum sphenoidale, the risk of contralateral optic nerve extension may warrant surgical excision, particularly in the face of severe visual loss. Observation is considered appropriate by many if there is no change in visual function or tumor size. Optic nerve sheath meningiomas in children may be more aggressive, with more rapid visual loss and more frequent recurrence after therapy. Therefore, children must be monitored with increased frequency and decisions made accordingly.

Andrews DW, Foroozan R, Yang BP, et al. Fractionated stereotactic radiotherapy for the treatment of optic nerve sheath meningiomas: preliminary observations of 33 optic nerves in 30 patients with historical comparison to observation with or without prior surgery. *Neurosurgery.* 2002;51(4):890–904.

Arnold AC. Optic nerve meningioma. *Focal Points. Clinical Modules for Ophthalmologists.* San Francisco: American Academy of Ophthalmology; 2004, module 7.

Dutton JJ. Optic nerve sheath meningiomas. *Surv Ophthalmol.* 1992;37(3):167–183.

Miller NR. New concepts in the diagnosis and management of optic nerve sheath meningioma. *J Neuroophthalmol.* 2006;26(3):200–208.

Turbin RE, Thompson CR, Kennerdell JS, Cockerham KP, Kupersmith MJ. A long-term visual outcome comparison in patients with optic nerve sheath meningioma managed with observation, surgery, radiotherapy, or surgery and radiotherapy. *Ophthalmology.* 2002;109(5): 890–900.

Optic glioma   Although optic gliomas (pilocytic astrocytomas) are generally uncommon (accounting for only about 1% of intracranial tumors), they are the most common primary tumor of the optic nerve. Whether the lesion is a true neoplasm or a hamartoma is controversial. Gliomas involving 1 optic nerve alone are termed *optic nerve glioma;* a lesion that involves the chiasm, with or without involvement of the optic nerves, is termed *optic chiasmal glioma.*

Approximately 70% of optic nerve gliomas are detected during the first decade of life and 90%, by the second; however, they may be seen at any age (Fig 4-25). There is

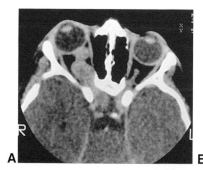

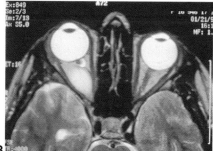

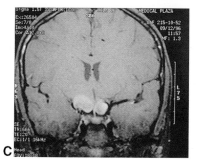

Figure 4-25 A, Axial contrast-enhanced orbital CT scan shows a right optic nerve glioma. The optic nerve is enlarged and kinked and demonstrates mild hypodense cystic change centrally. The tumor extends intracranially. **B,** Axial T2-weighted MRI scan (non–contrast-enhanced) of the orbits shows an enlarged, hyperintense, globular glioma of the right optic nerve. **C,** Coronal T1-weighted MRI scan shows prominent enlargement at the junction of the optic nerves and chiasm.

no definite sex predilection. The most common presenting findings are proptosis (94%), visual loss (87.5%), optic disc pallor (59%), disc edema (35%), and strabismus (27%). Patients infrequently present with asymptomatic isolated optic atrophy. An RAPD is usually present in unilateral or asymmetric cases, along with a typical optic nerve–related visual field defect (if the patient is cooperative enough for visual field testing). Optociliary shunt vessels may be present on the affected disc, although they are seen less commonly than with meningiomas. Diagnosis is confirmed by neuroradiologic findings (Table 4-6).

The relation of optic nerve glioma to neurofibromatosis type 1 (NF1) is incompletely understood. In patients with NF1, the incidence of optic nerve glioma is 7.8%–21%; in patients with optic nerve glioma, the incidence of NF1 is 10%–70%. The wide variance probably relates to referral bias, differences in neuroimaging detection rates, and criteria for diagnosis. Similarly, the relationship between NF1 and the behavior of the glioma is unclear. Several investigators suggest that optic nerve gliomas in patients with NF1 have a more benign prognosis, but this issue is unresolved. Neurofibromatosis is discussed in greater depth in Chapter 14.

As with optic nerve sheath meningiomas, biopsy of the mass is generally not required because

- the advent of high-resolution neuroimaging has raised diagnostic accuracy
- biopsy of the sheath alone may be inaccurate, with reactive meningeal hyperplasia in gliomas falsely suggesting meningioma
- biopsy of the optic nerve substance may produce additional visual loss
- the histopathologic appearance of the tumor is not necessarily predictive of biological behavior

There is no universally accepted management for optic nerve glioma. Observation is indicated for patients with relatively good vision and stable radiographic appearance. Most patients show stability or very slow progression over years and sometimes show spontaneous regression. Chemotherapy is emerging as the first-line treatment when visual loss is severe at presentation or there is evidence of progression. Combination carboplatin and vincristine (Oncovin) is the most accepted regimen, but other chemotherapeutic agents are used. Radiotherapy is controversial because of the inconclusive results and potential complications, including panhypopituitarism and mental retardation. Fractionated stereotactic radiotherapy for optic nerve gliomas was used successfully in one study without the secondary side effects after a median follow-up of 97 months. Surgical excision may

---

Table 4-6 Neuroradiologic Features of Optic Nerve Glioma

Fusiform or globular enlargement of the optic nerve
Thickening of both nerve and sheath by tumor
Kinking or buckling of the optic nerve
Regions of low intensity within the nerve (cystic spaces)
Smooth sheath margins (no extradural extension)
No calcification or hyperostosis on CT scan
Isointense or mildly hypointense to brain on T1-weighted MRI scan
Hyperintense on T2-weighted MRI scan
Variable-contrast (CT scan) and gadolinium (MRI scan) enhancement

be indicated in patients with severe visual loss in association with disfiguring proptosis. Surgery has been advocated to prevent advancement into the chiasm; however, extension to the chiasm is rare.

Gliomas involving the chiasm present with bilateral visual loss and may show bitemporal or bilateral optic nerve–related visual field defects. The optic discs are usually atrophic if visual loss is present but may appear normal or (less commonly) edematous. Involvement of brainstem pathways may produce see-saw nystagmus or a monocular nystagmus suggestive of spasmus nutans. Large tumors may cause obstructive hydrocephalus with elevated ICP, headache, and papilledema. Involvement of the hypothalamus may result in precocious puberty or the diencephalic syndrome.

An MRI scan is preferred to document the extent of the tumor, and that, along with the clinical course, indicates management. The relation of chiasmal glioma to NF1 is unclear, with 14%–60% of patients with chiasmal gliomas showing NF1, and 5.7% of patients with NF1 showing chiasmal gliomas. Occasionally, an exophytic component of the tumor may be surgically excised to relieve external compression on the chiasm, but otherwise surgical excision of the tumor is not indicated. Hydrocephalus may require surgical shunting. Apart from such circumstances, patients are generally observed for evidence of growth, progressive visual loss, or systemic complications from brain involvement; many cases remain stable for years. Radiotherapy is often recommended in these cases, although its efficacy is controversial and side effects (eg, mental retardation, psychiatric disorders, growth retardation, cerebral damage, and secondary tumors) may be severe, especially in children. Chemotherapeutic regimens, including vincristine, actinomycin D (Dactinomycin), nitrosourea agents, carboplatin, and etoposide, have been used with some success and may delay the need for irradiation.

Dutton JJ. Gliomas of the anterior visual pathway. *Surv Ophthalmol.* 1994;38(5):427–452.

Lee AG. Neuroophthalmological management of optic pathway gliomas. *Neurosurg Focus.* 2007; 23(5):E1.

Listernick R, Ferner RE, Liu GT, Gutmann DH. Optic pathway gliomas in neurofibromatosis-1: controversies and recommendations. *Ann Neurol.* 2007;61(3):189–198.

Listernick R, Louis DN, Packer RJ, Gutmann DH. Optic pathway gliomas in children with neurofibromatosis-1: consensus statement from the NF1 Optic Pathway Glioma Task Force. *Ann Neurol.* 1997;41(12):143–149.

Packer RJ, Ater J, Allen J, et al. Carboplatin and vincristine chemotherapy for children with newly diagnosed progressive low-grade gliomas. *J Neurosurg.* 1997;86(5):747–754.

Parsa CF, Hoyt CS, Lesser RL, et al. Spontaneous regression of optic gliomas: thirteen cases documented by serial neuroimaging. *Arch Ophthalmol.* 2001;119(4):516–529.

Malignant astrocytomas are rare neoplasms involving the anterior visual pathway that almost always occur in adulthood, with a mean age in the 60s; they are minimally more common in males (1.3:1). Patients present with acute onset of pain and either unilateral or bilateral visual loss, depending on whether the optic nerve or the chiasm is initially involved. With unilateral lesions, the second eye is invariably involved within weeks. The optic disc may be normal or pale at presentation, but in cases of more anterior tumors, retinal venous occlusive disease and disc edema are common secondary to obstruction of the central retinal vein within the intraorbital optic nerve.

An MRI scan most often shows diffuse intrinsic enlargement and enhancement of the affected optic nerves, chiasm, and optic tracts, with inhomogeneity due to cystic spaces within the tumor. Occasionally, a large exophytic component may encroach on the suprasellar cistern. Histologically, malignant optic nerve gliomas are classified as anaplastic astrocytomas or glioblastoma multiforme.

Visual loss is severe and rapidly progressive. Treatment is rarely successful, although radiotherapy and chemotherapy have been attempted, with blindness usually developing 2–4 months after onset of visual loss. The tumor is aggressively infiltrative, and death from hypothalamic and brainstem involvement usually occurs within 6–12 months.

Dario A, Iadini A, Cerati M, Marra A. Malignant optic glioma of adulthood. Case report and review of the literature. *Acta Neurol Scand.* 1999;100(5):350–353.

Hoyt WF, Meshel LG, Lessell S, Schatz NJ, Suckling RD. Malignant optic glioma of adulthood. *Brain.* 1973;96(1):121–132.

Millar WS, Tartaglino LM, Sergott RC, Friedman DP, Flanders AE. MR of malignant optic glioma of adulthood. *AJNR Am J Neuroradiol.* 1995;16(8):1673–1676.

Toxic/nutritional optic neuropathy

Optic neuropathy resulting from toxic exposure or nutritional deficiency is characterized by gradual, progressive, bilaterally symmetric, painless visual loss affecting central vision and causing central or cecocentral scotomata. At initial presentation, ophthalmic findings may be minimal or subtle. One detectable abnormality may be mild depression of visual sensitivity in the fixation region on Amsler grid testing or on perimetry focused within the central 10°. As the disturbance becomes progressively more severe, however, central visual loss worsens, with a decrease in visual acuity and color vision and a central scotoma on perimetry (Fig 4-26). A more rapid onset of decreased vision may occasionally occur. Optic atrophy eventually develops if the cause is not corrected. The optic discs rarely develop mild to moderate edema. Methanol and ethylene glycol toxicity result in a rapid onset of severe bilateral visual loss with prominent disc edema. Amiodarone (Cordarone) toxicity may present with visual loss and disc edema. It may be differentiated from NAION by its subacute onset, bilaterality, diffuse rather than altitudinal visual field loss, and slow resolution of optic disc edema over months after discontinuance of medication.

Diagnosis requires a careful history for possible medication or other toxic exposure, substance abuse, or dietary deficiency. The most commonly implicated medications include ethambutol, isoniazid, chloramphenicol, hydroxyquinolines, penicillamine, and the antineoplastic agents cisplatin and vincristine. Lead ingestion in children may result in optic neuropathy. Ethanol abuse probably is associated with optic neuropathy in that it may contribute to malnutrition. Dietary deficiencies of vitamin B_{12}, folate, and thiamine may cause optic neuropathy, but exact deficiencies are difficult to pin down in cases of so-called nutritional optic neuropathy. Epidemic nutritional optic neuropathies occurred in World War II and in Cuba in 1992–1993. Tobacco use has long been implicated in patients with optic nerve dysfunction, but the evidence is questionable.

Establishing the diagnosis may be difficult, particularly in patients with vague complaints and little objective abnormality. A careful and detailed dietary history may help, but ethanol abusers may obscure or falsify details of food and ethanol ingestion. Specific

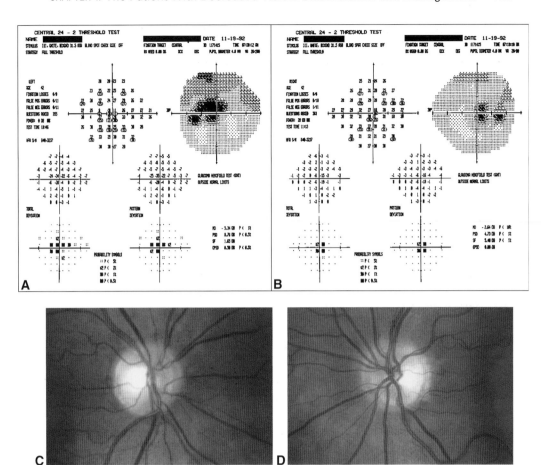

Figure 4-26 Nutritional optic neuropathy in a 42-year-old woman with a history of 4 bowel resections, who presented with bilateral blurred vision and trouble recognizing colors. Visual acuity was 20/70 OD and 20/200 OS, without an afferent pupillary defect. **A, B,** Visual fields demonstrate a cecocentral scotoma on the left and a relative central scotoma on the right. **C, D,** Fundus appearance shows mild temporal optic atrophy OU, with papillomacular nerve fiber layer dropout. After treatment with multivitamins and hydroxycobalamin injections, field defects resolved completely and acuity returned to 20/20. *(Courtesy of Steven A. Newman, MD.)*

vitamin deficiencies are detected only infrequently on blood testing. It may be challenging to implicate a specific medication in elderly patients using multiple medications. Differential diagnosis includes subtle maculopathies and hereditary, compressive, demyelinating, and infiltrative optic neuropathies. Fluorescein angiography, screening hematologic and serologic testing, and (rarely) CSF analysis are performed in questionable cases. Neuroimaging should be routinely performed to rule out a compressive etiology.

Treatment is directed at reversal of the inciting cause: stopping medication or substance abuse and replacement of dietary deficiencies. Prognosis for visual recovery is good if optic atrophy has not supervened, although the optic neuropathy is not invariably reversible. Visual recovery typically is slow, occurring over 3–9 months.

Epidemic optic neuropathy in Cuba: clinical characterization and risk factors. The Cuba Neuropathy Field Investigation Team. *N Engl J Med*. 1995;333(18):1176–1182.

Kumar A, Sandramouli S, Verma L, Tewari HK, Khosla PK. Ocular ethambutol toxicity: is it
reversible? *J Clin Neuro-Ophthalmol*. 1993;13(1):15–17.

Macaluso DC, Shults WT, Fraunfelder FT. Features of amiodarone-induced optic neuropathy.
Am J Ophthalmol. 1999;127(5):610–612.

Rizzo JF III, Lessell S. Tobacco amblyopia. *Am J Ophthalmol*. 1993;116(1):84–87.

Traumatic optic neuropathy

The optic nerve may be damaged by trauma to the head, orbit, or globe. *Direct traumatic optic neuropathy* results from avulsion of the nerve itself or from laceration by bone fragments (Fig 4-27) or other foreign bodies. Injuries may also produce compressive optic neuropathy secondary to intraorbital or intrasheath hemorrhage. *Indirect traumatic optic neuropathy* (without direct nerve trauma) may occur with severe or relatively minor head injury, often frontal, presumably related to shear forces on the nerve and possibly its vascular supply at its intracanalicular tethered point. Indirect trauma is the most common form and is discussed further here. Visual loss is typically immediate and often severe (24%–86% of patients have no light perception at presentation). External evidence of injury may be scarce. An afferent defect is invariably present, although the optic disc usually appears normal at onset and becomes atrophic within 4–8 weeks.

Management of suspected optic nerve injury requires neuroimaging to assess the extent of injury and to detect any associated intracranial and facial injury, intraorbital fragments, or hematoma. Orbital or cranial surgery may be necessary but may not affect the prognosis for the optic nerve. Therapy for indirect traumatic optic neuropathy is controversial. Although the prognosis for visual recovery has generally been regarded as poor, numerous reports describe spontaneous recovery of some visual function in a significant number of cases. Recommended therapies include high-dose intravenous corticosteroids (for both anti-inflammatory and neuroprotective [free radical–scavenging] effects) and transcranial or transethmoidal optic canal decompression. The International

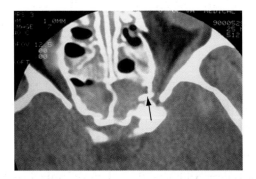

Figure 4-27 CT scan of an 18-year-old involved in a severe motor vehicle accident. He had noted decreased visual acuity on the left side. The CT scan shows fracture in the area of the left optic canal, with a bone fragment *(arrow)* impinging on the left optic nerve. Visual acuity improved following transethmoidal decompression of the canal. *(Courtesy of Steven A. Newman, MD.)*

Optic Nerve Trauma Study, a nonrandomized, multicenter, comparative analysis of treatment outcomes, found no clear benefit for either mode of therapy, and no consensus exists as to their use, either alone or combined.

A recent study of over 10,000 head injury victims compared the benefits of high-dose corticosteroids with placebo within an 8-hour window following trauma. The study was terminated early when the group treated with corticosteroids had a statistically significant higher rate of mortality compared to the placebo group. This raises the question of the safety of high-dose corticosteroids in the treatment of traumatic optic neuropathy, particularly in the setting of significant head trauma. However, one could consider using corticosteroids in an alert, cooperative patient without other contraindications as long as the patient is informed of its unproven benefit. Dosage recommendations vary from 1 g/day up to megadosages (30 mg/kg loading dose). If visual function improves on corticosteroid therapy, conversion to a tapering course of oral therapy after 48 hours can be considered. However, if there is no response, optic canal decompression might be considered.

Carta A, Ferrigno L, Salvo M, Bianchi-Marzoli S, Boschi A, Carta F. Visual prognosis after indirect traumatic optic neuropathy. *J Neurol Neurosurg Psychiatry.* 2003;74(2):246–248.

Cook MW, Levin LA, Joseph MP, Pinczower EF. Traumatic optic neuropathy. A meta-analysis. *Arch Otolaryngol Head Neck Surg.* 1996;122(4):389–392.

Edwards P, Arango M, Balica L, et al; CRASH trial collaborators. Final results of MRC CRASH, a randomised placebo-controlled trial of intravenous corticosteroid in adults with head injury—outcomes at 6 months. *Lancet.* 2005;365:1957–1959.

Lessell S. Indirect optic nerve trauma. *Arch Ophthalmol.* 1989;107(3):382–386.

Levin LA, Beck RW, Joseph MP, Seiff S, Kraker R. The treatment of traumatic optic neuropathy: the International Optic Nerve Trauma Study. *Ophthalmology.* 1999;106(7):1268–1277.

Steinsapir KD, Goldberg RA. Traumatic optic neuropathy. *Surv Ophthalmol.* 1994;38(6):487–518.

Posterior ischemic optic neuropathy

Acute ischemic damage of the retrobulbar portion of the optic nerve is characterized by abrupt, often severe, visual loss; an RAPD; and initially normal-appearing optic discs. *Posterior ischemic optic neuropathy (PION)* is considered rare and is a diagnosis of exclusion. It occurs in 3 distinct settings: perioperative (most commonly seen in spine, cardiac, and head/neck procedures); arteritic, or other vasculitides; and nonarteritic (with risk factors and clinical course similar to those of NAION). Perioperative PION has gained recent scrutiny because of the increasing number of reports that associate it with spinal surgery. In an attempt to identify the risks and thereby reduce the numbers of these cases, the Postoperative Visual Loss (POVL) Registry was started in 1999. In 93 patients who sustained POVL following spinal surgery, 83 had ischemic optic neuropathy, and 56 of these 83 (67%) had PION. Risk factors included being in the prone position during surgery, significant loss of blood (>1.0 L, median 2.0 L), and a long anesthesia time (>6 hours). Visual loss in perioperative PION is more commonly bilateral and profound. Without a history of previous surgery or trauma with significant hypovolemia, hypotension, or blood loss, a careful search for symptoms and laboratory evidence of GCA should be pursued. High-dose corticosteroid treatment is indicated for cases of proven GCA. Prognosis for visual recovery in PION is poor.

Buono LM, Foroozan R. Perioperative posterior ischemic optic neuropathy; review of the literature. *Surv Ophthalmol.* 2005;50(1):15–26.

Johnson MW, Kincaid MC, Trobe JD. Bilateral retrobulbar optic nerve infarctions after blood loss and hypotension. A clinicopathologic case study. *Ophthalmology.* 1987;94(12):1577–1584.

Lee LA, Roth S, Posner KL, et al. The American Society of Anesthesiologists Postoperative Visual Loss Registry: analysis of 93 spine surgery cases with postoperative visual loss. *Anesthesiology.* 2006;105(4):652–659.

Sadda SR, Nee M, Miller NR, Biousse V, Newman NJ, Kouzis A. Clinical spectrum of posterior ischemic optic neuropathy. *Am J Ophthalmol.* 2001;132(5):743–750.

Infiltrative optic neuropathy

Infiltration of the optic nerve by neoplastic or inflammatory cells results in progressive, often severe, visual loss. This visual failure progresses over days to weeks, either with or without other cranial nerve involvement, and is often associated with headache. Optic nerve involvement may be the presenting sign of systemic disease and may be unilateral or bilateral. With retrobulbar infiltration, the optic nerve head may appear normal initially; indeed, the combination of severe progressive visual loss and a normal disc appearance should raise the question of optic nerve infiltration. If the optic disc is affected, the cellular infiltrate creates a swollen appearance distinct from that of simple edema. The most common causes of infiltration include chiasmal and/or optic nerve glioma, leukemia, lymphoma, and granulomatous inflammation such as sarcoidosis, syphilis, tuberculosis, and fungal infections. Metastasis to the optic nerve is rare, usually occurring from breast or lung carcinoma. Carcinomatous infiltration of the meninges at the skull base may result in progressive involvement and dysfunction of multiple cranial nerves, including the optic nerves, which are affected in 15%–40% of cases. Onset may precede, coincide with, or follow diagnosis of the underlying malignancy.

Evaluation of cases of suspected infiltrative optic neuropathy should include neuroimaging (to rule out compressive lesions and to confirm parenchymal or meningeal infiltration), CSF analysis (for neoplastic or inflammatory cells or elevated protein), and screening tests for the myeloproliferative, inflammatory, and infectious disorders noted earlier. MRI of the brain and orbits (including the fat-suppression technique and intravenous gadolinium administration) is necessary to properly demonstrate optic nerve infiltration. MRI may show diffuse thickening and enhancement of the dura and the surrounding subarachnoid space in affected regions, including the optic nerve sheaths; however, abnormalities may not be visible in the early stages. Similarly, CSF analysis may reveal malignant cells and elevated protein but a single spinal tap may also be normal. Repeat testing is often necessary. Correct diagnosis is essential for the following reasons:

- Identification of the associated malignancy or systemic disease may be life-saving.
- In malignancies, palliative radiation therapy may significantly improve vision, even though the long-term prognosis is poor. Median survival for meningeal carcinomatosis ranges from 4 to 9 weeks, even with aggressive therapy; only a few patients survive past 1 year.
- In infectious or inflammatory disorders, antimicrobial or corticosteroid therapy may partially reverse damage resulting from infiltration and stabilize the systemic condition.

Grossman SA, Krabak MJ. Leptomeningeal carcinomatosis. *Cancer Treat Rev.* 1999;25(2): 103–119.

Mack HG, Jakobiec FA. Isolated metastases to the retina or optic nerve. *Int Ophthalmol Clin.* 1997;37(4):251–260.

Millar MJ, Tumuluri K, Murali R, Ng T, Beaumont P, Maloof A. Bilateral primary optic nerve lymphoma. *Ophthal Plast Reconstr Surg.* 2008;24(1):71–73.

Shields JA, Shields CL, Singh AD. Metastatic neoplasm in the optic disc: the 1999 Bjerrum Lecture. *Arch Ophthalmol.* 2000;118(2):217–224.

Yeung SN, Paton KE, Dorovini-Zis K, Chew JB, White VA. Histopathologic features of multiple myeloma involving the optic nerves. *J Neuroophthalmol.* 2008;28(1):12–16.

Optic Atrophy

The combination of visual loss, an RAPD, and optic atrophy is nonspecific and might represent the chronic phase of any of the optic neuropathies described earlier. When historical features and clinical signs do not suggest a specific cause, baseline studies of optic nerve function and a screening workup for treatable causes are usually undertaken. The level of optic nerve function is established by visual acuity, color vision testing, and quantitative perimetry. The degree and pattern of atrophy are documented by fundus photography, preferably in stereoscopic views, to detect subtle changes in contour over time. The role of optical coherence tomography in the evaluation and follow-up of optic atrophy is under investigation.

Neuroimaging, preferably MRI of the brain and orbits with gadolinium and fat suppression, is warranted in any case without a clear cause. In a study of 98 adult patients with isolated optic atrophy, 20% were discovered to harbor compressive lesions. There was little yield in screening for syphilis, vitamin B_{12} deficiency, folate deficiency, vasculitis, sarcoidosis, and heavy metal toxicity without a history or examination suggestive of these specific diseases. Laboratory evaluation, however, should be pursued in the appropriate clinical setting or if the history warrants it. If initial results are negative, observation is appropriate. However, if the condition worsens or new findings develop, reassessment of the initial testing or additional testing is necessary.

Lee AG, Chau FY, Golnik KC, Kardon RH, Wall M. The diagnostic yield of the evaluation for isolated unexplained optic atrophy. *Ophthalmology.* 2005;112(5):757–759.

Chiasmal Lesions

With segregation of nasal and temporal retinal fibers at the chiasm, visual field loss due to chiasmal and retrochiasmal lesions produce defects that align along the vertical meridian. The classic field abnormality associated with optic chiasmal disorders is a bitemporal hemianopia.

Bitemporal Visual Field Loss Patterns

Anterior chiasm

Lesions that injure 1 optic nerve at its junction with the optic chiasm produce the anterior chiasmal syndrome. Diminished visual acuity and central visual field loss in 1 eye accompany a superotemporal defect in the opposite eye as a result of damage to 1 optic nerve combined with early compression of the optic chiasm (the "junctional syndrome," referring to the junction of the optic nerve and chiasm) (Fig 4-28). The correlation of

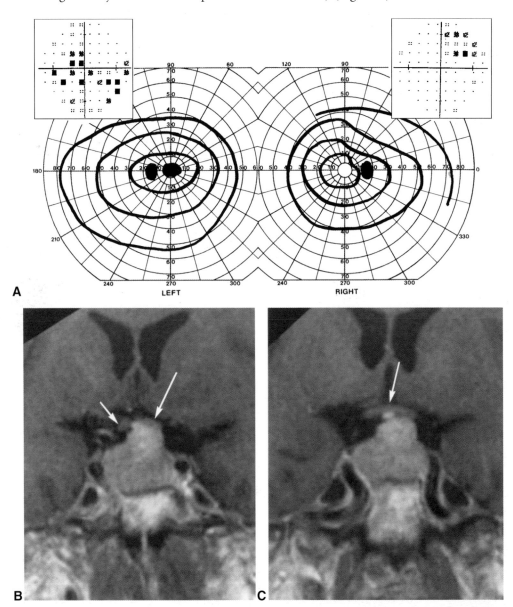

Figure 4-28 **A,** Visual fields from the Goldmann perimeter and the Humphrey 30-2 program *(insets).* Note the central scotoma in the patient's left eye along with the superotemporal depression in his right eye. **B, C,** Postcontrast, T1-weighted (TR = 650 msec, TE = 14 msec) MRI scans using a slice thickness of 3 mm. **B,** Coronal image of a section in front of the optic chiasm showing a tumor compressing the prechiasmic segment of the left optic nerve *(long arrow)* but not the right optic nerve *(short arrow).* **C,** Coronal image at the level of the optic chiasm showing minimal rostral displacement *(arrow)* but no notable direct mass effect. *(Reprinted with permission from Karanjia N, Jacobson DM. Compression of the prechiasmal optic nerve produces a junctional scotoma. Am J Ophthalmol. 1999;128(2):256–258. © 1999 Elsevier Inc.)*

this clinical syndrome with the so-called Wilbrand knee (a looping forward of crossing fibers into the contralateral optic nerve) is uncertain. In rare cases, a mass may compress the crossing (nasal) fibers of the intracranial optic nerve at the anterior chiasm, causing a temporal hemianopia that respects the vertical midline, with no involvement of the visual field in the opposite eye.

Mid chiasm

Lesions damaging the body of the chiasm produce a relative or absolute bitemporal hemianopia. Acuity may or may not be affected (Fig 4-29).

Posterior chiasm

Lesions at the posterior chiasm may compress only the crossing fibers derived from the macular region, producing a central bitemporal hemianopia respecting the vertical meridian.

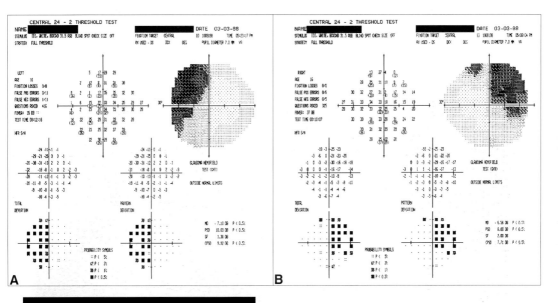

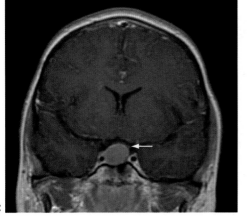

Figure 4-29 A, B, Visual fields in a patient with a pituitary tumor, showing bitemporal depression worse superiorly, with margination along the vertical midline. **C,** A T1-weighted coronal MRI scan shows an intrasellar enhancing mass, with extension into the suprasellar cistern and upward displacement and compression of the chiasm *(arrow)*. *(Parts A, B courtesy of Steven A. Newman, MD; part C courtesy of Sophia M. Chung, MD.)*

Horton JC. Wilbrand's knee of the primate optic chiasm is an artifact of monocular enucleation. *Trans Am Ophthalmol Soc.* 1997;95:579–609.

Parasellar Lesions Affecting the Chiasm

Parasellar lesions that involve the chiasm—whether compressing or infiltrating this area—produce gradually progressive, bilateral, often asymmetric visual loss. The peripheral (temporal) visual fields usually are involved first. In any case of bilateral visual field loss, the clinician must carefully evaluate perimetry for respect of the vertical midline, particularly if the depression is located superiorly. Any of the variations on bitemporal visual field loss described in the preceding discussion may occur. An affected optic nerve may produce more central loss, with impaired visual acuity, dyschromatopsia, and an RAPD on the affected side. Markedly asymmetric visual field loss without direct optic nerve damage may also produce an RAPD.

In chiasmal syndromes, the optic discs may show no visible abnormalities initially, even in the face of significant visual field loss. More commonly, there is subtle evidence of optic neuropathy, such as peripapillary retinal NFL dropout and mild disc pallor. With more damage, the optic discs show typical atrophy, often in the temporal portion of the disc corresponding to the papillomacular bundle of retinal nerve fibers and the nasal fibers (resulting in band atrophy). Cupping of the disc may increase. Most tumors that produce a chiasmal syndrome do not cause increased ICP and thus are not associated with papilledema.

The most common lesions producing the chiasmal syndrome include pituitary adenoma (see Fig 4-29), parasellar meningioma, craniopharyngioma (Fig 4-30), parasellar internal carotid artery aneurysm, and chiasmal glioma. Other, infrequent causes include inflammation (sarcoidosis, MS), frontal trauma with chiasmal contusion, and other CNS mass lesions that produce third-ventricle dilation and secondary posterior chiasmal compression.

Pituitary adenomas are the most common cause of chiasmal compression and may occur at any adult age; they are rare in childhood. These nonsecreting tumors typically present with visual loss, having reached a relatively large size without other symptoms; hormonally active tumors, however, are often detected prior to visual loss because of systemic symptoms related to hypersecretion. Prolactin-secreting tumors in males are the exception to this rule because the resultant decreased libido and impotence are not often reported early. Pituitary tumors may enlarge during pregnancy and produce chiasmal compression. Acute hemorrhage or infarction of the pituitary tumor, known as *pituitary apoplexy,* is a potentially life-threatening event heralded by severe headache, nausea, and altered consciousness and is often accompanied by diplopia and loss of vision or visual field (Fig 4-31). Sudden expansion of the tumor into the adjacent cavernous sinuses may cause compression of CNs III, IV, V, and VI, with CN III most commonly affected. Superior extension causes visual field loss but also may cause central visual loss to no light perception. Extravasation of blood into the subarachnoid space causes numerous symptoms, including a decreased level of consciousness and vasospasm with secondary stroke. The acute endocrine abnormalities may lead to numerous complications, including adrenal crisis. Therefore, the recognition of pituitary apoplexy is critical in efforts to initiate treatment emergently. Treatment includes immediate institution of corticosteroids, surgical decompression of

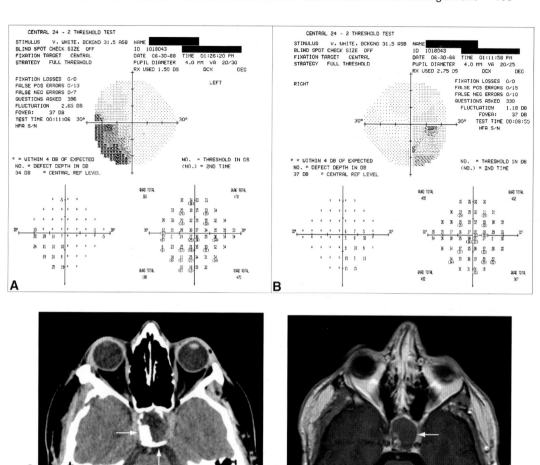

Figure 4-30 Patient with craniopharyngioma involving the suprasellar cistern, with compression of the chiasm from above. **A, B,** Visual fields show bilateral inferotemporal depression respecting the vertical midline. **C,** Axial CT scan without contrast shows cystic mass with peripheral calcification *(arrows)* within the suprasellar cistern. **D,** Axial MRI with contrast shows the same cystic mass *(arrow)*. *(Parts A, B courtesy of Steven A. Newman, MD; parts C, D courtesy of Sophia M. Chung, MD.)*

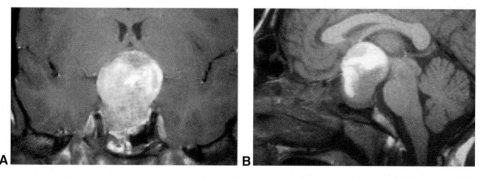

Figure 4-31 Acute compressive optic neuropathy in pituitary apoplexy. Coronal **(A)** and sagittal **(B)** MRI scans show a large pituitary tumor with suprasellar extension. Inhomogeneity within the tumor represents hemorrhage and infarction. *(Courtesy of Steven A. Newman, MD.)*

the sella, and appropriate supportive measures. Some authorities recommend conservative management in the setting of absent or mild neuro-ophthalmic signs.

Parasellar meningiomas occur most often in middle-aged females; arise most frequently from the tuberculum sella, planum sphenoidale, or clinoids; and often produce asymmetric bitemporal visual loss. Parasellar meningiomas may also enlarge and produce chiasmal compression during pregnancy.

Craniopharyngiomas are common in children but may present at any age, with a second incidence peak in adulthood. Often arising superiorly, these tumors more frequently produce *inferior* bitemporal visual field loss (see Fig 4-30), especially if the chiasm is relatively anteriorly placed ("prefixed").

Internal carotid artery aneurysms, particularly in the supraclinoid region, may produce a markedly asymmetric chiasmal syndrome, with optic nerve compression on the side of the aneurysm.

Chiasmal gliomas (described in detail earlier) are detected most often in children. They usually infiltrate affected structures and thus produce complex visual field abnormalities not limited to the crossing fibers. There may be evidence of bilateral optic nerve–related visual field defects, possibly worse in the temporal visual fields but often more diffuse and not aligned along the vertical midline. Chiasmal gliomas are also almost always accompanied by decreased central visual acuity.

Therapy of parasellar tumors is complex and depends on the age of the patient; the nature, location, and extent of the tumor; its hormonal activity; and the severity of symptoms. Modalities include observation only, surgery (transfrontal or transsphenoidal), medical therapy (primarily bromocriptine or cabergoline for prolactin-secreting pituitary tumors), and irradiation (either primary or as adjunctive therapy for incompletely resectable tumors). Visual recovery after surgical resection of the tumor and relief of anterior visual pathway compression is usually rapid (onset of improvement is within 24 hours) and may be dramatic, even with severe visual loss. Medical therapy for pituitary adenomas has a slower effect, taking days to weeks, but also produces tumor shrinkage and improved visual function in responsive cases. The ophthalmologist's role in the management of parasellar tumors is critical, in that the first sign of recurrence may be visual loss. Baseline visual field and visual acuity testing should be performed 2–3 months after treatment and at intervals of 6–12 months thereafter, depending on the course. Visual acuity and visual fields should be rechecked more often (immediately if necessary) if the patient feels any ongoing change. Periodic neuroimaging is essential.

Delayed visual loss following therapy for parasellar lesions should prompt the following considerations:

- tumor recurrence
- delayed radionecrosis of the chiasm or optic nerves
- chiasmal distortion due to adhesions or secondary empty sella syndrome, with descent and traction on the chiasm
- chiasmal compression from expansion of intraoperative overpacking of the sella with fat

Neuroimaging effectively differentiates among these entities and guides further management decisions.

Bianchi-Marzoli S, Rizzo JF III, Brancato R, Lessell S. Quantitative analysis of optic disc cupping in compressive optic neuropathy. *Ophthalmology.* 1995;102(3):436–440.

Chicani CF, Miller NR. Visual outcome in surgically treated suprasellar meningiomas. *J Neuroophthalmol.* 2003;23(1):3–10.

McCord MW, Buatti JM, Fennell EM, et al. Radiotherapy for pituitary adenoma: long-term outcome and sequelae. *Int J Radiat Oncol Biol Phys.* 1997;39(2):437–444.

Peter M, De Tribolet N. Visual outcome after transsphenoidal surgery for pituitary adenomas. *Br J Neurosurg.* 1995;9(2):151–157.

Verrees M, Arafah BM, Selman WR. Pituitary tumor apoplexy: characteristics, treatment, and outcomes. *Neurosurg Focus.* 2004;16(4):E6.

Retrochiasmal Lesions

As the fibers course in the retrochiasmal visual pathway (optic tract; lateral geniculate body; and temporal, parietal, and occipital lobe visual radiations), crossed nasal fibers from the contralateral eye and uncrossed temporal fibers from the ipsilateral eye are located together (see Chapter 1). Damage results in homonymous visual field defects that continue to respect the vertical midline. As fibers progress from the anterior to the posterior visual pathway, those from corresponding retinal regions of each eye tend to run closer and closer together. Historically, authorities have believed that anterior lesions produce dissimilar *(incongruous)* defects in the corresponding homonymous hemifields, whereas more posterior damage results in progressively more similar *(congruous)* defects as lesions approach the occipital lobes. However, this "rule" of congruity has been called into question recently. As many as 59% of optic radiation lesions and 50% of optic tract lesions were shown to cause congruent homonymous hemianopia in a series of 538 patients. Therefore, although one might reliably predict that a highly congruous homonymous hemianopia reflects occipital disease, it does not rule out the possibility of lesions anterior to the occiput. Lesions severe enough to produce complete hemianopic defects may occur at any anteroposterior retrochiasmal location; such defects do not help to localize lesions from the chiasm through the occipital cortex.

Stroke is the most common cause of homonymous hemianopias, followed by traumatic brain injury and tumor.

Kedar S, Zhang X, Lynn MJ, Newman NJ, Biousse V. Congruency in homonymous hemianopia. *Am J Ophthalmol.* 2007;143(5):772–780.

Zhang X, Kedar S, Lynn MJ, Newman NJ, Biousse V. Homonymous hemianopias: clinical-anatomic correlations in 904 cases. *Neurology.* 2006;66(6):906–910.

Optic Tract

Lesions of the optic tract tend to produce incongruous homonymous defects in the hemifields contralateral to the affected optic tract (Fig 4-32). Damage to the optic tract most commonly results from mass lesions; aneurysms are a relatively common etiology in this location. Inflammatory lesions occur occasionally. Ischemic lesions of the tract are uncommon but sometimes follow surgical disruption of the anterior choroidal artery. Because the fibers involved are primary neurons in the visual pathway (retinal ganglion cells), the

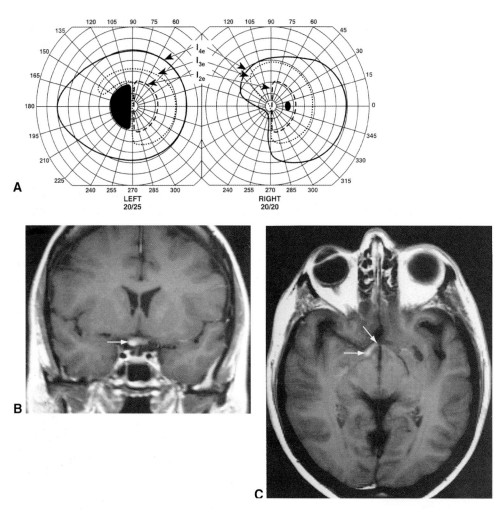

Figure 4-32 Chiasmal neuritis. A 40-year-old woman with sudden onset of visual field defect in the left eye. Visual acuity is 20/20 OD, 20/25 OS. Pupils, color vision, and fundi were normal. **A,** Visual field testing revealed an incongruous left homonymous hemianopia. A gadolinium-enhanced T1-weighted MRI scan revealed **(B)** enhancement and swelling *(arrow)* of the right side of the chiasm and **(C)** enhancement of the right optic tract *(arrows)*. *(Reprinted from Kline LB, Foroozan R, eds. Optic Nerve Disorders. 2nd ed. Ophthalmology Monograph 10. New York: Oxford University Press, in cooperation with the American Academy of Ophthalmology; 2007:75.)*

incongruous homonymous hemianopic visual field loss is accompanied by other findings that make up the *optic tract syndrome:*

- *Homonymous retinal NFL and optic disc atrophy.* Because the optic tract involves crossed fibers from the contralateral eye, the corresponding atrophy of crossed retinal fibers (those nasal to the macula) involves the papillomacular fibers and the nasal radiating fibers in the contralateral eye, producing atrophy in the corresponding nasal and temporal horizontal portions of the disc ("band" or "bow-tie" atrophy) (see Chapter 1, Fig 1-18). Atrophy in the ipsilateral eye involves only the arcuate temporal bundles, which enter the disc at the superior and inferior poles.

- *Mild RAPD in the contralateral eye.* This finding results when there are more crossed than uncrossed pupillary fibers in the tract, causing more pupillary fibers from the contralateral eye to be damaged by a tract lesion.

Newman SA, Miller NR. Optic tract syndrome: neuro-ophthalmologic considerations. *Arch Ophthalmol.* 1983;101(8):1241–1250.

Savino PJ, Paris M, Schatz NJ, Orr LS, Corbett JJ. Optic tract syndrome. A review of 21 patients. *Arch Ophthalmol.* 1978;96(4):656–663.

Lateral Geniculate Body

The *lateral geniculate body (LGB)* is a highly organized and layered retinotopic structure; lesions therefore can give highly localizing visual field defects. A very congruous horizontal sectoranopia results from damage in the distribution of the posterolateral choroidal artery, a branch of the posterior cerebral artery. Loss of the upper and lower homonymous quadrants (also called "quadruple sectoranopia") with preservation of a horizontal wedge occurs when the anterior choroidal artery, a branch off the middle cerebral artery, is disrupted (Fig 4-33; see Chapter 1, Fig 1-11). These visual field defects respect the vertical meridian, unlike the uncommon wedge defect seen in glaucoma. Very incongruous

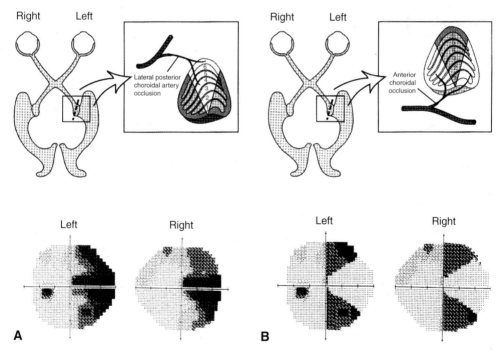

Figure 4-33 Visual field defects of the lateral geniculate body. Automated visual fields show **(A)** a central wedge-shaped homonymous sectoranopia caused by lateral posterior choroidal artery occlusion and **(B)** a loss of the upper and lower homonymous quadrants, with preservation of the horizontal wedge resulting from occlusion of the anterior choroidal artery. *(Reproduced with permission from Trobe JD. The Neurology of Vision. Contemporary Neurology Series. Oxford: Oxford University Press, 2001:130.)*

homonymous hemianopias also occur with lesions of the LGB. Sectoral optic atrophy occurs with LGB lesions, and, in rare cases, bilateral LGB lesions cause blindness.

Borruat FX, Maeder P. Sectoranopia after head trauma: evidence of lateral geniculate body lesion on MRI. *Neurology.* 1995;45(3 Pt 1):590–592.

Frisén L. Quadruple sectoranopia and sectorial optic atrophy: a syndrome of the distal anterior choroidal artery. *J Neurol Neurosurg Psychiatry.* 1979;42(7):590–594.

Frisén L, Holmegaard L, Rosencrantz M. Sectorial optic atrophy and homonymous, horizontal sectoranopia: a lateral choroidal artery syndrome? *J Neurol Neurosurg Psychiatry.* 1978;41(4):374–380.

Luco C, Hoppe A, Schweitzer M, Vicuña X, Fantin A. Visual field defects in vascular lesions of the lateral geniculate body. *J Neurol Neurosurg Psychiatry.* 1992;55(1):12–15.

Temporal Lobe

Inferior visual fibers course from the LGB anteriorly in the *Meyer loop* of the temporal lobe (approximately 2.5 cm from the anterior tip of the temporal lobe). Superior fibers tend to course more directly posteriorly in the parietal lobe. Lesions affecting the Meyer loop thus produce superior, incongruous, homonymous quadrantanopic defects contralateral to the lesion, which spare fixation (so-called *pie in the sky* defects) (Fig 4-34). Damage to the temporal lobe anterior to the Meyer loop does not cause visual field loss. Lesions affecting the radiations posterior to the loop produce homonymous hemianopic defects extending inferiorly.

Tumors within the temporal lobe are a common cause of visual field loss (see Chapter 3, Fig 3-7). Although the pattern of loss may be characteristic as noted, larger tumors may lead to a homonymous loss, and associated neurologic findings may be the only clue as to tumor location. Such findings may include seizure activity, including olfactory, and formed visual hallucinations. Surgical excision of seizure foci in the temporal lobes may lead to visual field defects.

Parietal Lobe

Lesions of the parietal lobe tend to involve superior fibers first, resulting in contralateral inferior homonymous hemianopic defects. More extensive lesions involve the superior visual fields but remain denser inferiorly. Lesions in the parietal lobe usually are due to stroke. Parietal lobe syndromes encompass a wide variety of other neurologic complaints, including perceptual problems (agnosia) and apraxia. Lesions of the dominant parietal lobe cause Gerstmann syndrome, a combination of acalculia, agraphia, finger agnosia, and left-right confusion.

Damage to pursuit pathways that converge in the posterior parietal lobes (near the visual radiations) may cause abnormalities in optokinetic nystagmus (OKN). The examiner elicits the impaired OKN response by moving targets toward the lesion, inducing attempts to use the damaged pursuit pathway. Thus, a patient with a homonymous hemianopia due to a parietal lobe lesion will have a reduced OKN response with the target moving toward the affected side, whereas a homonymous hemianopia due to a lesion of the optic tract or occipital lobe will have an intact OKN response.

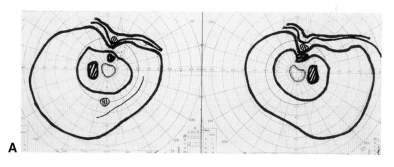

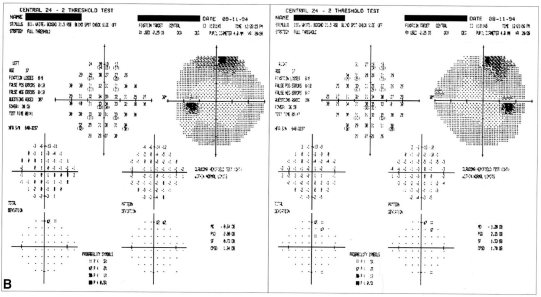

Figure 4-34 Visual fields after partial left temporal lobectomy for seizure disorder. **A,** Goldmann visual fields show a predominantly peripheral right superior homonymous quadrantanopia sparing fixation. **B,** Humphrey central 30° perimetry detects a minimal portion of the field defects. *(Courtesy of Steven A. Newman, MD.)*

This response was once thought to indicate a mass lesion rather than a vascular lesion but is more likely related to the extent of the lesion. Asymmetry in the pursuit system likely indicates involvement of area V5 or MT. Homonymous hemianopia should prompt OKN testing; only rarely do occipital lobe lesions cause such abnormalities.

Occipital Lobe

As fibers approach the occipital lobes, congruity becomes more important. Central fibers become separate from peripheral fibers, the former coursing to the occipital tip, the latter to the anteromedial cortex. Because of the disparity in crossed versus uncrossed fibers, some of the peripheral nasal fibers leading to the anteromedial region are not matched with corresponding uncrossed fibers; they subserve a monocular "temporal crescent" of visual field in the far periphery (60°–90°). Finally, fibers localize within the occipital cortex superior and inferior to the calcarine fissure. Thus, visual field defects from occipital lobe lesions may have the following characteristics in the hemifields contralateral to the lesion:

- congruous homonymous hemianopia, possibly sparing the fixational region (Fig 4-35)
- bilateral occipital lobe disease with preservation of the occipital tips, creating macular sparing (or preserved central islands of visual field) of different sizes in the 2 hemifields and "keyholes" with a detectable notch along the vertical midline
- homonymous hemianopic lesions involving only the fixational region (homonymous hemianopic scotomata) (Fig 4-36)

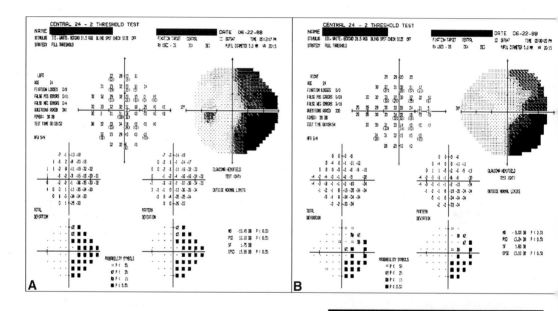

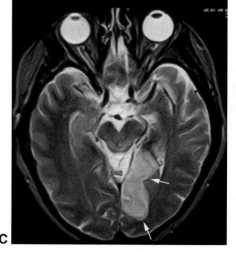

Figure 4-35 Occipital lobe infarction. **A, B,** Visual fields show congruous right homonymous hemianopia respecting the vertical meridian and sparing fixation. **C,** T2-weighted axial MRI scan showing left parieto-occipital stroke *(arrows)* sparing the occipital tip. *(Parts A, B courtesy of Steven A. Newman, MD; part C courtesy of Anthony C. Arnold, MD.)*

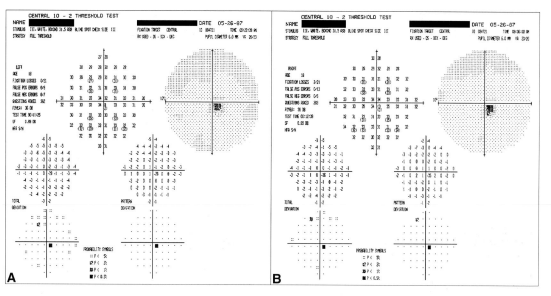

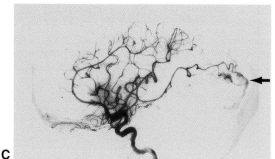

Figure 4-36 An 18-year-old woman with an 8-day history of sharp left-sided headaches. Visual acuity was 20/20 bilaterally. **A, B,** She was noted to be losing letters to the right, and bilateral 10-2 programs demonstrated a tiny 1° homonymous scotoma just below and to the right of fixation in both eyes. **C,** Her angiogram revealed an arteriovenous malformation involving the occipital tip *(arrow). (Courtesy of Steven A. Newman, MD.)*

- a monocular defect of the temporal crescent only or a homonymous lesion sparing the temporal crescent (Fig 4-37) (detected only on testing the peripheral 60°–90° visual field with Goldmann perimetry) in the eye contralateral to the lesion
- bilateral altitudinal defects or checkerboard patterns related to superior/inferior separation in bilateral incomplete homonymous hemifield involvement (eg, right superior and left inferior homonymous quadrantanopias)

Most occipital lobe lesions seen by ophthalmologists result from stroke and cause no other neurologic deficits. These deficits were described earlier, but several specific categories are important in clinical practice.

A macula-sparing homonymous hemianopia suggests a stroke involving the portion of the primary visual cortex supplied by the posterior cerebral artery. The tip of the occipital lobe receives a dual blood supply from both the middle cerebral artery and the posterior cerebral artery. Occlusion of the posterior cerebral artery damages the primary visual cortex except for the region representing the macula at the posterior tip of the occipital lobe; this region is spared because it remains perfused by the middle cerebral artery.

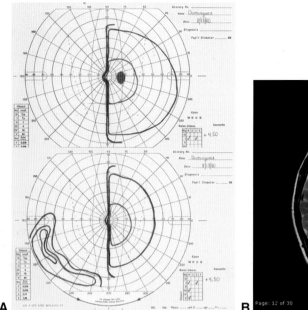
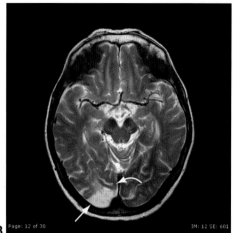

Figure 4-37 This 60-year-old woman presented with 3 episodes of transient visual loss to the left side. When evaluated, visual acuity was 20/20 bilaterally, but visual fields demonstrated a left homonymous hemianopia **(A)**. Her temporal crescent was intact on the left side, and an MRI scan **(B)** confirmed the presence of a right occipital lobe stroke *(straight arrow)* compatible with an infarct and sparing of the anterior visual cortex *(curved arrow)*. *(Part A courtesy of Steven A. Newman, MD; part B courtesy of Sophia M. Chung, MD.)*

Systemic hypoperfusion often damages the occipital tip because the tip is supplied by the endarterial branches of the posterior and middle cerebral artery systems. This highly vulnerable region may be the only injured area, resulting in homonymous paracentral hemianopic scotomata. Such scotomata are most common after surgery and other instances of blood loss with severe hypotension.

Cortical blindness results from bilateral occipital lobe destruction. Normal pupillary responses and optic nerve appearance distinguish cortical blindness from total blindness caused by bilateral prechiasmal or chiasmal lesions. Anton syndrome (denial of blindness), though classically associated with cortical blindness, can be due to a lesion at any level of the visual system severe enough to cause blindness. Bilateral occipital lobe lesions occasionally permit some residual visual function.

Lesions of the primary visual cortex may also produce *unformed visual hallucinations* from tumors, migraine, or drugs. *Formed hallucinations* (see Chapter 6) are usually attributed to lesions of the extrastriate cortex or temporal lobe. Patients with injury of the occipital cortex sometimes perceive moving targets but not static ones; this *Riddoch phenomenon* may also occur with lesions in other parts of the visual pathway. The Riddoch phenomenon probably reflects the fact that cells in the visual system respond better to moving stimuli than to those that are static.

Riddoch G. Dissociation of visual perceptions due to occipital injuries, with especial reference to appreciation of movement. *Brain.* 1917;40:15–57.

CHAPTER 5

The Patient With Transient Visual Loss

Transient visual loss is the sudden loss of visual function (partial or complete) in 1 or both eyes that lasts less than 24 hours. It most often stems from transient vascular compromise to the eye or afferent visual pathways in the brain. A systematic approach to patients with transient visual loss is imperative. To begin, several questions can guide appropriate clinical testing and patient management:

- Is the visual loss monocular or binocular?
- How old is the patient?
- What was the duration of visual loss?
- What was the pattern of visual loss and recovery?
- Does the patient report associated symptoms or demonstrate additional signs?

Answers to these questions ultimately dictate correct diagnosis and appropriate therapy.

Is the visual loss monocular *or* binocular*?*

Establishing transient visual loss as monocular or binocular is important for localizing the lesion: monocular implies a prechiasmal problem, whereas binocular is chiasmal or retrochiasmal. One setting in which the patient's perception of monocular vs binocular may be faulty is homonymous visual loss. If the patient describes having had temporal hemifield loss in only 1 eye, consider that the deficit may actually have been a transient homonymous hemianopia on the side of the eye mentioned.

How old *is the patient?*

In a patient younger than 50 years, migraine or vasospasm is the most likely cause of transient visual loss. One important exception in pregnant women is eclampsia, in which transient visual loss may be a harbinger of more serious and permanent visual loss, usually within days of delivery (see Chapter 14). In older patients, cerebrovascular disease and giant cell arteritis should be considered.

What was the duration *of visual loss?*

Cerebrovascular disease typically causes transient visual loss lasting less than 15 minutes. The Dutch Transient Monocular Blindness Study Group (2001) found that onset of visual loss within seconds and duration of symptoms between 1 and 10 minutes were associated with ipsilateral internal carotid artery stenosis of 70%–99%. In contrast, transient visual loss (monocular or binocular) lasting seconds and often precipitated by a change in posture (called "transient obscurations of vision") is common in patients with optic disc drusen or papilledema. Visual loss from vasospasm or migraine may last from seconds to an hour and may be accompanied by positive visual phenomena such as flashes, sparkles, or heat waves. The typical scintillating scotoma of migraine is binocular and lasts 20–30 minutes.

What was the pattern of visual loss and recovery?

Transient monocular visual loss (TMVL) from carotid artery disease is classically de-scribed as a curtain coming down over the vision and eventually lifting. However, others describe a closing in of vision or sudden loss of vision in the affected eye. The Dutch Tran-sient Monocular Blindness Study Group reported that attacks with an altitudinal onset and disappearance of symptoms were strongly associated with ipsilateral carotid artery stenosis. Conversely, attacks in which patients could not remember the nature or timing of the visual loss were associated with normal carotid arteries. Transient visual loss due to vasospasm or migraine may resemble that of carotid disease. The attacks are sometimes precipitated by exercise. *Uhthoff symptom* (transient visual blurring with physical activ-ity or elevation in body temperature) occurs in the setting of a previous episode of optic neuritis (see Chapter 14). Posterior circulation ischemia typically causes an abrupt change in vision, either a homonymous hemianopia or complete, bilateral visual loss, that is as-sociated with brainstem and cerebellar symptoms.

A transient geometric pattern in both eyes (eg, a hexagonal "chicken wire" pattern) that precedes or dominates visual loss strongly suggests occipital lobe dysfunction (eg, mi-graine, ischemia, or seizure). Whiteout of vision in both eyes simultaneously or a gradual peripheral constriction ("closing in") of vision without positive visual phenomena results from occipital lobe ischemia.

Does the patient report associated symptoms or demonstrate additional signs?

Positive visual phenomena and headache accompanying transient visual loss suggest mi-graine, although neither symptom need be present. Persistent headaches and intracranial noises are typical for increased intracranial pressure. In an elderly patient, transient visual loss associated with headaches, weight loss, fever, malaise, and scalp tenderness strongly suggests giant cell arteritis. Other neurologic symptoms and signs can help localize the vascular territory involved. Loss of consciousness, dizziness, diplopia, dysarthria, or focal weakness accompanying the visual loss suggests global perfusion problems, often involv-ing the brainstem or cortex. Skin or joint changes or Raynaud phenomenon (poor cir-culation in the fingertips, often exacerbated by cold exposure) may accompany collagen vascular disease.

Donders RC; Dutch TMB Study Group. Clinical features of transient monocular blindness and the likelihood of atherosclerotic lesions of the internal carotid artery. *J Neurol Neurosurg Psychiatry.* 2001;71(2):247–249.

Examination

With any patient who reports transient visual loss, it is important to document the cur-rent status of the afferent visual system. This requires assessment of best-corrected visual acuity (refraction), analysis of the extrafoveal visual system (perimetry), and identification of an afferent pupillary defect. The fundus examination is also critical. The optic disc may show evidence of anomalies (optic nerve head drusen or coloboma); there may be nerve fiber bundle dropout (optic atrophy) or signs of vascular occlusive disease such as emboli (Fig 5-1), cotton-wool spots, hemorrhage, or vascular attenuation. Occasionally, more detailed ocular and orbital examination may be appropriate, as discussed in the following sections. A photostress test may indicate macular ischemia.

Transient Monocular Visual Loss

Table 5-1 outlines the most common ocular, orbital, and systemic disorders leading to TMVL.

Ocular

Patients with blepharospasm who cannot keep their eyes open may experience moments of visual loss (see Chapter 11, Fig 11-14). Blurred vision caused by irregularity of the corneal tear film usually improves with a blink or application of a tear supplement, as well as with viewing through a pinhole. The slit lamp may reveal an abnormal-appearing tear film and cornea, with rapid tear breakup time and punctate keratopathy suggestive of keratitis sicca. A Schirmer test may confirm inadequate tear production.

Opacities in the media of the anterior chamber or the vitreous can mimic amaurosis fugax. For example, recurrent hyphema occasionally causes transient monocular blindness in patients with anterior chamber lenses who develop uveitis-glaucoma-hyphema

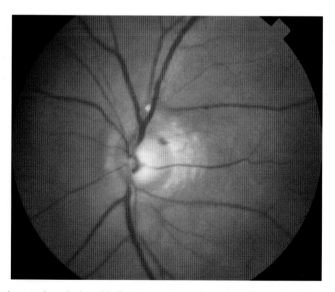

Figure 5-1 Cholesterol embolus (Hollenhorst plaque) at the bifurcation of a retinal arteriole. *(Courtesy of Karl C. Golnik, MD.)*

Table 5-1 Causes of Transient Molecular Visual Loss

Ocular pathology (nonvascular causes)
Tear film abnormalities
Corneal disease (eg, keratoconus)
Recurrent hyphema
Intermittent angle-closure glaucoma
Vitreous debris
Macular disease and photostress

Optic nerve disorders
Acquired or congenital disc disease (eg, papilledema, drusen)
Compressive lesions of the intraorbital optic nerve
Demyelinating disease

Vascular disease
Ocular hypoperfusion (ocular ischemic syndrome)
Embolic phenomenon
  Carotid
  Cardiac
  Great vessels
Carotid artery dissection
Vasculitis (eg, giant cell arteritis)
Vasospasm
Migraine
Systemic hypotension
Hyperviscosity/hypercoagulability states (eg, venous stasis or antiphospholipid antibody
  syndrome)

Nonorganic visual loss

(UGH) syndrome. Inflammation or recurrent bleeding may correlate with episodes of decreased vision. Large vitreous debris sometimes obscures vision.

Transient monocular visual obscurations accompanied by halos and pain should always prompt gonioscopy of the anterior chamber angle in a search for angle-closure glaucoma. The anterior lens should be inspected for glaukomflecken, which indicates prior episodes of angle closure.

Transient visual loss or prolonged afterimages following exposure to bright light (eg, sunlight) may indicate macular disorders, such as detachment or age-related macular degeneration or ocular ischemia. In such patients, performing the photostress test (10 seconds of exposure to a bright light) shows that return of normal central acuity is abnormally prolonged (>45 seconds).

At times, patients with well-developed papilledema experience "grayouts" or "blackouts" of vision. These episodes are typically brief (<10 seconds) and are often precipitated by changes in posture, although they may occur spontaneously. Dimming of vision lasts a few seconds, may involve 1 eye at a time, and clears completely. These obscurations are not a harbinger of impending visual failure and are not prognostic of optic nerve damage in patients with pseudotumor cerebri (see Chapter 4).

Disc anomalies, such as optic nerve head drusen, high myopia, and colobomas, have been reported in patients who experience brief (10–30-second) episodes of visual loss.

Kaiboriboon K, Piriyawat P, Selhorst JB. Light-induced amaurosis fugax. *Am J Ophthalmol.* 2001;131(5):674–676.

Orbital

Patients with orbital masses such as hemangioma or meningioma—especially those with an intraconal mass accompanied by disc swelling—may experience transient obscurations of vision in certain fields of gaze, especially downgaze. These obscurations presumably result from positional vascular obstruction. There is often a clue to orbital involvement (eg, proptosis, restriction in motility).

> Otto CS, Coppit GL, Mazzoli RA, et al. Gaze-evoked amaurosis: a report of five cases. *Ophthalmology.* 2003;110(2):322–326.

Systemic

After ocular and orbital causes of TMVL have been ruled out, retinovascular and cardiovascular causes must be considered. Amaurosis fugax ("fleeting blindness") is a subtype of TMVL attributed to ischemia or vascular insufficiency. Amaurosis fugax is characterized as sudden, painless, temporary visual loss lasting 2–30 minutes, followed by complete recovery. Between episodes, ocular examinations reveal normal anatomy or abnormalities confined to the retinal vasculature. (See also Cerebrovascular Disorders in Chapter 14.)

Emboli

In the late 1950s, C. Miller Fisher called attention to retinal emboli as a significant cause of TMVL when he observed embolic material passing through the retinal circulation. The patient with TMVL typically reports that a curtain of darkness descends over 1 eye, resulting in loss of vision lasting 2–30 minutes. In patients with some residual circulation from a retinal or cilioretinal artery, the curtain may extend only partially. At resolution, the curtain may either ascend or dissolve like a clearing fog.

Emboli that cause TMVL usually travel to and lodge within blood vessels that supply the optic nerve, retina, or both. Because emboli can be visualized with an ophthalmoscope and often appear distinctive, their probable site of origin can often be inferred. This inference may be crucial in directing appropriate patient evaluation.

The three most common types of emboli—cholesterol (see Fig 5-1), platelet-fibrin (Fig 5-2), and calcium (Fig 5-3)—are reviewed in Table 5-2. Other, less common varieties include emboli from cardiac tumors (myxoma), fat (long bone fractures, pancreatitis), sepsis, talc, air, silicone, and depot drugs (corticosteroids).

An embolic cause of TMVL necessitates careful vascular and cardiac evaluation. A search for atherosclerotic disease, the most likely cause of TMVL, is where the workup begins.

Atheroma formation is most common at the bifurcation of the common carotid artery into the internal and external carotid arteries and in the carotid siphon (Fig 5-4). Atheromas can remain stationary, become fibrotic, regress, ulcerate, narrow and occlude the lumen, or release emboli. It is thought that the normal internal carotid lumen must be reduced by 50%–90% before distal flow is affected. Hypertension, diabetes, hypercholesterolemia, and smoking are treatable risk factors.

Cardiac emboli arise from many causes, including ventricular aneurysms; hypokinetic wall segments; endocarditis (infectious [associated with subacute bacterial endocarditis] or noninfectious [marantic]); and valvular heart disease, including mitral valve prolapse

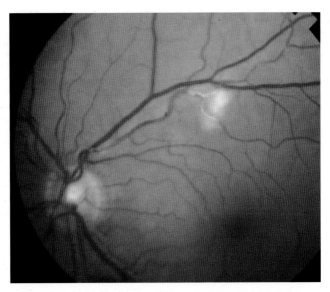

Figure 5-2 Platelet-fibrin embolus. *(Courtesy of Karl C. Golnik, MD.)*

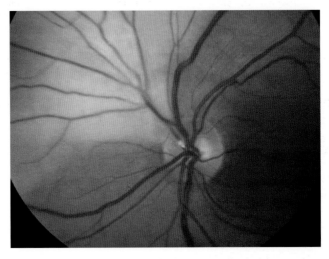

Figure 5-3 Calcific embolus with branch retinal artery occlusion. *(Courtesy of Karl C. Golnik, MD.)*

and atrial myxoma. Other cardiac causes include cardiac arrhythmia, particularly atrial fibrillation and other paroxysmal arrhythmias, and unsuspected patent foramen ovale with right-to-left cardiac shunt.

Other possible causes of transient monocular blindness and carotid territory ischemia are ophthalmic artery disease, giant cell arteritis, Raynaud disease, vasculitis, hyperviscosity syndromes, antiphospholipid antibody syndrome, and vasospasm (migraine). Carotid dissection should be considered in patients with ipsilateral monocular visual loss, particularly if associated with Horner syndrome, pain in the face or neck, and contralateral neurologic signs (see Fig 10-4).

Table 5-2 Clinical Aspects of Common Retinal Emboli

Type	Appearance	Source	Evaluation
Cholesterol (see Fig 5-1)	Yellow-orange or copper color Refractile Globular or rectangular Usually located at major bifurcation	Usually from common or internal carotid artery Rarely, from aorta or innominate artery	General medical examination Noninvasive studies of carotid patency Angiography, including aortic arch Cardiac assessment*
Platelet-fibrin (see Fig 5-2)	Dull gray-white color Long, smooth shape Concave meniscus at each end Usually mobile Lodge along course of vessel	From wall of atherosclerotic vessel From heart, especially valves	General medical evaluation Cardiac assessment, including Holter monitor and echocardiography Noninvasive studies of carotid patency Hematologic studies
Calcium (see Fig 5-3)	Chalky white Large Round or ovoid Lodge in first or second bifurcation May overlie optic disc	From heart or great vessels Rheumatic heart disease Calcific aortic stenosis Calcification of mitral valve annulus	General medical evaluation Cardiac assessment, including echocardiogram Angiogram of aortic arch

* Not for source of embolus but because these emboli increase the risk of cardiac disease and death from cardiac dysfunction.

From Miller NR. Embolic causes of transient monocular visual loss. *Ophthalmol Clin North Am.* 1996;9:359–380.

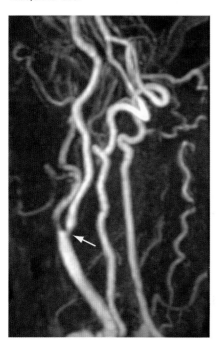

Figure 5-4 High-grade stenosis *(arrow)* of the cervical internal carotid artery at the bifurcation, as seen on MR angiogram. *(Courtesy of Aki Kawasaki, MD.)*

Biousse V, Touboul PJ, D'Anglejan-Chatillon J, Lévy C, Schaison M, Bousser MG. Oph-thalmologic manifestations of internal carotid artery dissection. *Am J Ophthalmol.* 1998; 126(4):565–577.

Fisher CM. Observation of the fundus oculi and transient monocular blindness. *Neurology.* 1959;9(5):333–347.

Hollenhorst RW. Significance of bright plaques in the retinal arterioles. *JAMA.* 1961;178:23–29.

Trimble M, Bell DA, Brien W, et al. The antiphospholipid syndrome: prevalence among pa-tients with stroke and transient ischemic attacks. *Am J Med.* 1990;88(6):593–597.

Clinical and laboratory evaluation   Presumed carotid territory ischemia warrants mea-surement of blood pressure, cardiac auscultation, and auscultation for carotid bruits (best heard at the angle of the jaw, where the bifurcation is located). The presence or absence of a bruit, however, is not a reliable indicator of carotid disease. A bruit indicates turbulent flow within the vessel, and it may be heard with narrowing of the external or internal ca-rotid artery. However, a bruit will be absent if flow is undisturbed *or* if carotid occlusion is complete.

Angiography remains the gold standard for quantifying the degree of carotid stenosis. The test is invasive, requiring intra-arterial injection of iodinated contrast dye. In centers where angiography is performed regularly, the risk of serious complication (such as stroke or death) is less than 1%.

Because of the time, expense, and morbidity associated with conventional angiography, noninvasive imaging modalities are often used, especially for screening tests. The 3 most popular modalities are carotid ultrasonography (duplex scanning), magnetic resonance angiography (MRA), and computed tomographic arteriography (CTA). Ultrasonography is a sensitive method of detecting ulcerated plaques, but reliability varies. MRA and CTA tend to overestimate the degree of carotid stenosis, especially those of moderate to high grade, compared to conventional angiography. However, besides being noninvasive, MRA and CTA have the advantage of visualizing and characterizing the plaque in question, as well as the surrounding arterial wall. MRA, along with MRI, is extremely useful for detect-ing carotid artery dissection.

Echocardiography is useful for detecting valvular and cardiac wall defects, intracar-diac tumors, and large thrombi. Transesophageal echocardiography is more sensitive than conventional transthoracic echocardiography. A normal-appearing echocardiogram does not exclude the possibility of emboli, because very small particles are not visualized. With carotid artery disease, a routine echocardiogram is mandatory. Coincident myocardial and cerebral ischemia should always be considered. Prolonged inpatient cardiac moni-toring or ambulatory Holter monitoring may document previously undetected cardiac arrhythmias. Suspected endocarditis should prompt blood cultures.

If a cardiac or carotid source is not found, other systemic processes may be con-tributing to stroke. Major risk factors include age, hypertension, hypotension and syn-cope (possibly iatrogenic from overly vigorous treatment of hypertension or from other medications), ischemic heart disease, diabetes, hypercholesterolemia, smoking, and sleep apnea. Most of these conditions are treatable. Laboratory studies should be obtained to look for these conditions and any others under clinical suspicion such as thyroid disease, hypercoagulable states, collagen vascular diseases, vasculitis, or syphilis.

Biousse V, Trobe JD. Transient monocular visual loss. *Am J Ophthalmol.* 2005;140(4):717–721.

Newman NJ. Evaluating the patient with transient monocular visual loss. The young versus the elderly. *Ophthalmol Clin North Am.* 1996;9:455–465.

Prognosis   Symptoms produced by carotid stenosis and those produced by carotid occlusion may be clinically indistinguishable. More than 40% of patients with carotid artery disease have transient ischemic attack (TIA) symptoms before a permanent deficit develops. With cerebral hemisphere TIAs, 20% of subsequent strokes occur within 1 month of the TIA, 50% within 1 year. The stroke rate drops to 5%–8% per year thereafter. It is impossible to predict which patients with TIA will have major strokes, although severe ipsilateral carotid stenosis is associated with higher risk. The major cause of death following TIA or stroke is myocardial infarction.

The annual risk of stroke following transient monocular blindness (~2%) is lower than that following cerebral TIA (~8%) (Table 5-3). TMVL occurs in 30%–40% of patients with ipsilateral atherosclerotic carotid disease. Carotid stenosis or occlusion may be demonstrated in about 53%–83% of patients with transient monocular blindness.

Biousse V. Carotid disease and the eye. *Curr Opin Ophthalmol.* 1997;8(6):16–26.

Kline LB. The natural history of patients with amaurosis fugax. *Ophthalmol Clin North Am.* 1996;9:351–357.

The presence of retinal emboli has important clinical implications whether the patient reports TMVL, develops a retinal artery occlusion, or is asymptomatic. The risk of stroke increases in patients with retinal emboli and the mortality rate increases (2%–4%/yr without emboli; 4%–8%/yr with emboli).

Bruno A, Jones WL, Austin JK, Carter S, Qualls C. Vascular outcome in men with asymptomatic retinal cholesterol emboli: a cohort study. *Ann Intern Med.* 1995;122(4):249–253.

Treatment   In the 1990s, 2 large trials (the North American Symptomatic Carotid Endarterectomy [NASCET], 1991, and the European Carotid Surgery Trial [ECST], 1995) compared medical therapy to *carotid endarterectomy (CEA)* in patients with symptomatic carotid stenosis (TMVL, hemispheric TIA, mild stroke). Both studies found that CEA was superior (≥70%) for reducing the risk of ipsilateral stroke in patients with severe carotid stenosis. Surgery was not better than medical therapy in patients with moderate (50%–69%) stenosis.

Table 5-3 Spectrum of Stroke Risk

Patient Group	Risk of Stroke per Year (%)
No carotid disease	0.1
Asymptomatic carotid bruit	0.1–0.4
Amaurosis fugax	2.0
Asymptomatic carotid stenosis	2.5
Retinal infarcts, emboli	3.0
Transient cerebral ischemic attack	8.0

From Trobe JD. Carotid endarterectomy: who needs it? *Ophthalmology.* 1987;94:725–730.

In 2001, a retrospective analysis of a subset of the NASCET data found that, among the patients with TMVL, the degree of carotid stenosis did not change the risk of stroke, which was about 10% overall. However, other risk factors were important in this subset of patients:

- male gender
- age 75 years or older
- history of hemispheric TIA or stroke
- intermittent claudication
- ipsilateral internal carotid artery stenosis of 80%–94%
- absence of collateral vessels on angiography

Having a greater number of risk factors was associated with a higher risk of stroke. Patients with none or only 1 of these risk factors had a very low 3-year risk of ipsilateral stroke (1.8%). For patients with 2 risk factors, it was 12.3%, and for patients with 3 or more risk factors, the stroke risk reached 24.2%. Thus, the NASCET data support the use of CEA in patients with TMVL who have 3 or more of the aforementioned risk factors.

Based on independent cases or series, CEA is sometimes performed for ophthalmic conditions other than TMVL, such as ocular ischemic syndrome or retinal artery occlusion. However, there are no definitive data on the efficacy of CEA in these conditions.

Medical treatment of TMVL due to carotid artery stenosis begins with aspirin. Although the addition of dipyridamole is controversial, an aspirin-dipyridamole combination (Aggrenox) is often prescribed. Clopidogrel bisulfate (Plavix) is useful for patients who are intolerant of or allergic to aspirin. A selective cAMP phosphodiesterase inhibitor, cilostazol (Pletal), inhibits platelet aggregation and is a direct arterial vasodilator; it may be more protective than aspirin alone or clopidogrel. Once antiplatelet therapy is maximized, consideration should be given to adding a statin or increasing the dose of a statin that the patient is already taking. There is some evidence that large doses of statins can reduce plaques and the frequency of stroke. Finally, angiotensin-converting enzymes (ACE) inhibitors and ACE receptor blockers may be given for their favorable effects on endothelial tissue.

Bucher HC, Griffith LE, Guyatt GH. Effect of HMGcoA reductase inhibitors on stroke: a meta-analysis of randomized, controlled trials. *Ann Intern Med.* 1998;128(2):89–95.

Crouse JR III, Byington RP, Bond MG, et al. Pravastatin, lipids, and atherosclerosis in the carotid arteries (PLAC II). *Am J Cardiol.* 1995;75(7):455–459.

Furberg CD, Adams HP Jr, Applegate WB, et al. Effect of lovastatin on early carotid atherosclerosis and cardiovascular events. Asymptomatic Carotid Artery Progression Study (ACAPS) Research Group. *Circulation.* 1994;90(4):1679–1687.

Hodis HN, Mack WJ, LaBree L, et al. Reduction in carotid arterial wall thickness using lovastatin and dietary therapy: a randomized controlled clinical trial. *Ann Intern Med.* 1996;124(6): 548–556.

Recently, there has been growing enthusiasm for *carotid artery stenting (CAS)* as a less invasive alternative procedure to CEA. Various reports have suggested a high efficacy and low complication rate for CAS. The Carotid Revascularization Endarterectomy Versus Stent Trial (CREST) is a multicenter, randomized prospective clinical trial designed to compare the efficacy of CEA and CAS for carotid stenosis in symptomatic patients and asymptomatic patients with high-grade (>70%) stenosis. Enrollment of patients continued into 2008. No results have yet been disclosed for randomized patients, but a report on the complication rate of CAS during the credentialing phase found the 30-day stroke or death rate to be 3.9% (5.6% for symptomatic patients, 3.4% for asymptomatic patients), rates similar to those reported for CEA in symptomatic patients in NASCET.

Hobson RW II. Update on the Carotid Revascularization Endarterectomy versus Stent Trial (CREST) protocol. *J Am Coll Surg.* 2002;194(1 suppl):S9–S14.

Vasculitis

TMVL in elderly patients (usually over age 50) can also be caused by giant cell arteritis. Therefore, the diagnostic workup must include a Westergren sedimentation rate and C-reactive protein. The patient also should be questioned about symptoms of headache, scalp tenderness, jaw claudication, weight loss, depressed appetite, proximal joint pain, muscle aches, myalgias, and malaise. Evidence of choroidal hypoperfusion (low intraocular pressure [IOP] or changes on fluorescein angiogram) may be particularly suggestive. Unless treated immediately with high-dose corticosteroids, giant cell arteritis heralded by TMVL may lead to permanent blindness in 1 or both eyes, which sometimes, but not always, can be averted or reversed by immediate treatment with high-dose intravenous corticosteroids. See also BCSC Section 1, *Update on General Medicine.*

Siatkowski RM, Gass JD, Glaser JS, Smith JL, Schatz NJ, Schiffman J. Fluorescein angiography in the diagnosis of giant cell arteritis. *Am J Ophthalmol.* 1993;115(1):57–63.

Hypoperfusion

Hypoperfusion may lead to TMVL in several situations. The first is in the setting of occlusive disease of the retinal venous system. Although a sudden decline in central vision is not a common complaint of patients with central retinal vein occlusion, some report transient visual impairment lasting seconds to minutes, with recovery to normal vision. Such symptoms may predate more lasting visual loss by days or weeks, or the symptoms may cease when collateral vessels develop.

The second type is progressive restriction of vision from the periphery ("iris diaphragm pattern"), lasting from seconds to 1–2 minutes. This form of TMVL may be precipitated by a change in posture from a sitting to a standing position. Hypoperfusion can be caused by cardiac arrhythmia or severe stenosis of the great vessels.

The third entity in which hypoperfusion leads to TMVL is the *ocular ischemic syndrome.* This syndrome is characterized in part by a hypotensive, ischemic retinopathy with low retinal artery pressure, poor perfusion, and midperipheral retinopathy. Recurrent orbital or facial pain that improves when the patient lies down is highly suggestive of carotid occlusive disease. In the early stages, there may be transient or persistent blurred vision or transient visual loss upon exposure to bright light. Dot-and-blot retinal hemorrhages characterize early ocular ischemia. At times, these hemorrhages may resemble the diabetic variety.

Severe ischemia causes anterior segment changes that may be confused with intraocular inflammation. The patient may have decreased visual acuity; a red, painful eye with episcleral vascular injection; and aqueous flare (ischemic uveitis). Even though neovascularization of the chamber angle and iris is common, IOP may be low, normal, or high. Low or normal IOP in this setting is the result of impaired ciliary body perfusion. Fundus changes may include dilated and retinal veins, narrowed retinal arteries with microaneurysm formation, midperipheral dot-and-blot hemorrhages, and macular edema (Fig 5-5). These changes have been termed *venous stasis retinopathy (VSR)* and may be caused by vascular occlusion anywhere between the heart and the eye.

Treatment of ocular ischemic syndrome includes CEA, IOP-lowering agents, corticosteroids for pain, and panretinal photocoagulation. If the preoperative IOP is low, restoration of blood flow by CEA may precipitate dangerously high IOP. Once the patient develops signs of chronic hypoperfusion, however, improvement is unlikely. In other patients, carotid occlusion may be too advanced for surgical correction. Early detection is critical because neovascularization and progressive ocular ischemia occur with prolonged hypoperfusion. See also BCSC Section 12, *Retina and Vitreous.*

Mizener JB, Podhajsky P, Hayreh SS. Ocular ischemic syndrome. *Ophthalmology.* 1997;104(5): 859–864.

Vasospasm/Hyperviscosity/Hypercoagulability

Vasospasm is the presumed cause of TMVL in 2 clinical circumstances. The first is the patients who experience stereotypic episodes of severe monocular visual loss and have a strong personal or family history of migraine. These patients are generally young (<50 years), and their episodes of transient visual loss have been designated *retinal* or *ocular migraine.* The second type is patients with no history of migraine but whose examination during attacks of visual loss reveals constriction of the retinal arteries. In either circumstance, other causes of transient visual loss should be excluded before a diagnosis of vasospasm is accepted. The workup should include complete blood count, Westergren sedimentation rate, and cardiac and carotid evaluation. It is also necessary to rule out

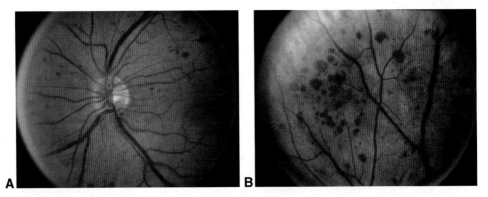

Figure 5-5 Ocular ischemic syndrome. **A,** Fundus demonstrates retinal venous dilation, scattered hemorrhages, and mild optic disc edema. **B,** Midperipheral dot-and-blot hemorrhages. *(Reprinted with permission from John E. Carter, MD. From Carter JE. Panretinal photocoagulation for progressive ocular neovascularization secondary to occlusion of the common carotid artery. Ann Ophthalmol. 1984;16(6):572–576.)*

hyperviscosity syndrome and hypercoagulable states, particularly in a young patient. Tests should include anticardiolipin antibody, antiphosphotidyl choline and serine, antinuclear antibody, serum protein electrophoresis, partial thromboplastin time, Venereal Disease Research Laboratory (VDRL), protein S, and protein C. Whether vasospasm can truly cause transient visual loss is debated, but calcium channel blockers that prevent vasospasm seem to provide relief from attacks of amaurosis in some patients.

Hyperviscosity is a rare cause of transient visual loss. Approximately 10% of patients with polycythemia vera complain of episodes of TMVL.

Glueck CJ, Goldenberg N, Bell H, Golnik K, Wang P. Amaurosis fugax: associations with heritable thrombophilia. *Clin Appl Thromb Hemost.* 2005;11(3):235–241.

Winterkorn JMS, Burde RM. Vasospasm—not migraine—in the anterior visual pathway. *Ophthalmol Clin North Am.* 1996;9:393–405.

Transient Binocular Visual Loss

Common causes of transient binocular visual loss include

- migraine
- occipital mass lesions: tumor, arteriovenous malformation
- occipital ischemia: embolic, vasculitic, hypoperfusion
- occipital seizures

Migraine

The most common cause of transient binocular loss is the homonymous hemianopic defect caused by migraine. On occasion, this may progress to a fixed visual field defect and be classified as complicated migraine. Patient evaluation, including cranial MRI, is mandatory in such cases (see Chapter 12).

Occipital Mass Lesions

In a patient with episodic headaches and visual loss, if attacks always occur on the same side or if visual symptoms *follow* rather than *precede* the onset of headache, a structural lesion must be ruled out—usually an occipital arteriovenous malformation or tumor. Such patients require contrast-enhanced cranial MRI and possibly cerebral angiography.

Occipital Ischemia

As the patient with migraine grows older, the intensity of the headaches may diminish or the headaches may not occur at all after visual symptoms. A diagnostic dilemma is presented by the elderly patient who experiences a migraine-like aura for the first time but no headache. Differentiating between migrainous vasospasm and vertebrobasilar insufficiency may be difficult. Treatable causes of cerebrovascular disease or a source of emboli should be excluded. Patient evaluation should include hematologic studies (eg, complete blood count, Westergren sedimentation rate), as well as MRI and MRA to evaluate the vertebrobasilar circulation. If the evaluation is negative, the prognosis is usually good, and treatment of a presumed migrainous syndrome may be warranted.

Transient recurrent bilateral visual blurring is one of the most frequent symptoms of vertebrobasilar insufficiency. Composed of the vertebral, basilar, and posterior cerebral arteries (see Chapter 1), the vertebrobasilar system supplies the occipital cortex, brainstem, and cerebellum. Patients with vertebrobasilar insufficiency often present to the ophthalmologist first because of prominent ocular motor and visual symptoms. Nonophthalmic symptoms of TIAs in the vertebrobasilar system are discussed in Chapter 14.

Occipital Seizures

Occipital seizures typically produce unformed positive visual phenomena, such as colored or swirling lights or a whiting out of vision, "like a flashbulb going off." However, some patients experience purely negative visual spells, usually described as a blacking out of vision. The episodes usually last 1–2 minutes, although they may persist for many hours (status epilepticus amauroticus). Most adults with occipital seizures harbor a structural lesion (tumor, arteriovenous malformation, trauma); in children, such seizures are more often benign. A normal electroencephalogram (EEG) does not rule out an underlying seizure disorder, and, in appropriate cases, prolonged EEG monitoring may be required. Treatment consists of anticonvulsant therapy.

Kun Lee S, Young Lee S, Kim DW, Soo Lee D, Chung CK. Occipital lobe epilepsy: clinical characteristics, surgical outcome, and role of diagnostic modalities. *Epilepsia.* 2005;46(5):688–695.

CHAPTER 6

The Patient With Illusions, Hallucinations, and Disorders of Higher Cortical Function

Patients are often reluctant to complain of "seeing things" lest they be dispatched to a psychiatrist. However, most visual hallucinations or illusions are a harbinger not of psychiatric disease but of ocular, optic nerve, or brain pathology. The clinician should ask about these symptoms because patients may be reluctant to volunteer such information. *Illusions* are the false perceptions of visual information that is present in the external environment. For example, a person looking at stationary high-contrast borders may perceive the illusion of movement. A *hallucination* is the subjective perception of an object or event when no sensory stimulus is present. Illusions should disappear with eye closure; hallucinations usually do not.

The first step in assessing patients with such visual disorders is to ascertain their mental status and the status of their afferent visual pathways. Patients with dementia or altered sensorium (delirium, hypnosis) are prone to hallucinations. Reduced visual acuity or visual field loss often leads to positive visual phenomena. Best-corrected visual acuity, assessment of color perception, and perimetry should be performed. The primary goal is to anatomically localize the disorder, which helps establish a likely pathophysiology or at least a differential diagnosis.

Norton JW, Corbett JJ. Visual perceptual abnormalities: hallucinations and illusions. *Semin Neurol*. 2000;20(1):111–121.

The Patient With Illusions

The alterations of perception that make up the spectrum of illusions can arise at various parts of the visual system. Nonvisual causes of illusions and hallucinations are shown in Table 6-1.

Ocular Origin

Many illusions have an ocular basis. Such illusions may be classified into those due to optical causes and those due to alterations in photochemical transduction in the retina.

Table 6-1 Nonvisual Causes of Illusions and Hallucinations

Medications
Anticholinergic and dopaminergic drugs
Indomethacin, digoxin, cyclosporine, lithium, lidocaine
Topical scopolamine, atropine, homatropine
Lysergic acid (LSD), mescaline, psilocybin, amphetamines, cocaine

Medical Conditions
Alzheimer disease, Parkinson disease, narcolepsy, Huntington chorea,
   Lewy body dementia, epilepsy

Psychiatric Conditions
Schizophrenia, affective disorders, conversion disorders

Toxic and Metabolic Conditions
Uremia, hepatic disease, infection (fever)
Alcohol withdrawal (delirium tremens)

Miscellaneous
Entoptic imagery
Dreams and imaginary childhood companions
Sensory deprivation, sleep deprivation, hypnosis
Intense emotional experience

Optical causes

The tear film is the primary refracting surface of the eye. Any alteration in the tear film (early tear breakup time, dry eye syndrome, abnormalities in blink) can distort vision. Irregularities in the corneal surface (eg, keratoconus, corneal scarring) may also result in distortions of vision. The lens may produce irregularities, especially with early oil-droplet changes of nuclear sclerosis or posterior subcapsular scattering. The lens also acts as a filter, changing the spectrum of the light transmitted; thus, spectral changes may be seen as alterations of shape and color. Images may be multiplied (monocular diplopia), especially when related to high astigmatism induced by changes in the lens or cornea. Cataract extraction often causes changes in visual perception, especially of color and brightness.

Retinal causes

Changes in the position of the retinal receptors can cause various alterations in vision. This repositioning usually results from macular changes, which may be due to pathology on the surface of the retina (epiretinal membrane), within the retina (macular edema, macular hole), or below the retina (changes in the retinal pigment epithelium [RPE] or choroid).

Metamorphopsia

With *metamorphopsia* (perceptual distortion), the patient reports that linear objects appear curved or discontinuous. This symptom is characteristic of macular disease and may occur with epiretinal, intraretinal, or subretinal pathology (eg, proliferative vitreo-retinopathy, cystoid macular edema, retinal pigment epithelial detachments, subretinal neovascular membranes, or choroidal circulatory problems).

With intraretinal edema, the retinal elements are often pushed apart, causing perceived image shrinkage *(micropsia)*. *Macropsia* (perceived image enlargement) can occur if the photoreceptors are pushed together.

The retina may be the source of changes in color perception associated with drug effects (eg, digoxin-induced yellowing of vision, sildenafil citrate (Viagra)-induced blue tinge). Other changes of color perception may be related to choroidal or retinal ischemia (eg, giant cell arteritis), which can also lead to persistent afterimages.

Optic Nerve Origin

Conduction delay in 1 optic nerve following an episode of optic neuritis (demyelination) may lead to an altered perception of motion. Because of the disparity in neuronal transmission, a pendulum, for example, may appear to trace an elliptical pathway instead of its true single-plane oscillation *(Pulfrich phenomenon)*.

Cortical Origin

Perception is a cortical phenomenon; thus, it is not surprising that cortical pathology may be responsible for illusory changes. In addition to altering perceived shape and position, cortical abnormalities may change the perception of motion. Cortical pathology may cause loss of color vision or multiplicity of images. Cortical pathology may be located in the primary visual cortex (V1) or the associative areas (V2, V3, V4) (see Chapter 1). Disorders of visual perception are common with parietal lobe abnormalities, such as micropsia, macropsia, *teleopsia* (objects appear too distant), and *pelopsia* (objects appear too close).

The Patient With Hallucinations

Hallucinations consist of perception unrelated to active stimuli. Like illusions, hallucinations may originate anywhere along the visual pathway but most commonly do so within the globe or cortex. Hallucinations may be of objects (eg, animals, flowers, cars) or people; if so, they are called *formed hallucinations*. If the hallucinations are of lights, spots, dots, or geometric patterns (eg, chain-link fences), they are termed *unformed hallucinations*.

Ocular Origin

Unlike illusions, hallucinations have no optical causes. Vitreous detachment with persistent vitreoretinal adhesions may produce colored shapes or vertical white flashes (socalled *lightning streaks of Moore*). Such hallucinations are often most apparent in a dark environment. Retinal detachment may produce persistent flashes and floaters with or without visual loss.

Zaret BS. Lightning streaks of Moore: a cause of recurrent stereotypic visual disturbance. *Neurology*. 1985;35(7):1078–1081.

Outer retinal diseases may result in continuous flashing lights that tend to persist (unlike the transient flashes of migraine). These flashes may be simple white lights, but often they form geometric webs that may take on colors, including silver and gold. Flashing dots and spots of light often accompany the onset of cancer-associated retinopathy, a paraneoplastic process. Similarly, flashing lights may accompany a variety of retinal, RPE, and choroidal abnormalities (multiple evanescent white dot syndrome, acute zonal occult outer retinopathy, birdshot chorioretinopathy). For a complete description of these conditions, see BCSC Section 12, *Retina and Vitreous*.

Retinal vasospasm (migraine) may produce visual loss or unformed monocular images—colors, lines, or *phosphenes* (fleeting, bright flashes of light)—that last up to 45 minutes and may be followed by a headache. Sequelae are unusual, although a permanent scotoma may, rarely, develop.

Alabduljalil T, Behbehani R. Paraneoplastic syndromes in ophthalmology. *Curr Opin Ophthalmol.* 2007;18(6):463–469.

Gass JD, Agarwal A, Scott IU. Acute zonal occult outer retinopathy: a long-term follow-up study. *Am J Ophthalmol.* 2002;134(3):329–339.

Headache Classification Subcommittee of the International Headache Society. The International Classification of Headache Disorders. 2nd ed. *Cephalalgia.* 2004;24(Suppl 1):9–160.

Optic Nerve Origin

Optic neuritis often produces phosphenes induced by eye movement or a dark setting. Patients with subacute or long-standing optic neuropathy may experience sound-induced *photisms* (sensations of color or light associated with noise, touch, taste, or smell). These phenomena tend to be unformed and are triggered by various sounds heard in the ipsilateral ear. Sound-induced photisms are attributed to discharges from the lateral geniculate nucleus, which is also responsive to sound and is adjacent to the medial geniculate nucleus of the auditory system.

Cortical Origin

It is often taught that lesions affecting the anterior optic radiations (the temporal lobe) cause formed hallucinations and that more posterior lesions (in the parietal and occipital lobes) produce unformed hallucinations. However, these guidelines have many exceptions. In rare cases, lesions involving the mesencephalon may cause hallucinations (peduncular hallucinosis). These hallucinations are formed and can be constant. They are usually associated with an inverted sleep-wake cycle. Associated symptoms may occur if adjacent structures are affected (eg, oculomotor nerve fascicle[s], corticospinal tract[s]).

Temporal/parietal/occipital lobes

Temporal lobe lesions most often produce olfactory and gustatory hallucinations. Visual phenomena from this area are usually complex, formed hallucinations in either the ipsilateral or the contralateral visual field. Epilepsy is the most common setting for hallucinations traced to this region. A visual aura implies that the seizure began focally.

In the parietal lobe, hallucinations may be either formed or unformed.

Unformed hallucinations are common with disorders of the occipital lobe. Patients may describe white or colored flashes of light, kaleidoscopic colors, moving discs, flickering, or a hexagonal array (chickenwire or honeycomb pattern). A complete whiteout of vision suggests bilateral occipital lobe ischemia.

Patients sometimes describe hallucinations within a homonymous hemianopia or quadrantanopia. These images are generally complex and may be static or move throughout the visual field. *Hallucinatory palinopsia* (see the following section) is the apparition of objects or persons seen earlier. It may occur with temporal, parietal, or occipital involvement, particularly with posterior circulation ischemia.

Palinopsia

Interesting cortical phenomena may occur with disorders of the nondominant parietooccipital area. *Palinopsia* is visual perseveration after the removal of the original stimulus (multiple afterimages). The afterimages may be associated with a homonymous hemianopia in which the palinoptic images appear in the blind hemifield. Visual hallucinations may also be present. Migraine and medications (clomiphene [Clomid], trazodone [Desyrel], nafazodone [Serzone]) can produce similar symptoms.

Lepore FE. Spontaneous visual phenomena with visual loss: 104 patients with lesions of retinal and neural afferent pathways. *Neurology.* 1990;40(3 pt 1):444–447.

Vaphiades MS, Celesia GG, Brigell MG. Positive spontaneous visual phenomena limited to the hemianopic field in lesions of central visual pathways. *Neurology.* 1996;47(2):408–417.

Migraine

The visual phenomena of migraine are thought to be caused by abnormal excitatory activity in the cerebral cortex, followed by a wave of depressed neuronal function *(spreading depression of Leão)*. In migraine with aura, the visual phenomena typically last 10–30 minutes and are followed by a typical headache (see Chapter 12). The hallucinations are binocular. Besides the classic fortification spectra, patients may experience the "Alice in Wonderland effect" (micropsia/macropsia), formed or unformed images, or visual distortion. Common descriptions include heat waves, cracked glass, kaleidoscopic vision, or fragmented vision. Patients may also experience the visual phenomena without a headache.

Charles Bonnet syndrome

The *Charles Bonnet syndrome* is the triad of visual hallucinations, ocular pathology causing bilateral visual deterioration, and preserved cognitive status. With this syndrome, hallucinations may be elementary or highly organized and complex. Patients may have formed or unformed hallucinations that either are persistent or come and go abruptly. Patients with Charles Bonnet syndrome have a clear sensorium and are aware that the visions are not real. If the cause of visual loss is known, neuroimaging is not necessary. A variety of medical treatments have been used, but with mixed success.

Menon GJ, Rahman I, Menon SJ, Dutton GN. Complex visual hallucinations in the visually impaired: the Charles Bonnet syndrome. *Surv Ophthalmol.* 2003;48(1):58–72.

Rovner BW. The Charles Bonnet syndrome: a review of recent research. *Curr Opin Ophthalmol.* 2006;17(3):275–277.

The Patient With Disorders of Higher Cortical Function

The visual information that reaches the occipital striate cortex (area V1) represents the beginning of the process of "seeing." This information must be processed by the associative cortical visual areas for visual awareness to occur (see Chapter 1). Visual information that reaches the primary occipital cortex is projected through 2 pathways (see Chapter 1, Fig 1-22): a ventral occipitotemporal pathway and a dorsal occipitoparietal pathway. The ventral pathway is involved with processing the physical attributes of an image (the "what") such as color, shape, and pattern. The dorsal pathway is important for visuospatial analysis (the "where," or the localization of items in space) and for guiding movements toward items of interest. In addition, interconnecting pathways are critical to the transfer of information from the primary cortex to the associative areas (areas V2–V5).

In general, *cortical syndromes* due to abnormalities in visual processing can result through 2 mechanisms: (1) specific cortical areas responsible for processing information may be damaged, or (2) the flow of information between such areas may be interrupted *(disconnection syndromes)*. The disorders of higher cortical visual function may be divided into problems with object recognition, difficulty with visual–spatial relationships, and awareness of visual deficit (Table 6-2).

Girkin CA, Miller NR. Central disorders of vision in humans. *Surv Ophthalmol.* 2001;45(5): 379–405.

Disorders of Recognition

Object agnosia

Interruption of signal flow from the occipital lobe to the area of the temporal lobe involved in object identification results in an inability to recognize objects (eg, pen, bottle, car) called *object agnosia,* a form of visual–visual disconnection. This often results from a bilateral occipitotemporal (ventral pathway) dysfunction affecting the inferior longitudinal fasciculi. Patients can identify objects by touch or by description but not by sight.

Table 6-2 Disorders of Higher Cortical Function

Disorders of Recognition
Object agnosia
Prosopagnosia
Akinetopsia
Alexia without agraphia
Cerebral achromatopsia

Disorders of Visual–Spatial Relationships
Simultanagnosia
Optic ataxia
Acquired ocular motor apraxia
Balint syndrome
Visual allesthesia

Disorders of Awareness of Vision or Visual Loss
Anton syndrome
Riddoch phenomenon
Blindsight
Hemispatial neglect

Prosopagnosia

Prosopagnosia, the inability to recognize familiar faces, is a more specific form of visual–visual disconnection. These patients usually have difficulty with other visual memory tasks. The condition usually occurs with bilateral occipital lobe damage but may also occur with right inferior occipital lobe damage. Superior homonymous visual field defects are common. It is thought that this form of agnosia is the reason patients with advanced Alzheimer disease do not recognize their relatives.

Barton JJ. Disorders of face perception and recognition. *Neurol Clin.* 2003;21(2):521–548.

Akinetopsia

Patients with pathology affecting the dorsal pathway (area V5/MT) may lose the perception of visual motion *(akinetopsia)* but still be able to perceive form, texture, and color.

Alexia without agraphia

The interruption of visual information between the occipital lobe and the dominant angular gyrus causes visual–verbal disconnection. During the act of reading, visual information from the left visual field is received in the right occipital lobe and is transferred to the left side of the brain through the corpus callosum, where the information is relayed anteriorly to the angular gyrus of the parietal lobe for comprehension. However, the information from the left field cannot cross from the right to the left occipital lobe if the splenium of the corpus callosum is damaged (Fig 6-1). Typically, there is also damage to the left occipital lobe, and this combination results in *alexia without agraphia* (ie, the patient can write but not read). This is usually due to the infarction of the left occipital lobe and to fibers

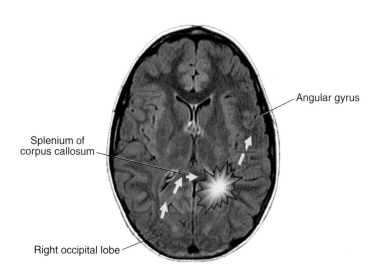

Figure 6-1 Alexia without agraphia. The diagram depicts the flow of information from the right occipital lobe through the splenium of the corpus callosum to the angular gyrus. A lesion in the left occipital lobe obstructs this flow. *(Courtesy of Eric Eggenberger, DO.)*

crossing in the splenium of the corpus callosum. However, because the structures anterior to the splenium are intact, these patients can produce language and write. Interestingly, they cannot read what they have just written! If the left angular gyrus itself is damaged, then both reading and writing will be affected *(alexia with agraphia)*. These patients also often have acalculia, right–left confusion, and finger agnosia *(Gerstmann syndrome)*.

Biran I, Coslett HB. Visual agnosia. *Curr Neurol Neurosci Rep.* 2003;3(6):508–512.

Cerebral achromatopsia

Color discrimination may be abnormal with bilateral parietal or occipital lobe lesions (lingual and fusiform gyrus; see Chapter 1). Affected patients cannot match colors or order them in a series according to hue. Bilateral occipital ventromedial cortex damage may cause complete achromatopsia; unilateral damage may cause only hemiachromatopsia. Superior homonymous visual field defects are often present.

Heywood CA, Kentridge RW. Achromatopsia, color vision, and cortex. *Neurol Clin.* 2003;21(2): 483–500.

Disorders of Visual–Spatial Relationships

Simultanagnosia

Simultanagnosia is the failure to integrate multiple elements of a scene to form the total picture. The clinician may assess for simultanagnosia by asking patients to describe a picture scene (Fig 6-2). The description of only part of the picture adds evidence of a problem with visual analysis. The patient will not describe other portions of the picture unless the examiner identifies them. Testing color vision with the Ishihara pseudoisochromatic color plates may suggest simultanagnosia if the patient can identify colors but not the shapes of numbers (the patient does not see the whole picture as the sum of its parts).

Brazis PW, Graff-Radford NR, Newman NJ, Lee AG. Ishihara color plates as a test for simultanagnosia. *Am J Ophthalmol.* 1998;126(6):850–851.

Optic ataxia

Patients with *optic ataxia* reach for an object as if they were blind; there is a disconnect between visual input and the motor system. The anatomical localization is complex, involving the posterior parietal cortex, premotor cortex, motor areas, ventromedial cortical areas, and subcortical structures.

Acquired ocular motor apraxia

Also known as "spasm of fixation" or "psychic paralysis of gaze," *acquired ocular motor apraxia* involves the loss of voluntary movement of the eyes while fixating on a target. Frontal eye field damage is thought to be responsible.

Balint syndrome

A rare phenomenon resulting from bilateral occipitoparietal lesions is *Balint syndrome,* which consists of the triad of simultanagnosia, optic ataxia, and acquired oculomotor apraxia. Clinically, this triad of findings rarely occur together and they are thus considered individually, as just described.

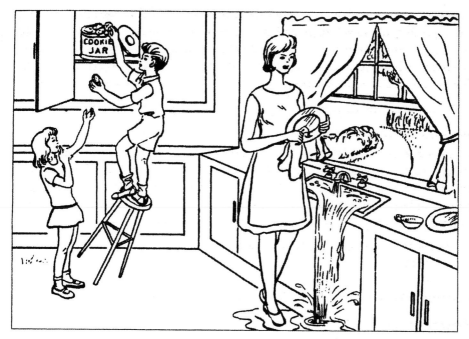

Figure 6-2 The patient is asked to describe what is occurring in this drawing, the "cookie theft picture," modified from the Boston Diagnostic Aphasia Examination. The patient with simultanagnosia will describe one part of the scene and not see anything else. *(Used with permission from Kline LB, Bajandas FJ. Neuro-Ophthalmology Review Manual. Rev. 5th ed. Thorofare, NJ: Slack; 2004:227.)*

Visual allesthesia

Patients with *visual allesthesia* see their environment rotated, flipped, or inverted. This localizes the damage to either the lateral medullary region *(Wallenberg syndrome)* or the occipitoparietal area.

Disorders of Awareness of Vision or Visual Deficit

Anton syndrome

A patient with cortical blindness may deny that there is any visual problem; this is termed *Anton syndrome.* Patients with Anton syndrome have no demonstrable visual behavior, but they hallucinate and confabulate visual images, claiming the ability to see. Anton syndrome is most common with bilateral occipital infarctions and has been described in patients with blindness from bilateral optic nerve lesions.

Stasheff SF, Barton JJS. Deficits in cortical visual function. *Ophthalmol Clin North Am.* 2001; 14(1):217–242.

Riddoch phenomenon

The preservation of motion perception in a blind hemifield is called the *Riddoch phenomenon.* If present in an otherwise complete homonymous hemianopsia, it is thought to portend better visual prognosis.

Blindsight

Cortically blind patients may have an unconscious rudimentary visual perception *(blindsight)*. This may be due to either visual pathways through the superior colliculus or connections between the lateral geniculate body and the extrastriate visual cortex.

Hemispatial neglect

Patients with *hemispatial neglect* (hemineglect) will not acknowledge seeing objects in an area of vision known to be intact. Confrontation testing using double simultaneous stimulation may be used to verify this condition (see Chapter 3 for the description of confrontation visual field testing). Hemispatial neglect is usually due to damage in the right hemisphere (posterior parietal cortex, frontal eye fields, cingulate gyrus) that mediates attention in both hemifields.

Kline LB, Bajandas FJ. *Neuro-Ophthalmology Review Manual.* Rev. 5th ed. Thorofare, NJ: Slack; 2004:chap 18.)

CHAPTER 7

The Patient With Supranuclear Disorders of Ocular Motility

The *efferent visual system* controls ocular movements. (The anatomy of this system is introduced in Chapter 1.) Basically, the efferent ocular motor system (like all efferent systems) can be divided into supranuclear and infranuclear pathways. This distinction is clinically significant in that supranuclear disorders almost always affect both eyes similarly, whereas infranuclear disorders affect the eyes differently. The patterns of symmetric dysfunction that occur with supranuclear disorders typically do not produce diplopia (although there are exceptions, such as skew deviation). Conversely, infranuclear lesions usually do produce diplopia. The former is discussed in this chapter, and the latter is discussed in Chapter 8.

Supranuclear pathways include all premotor and motor regions of the frontal and parietal cortices; cerebellum; basal ganglia; superior colliculi; thalamus (dorsal lateral geniculate nucleus and pulvinar); and brainstem centers, including the paramedian pontine reticular formation, neural integrators, and vestibular nuclei. *Infranuclear pathways* include ocular motor nuclei, the intramedullary segments of the ocular motor nerves, the peripheral segments of the ocular motor nerves (as they course through the subarachnoid space, cavernous sinus, superior orbital fissure, and orbit), the neuromuscular junction, and the extraocular muscles.

Fundamental Principles of Ocular Motor Control

The afferent visual system of primates is broadly designed to achieve 2 fundamental goals: (1) to detect objects and motion within the environment; and (2) to provide a high level of spatial resolution for those objects that command our attention. The entire retina outside the fovea is devoted essentially to the detection of objects. Only the fovea, which occupies a tiny fraction of the total retinal area, provides the fine-quality images that allow us to read or perform highly precise visual motor tasks.

Our attention to peripherally placed objects is usually driven by the perception of a changing stimulus (eg, one that moves, becomes brighter or larger). It is a basic principle of all sensory systems that any persistent, unchanging stimulus gradually produces an attenuated neural response. This explains, for instance, why one does not attend to the constant tactile stimulus of a wristwatch or clothes that are worn. This physiologic design improves the efficiency of neural communication.

Movement is an especially strong stimulus that generates the conscious awareness of an object in our environment. When we wish to fixate on them, however, moving objects present a special challenge. Any imprecision in maintaining alignment of the fovea on the moving target degrades the appearance of the image. In the natural environment, the task is complicated by the simultaneous but usually unrelated movement of the viewer and object. The need to maintain high-quality vision despite such "relative movement" is addressed by multiple ocular motor systems that have evolved to meet this challenge. These systems provide a seamless flow for object tracking over a wide range of relative velocities (Table 7-1).

Relatively slow-moving targets (less than 30° per second) are tracked by the *pursuit system.* (Consider that a target moving at this speed would cover one third the distance from the primary position to the far extent of one's temporal visual field in 1 second.) An object moving at this speed can be tracked even if head movements are occurring simultaneously because of the influence of the *vestibular ocular reflexes (VOR),* which produce eye movements in a direction opposite to that of head acceleration. The VOR, however, attenuates fairly quickly (ie, within seconds) during a persistent period of stable head velocity. Any attenuation of the VOR response would reduce the capability of the subject to follow a moving target, which would cause visual blurring. The ability to follow objects over a sustained period of motion is supplemented by the *optokinetic nystagmus (OKN) system,* which uses smooth pursuit to track a moving object but then introduces a saccade in the opposite direction when the maximal amplitude of the pursuit movement is reached or when the speed of the moving object exceeds the maximal velocity of the pursuit system. These vestibular responses can be suppressed by visual fixation on a target (eg, the discomfort of motion sickness can be lessened by visual fixation on a nonmoving target).

Faster-moving targets cannot be tracked by the pursuit system but can be followed by the use of relatively fast, back-to-back eye movements generated by the *saccadic system.* These eye movements, known as *saccades,* are "ballistic" movements—ones that generally cannot be altered once initiated. Relative movement of objects toward or away from us activates one of the *vergence* systems. *Convergence,* which rotates both eyes inward, is activated by relative movement that brings an object closer to us. *Divergence* is activated by movement that produces increasing separation of the object from the viewer.

Table 7-1 Eye Movements

Class	Main Function
Vestibular	Holds retinal image steady during brief head rotation or translation
Visual fixation	Holds stationary object image steady by minimizing ocular drifts
Optokinetic	Holds images steady on the retina during sustained head rotation
Smooth pursuit	Holds target image steady during linear motion of object or self
Nystagmus quick phases	Reset eyes during prolonged rotation to direct gaze toward oncoming scene
Saccades	Rapidly bring object of interest to the fovea
Vergence	Moves the eyes in opposite directions so a single image is simultaneously held on each fovea

Abnormalities in any of these systems may result in degradation of visual acuity, visual blur, oscillopsia, or possibly some degree of motion sickness.

The pursuit, OKN, and saccadic systems are each controlled by different anatomical pathways. However, at the level of the brainstem, the pursuit and saccadic systems share the same supranuclear neurons (including the paramedian pontine reticular formation for horizontal movements and the rostral interstitial nucleus of the medial longitudinal fasciculus for vertical movements), which then innervate the ocular motor cranial nerve nuclei. The anatomical divergence among these pathways makes possible selective disruption of these ocular motor functions by a disease process. Likewise, clinical examination of these systems allows the clinician to appreciate which nervous system components and their anatomy are involved and which can provide important insight into the interpretation of which disease might be responsible for the dysfunction.

Fixation of the fovea onto a target provides the greatest degree of spatial detail. Persistent foveation, however, causes attenuation of neuronal responses in the retina, as described earlier. The degradation of image quality that results is countered by *microsaccadic refixation movements.* These eye movements are continuous, very small amplitude (0.1°– 0.2° of visual angle) "square-waves." The term *square waves* derives from the appearance of eye movement tracings, in which eye movements that are equal in amplitude and speed to the left and right and have a brief intersaccadic interval produce tracings with the shape of square waves (see Chapter 9). The to-and-fro movements are small enough that the image is maintained within the field of the fovea but large enough to provide a constantly changing image to photoreceptors, which enhances perceptual quality. As is true for most saccadic movements, there is a slight pause (180–200 msec) between movements (ie, an intersaccadic interval).

Anatomy and Clinical Testing of the Functional Classes of Eye Movements

Clinical examination of the central eye movement system includes assessment of fixation, VOR, OKN, saccadic and pursuit eye movements, and convergence (see Table 7-1). Each of these movements is controlled by dedicated anatomical pathways, the collective goals of which are to maintain the position of both eyes on targets of interest and to permit accurate eye movements to desired locations in space. Methods of assessing each subsystem are described in the following sections. A complete assessment of ocular motility also requires the search for nystagmus, which is discussed in Chapter 9.

Ocular Stability

Visual fixation is required to hold the image of an object on the fovea. The system maintaining this alignment while an object or person moves is supplemented by the pursuit system. There is evidence that these 2 systems are controlled by separate anatomical pathways, although the structures involved in visual fixation are not well known.

The most straightforward test of ocular stability is performed simply by observing a patient's ability to maintain fixation on a target when the head and body are held stationary.

Testing the patient's ability to fixate on a target may also reveal spontaneous nystagmus, which is most frequently caused by an imbalance of vestibular input to the ocular motor nuclei. Abnormal eye movements that occur secondary to vestibular dysfunction can be suppressed by visual fixation (and will worsen in the absence of visual input; see Chapter 9).

During tasks of viewing an object, fixation is used to suppress any unwanted eye movements. Saccades that are undesirable and that cannot be suppressed by the normal fixation mechanisms are known as *saccadic intrusions;* the most common of these are *square-wave jerks* (which lead the eyes off and then back onto a target with symmetric left and right movements; see Chapter 9). Small movements of this type may be seen in normal individuals, but they are more frequent in patients with *progressive supranuclear palsy (PSP)* and certain cerebellar diseases.

Vestibular Ocular Reflex

The function of the VOR is to hold visual images stably on the retina during *brief, high-frequency* rotations of the head, as routinely occur during walking. VOR responses are driven both by semicircular canals (for angular movements) and by the otoliths of the utricle and saccule (for linear acceleration). Neural activity (excitatory and inhibitory) from these structures passes along the vestibular nerves to the vestibular nuclei in the medulla of the brainstem, which then project to the ocular motoneurons (ie, the vestibular ocular reflex pathway; see Chapter 1, Fig 1-32). The vestibular nuclei are strongly interconnected with the cerebellum, especially the anterior vermis, nodulus, and flocculus. Each of the semicircular canals innervates 1 pair of yoked extraocular muscles, which move the 2 eyes in the same plane as the canal. Each semicircular canal monitors rotational movements in both directions within its plane; these movements are controlled by 2 populations of neurons that show mutually antagonistic activity, depending on the direction of movement. The VOR response attenuates fairly quickly, but a "velocity storage" mechanism provides the VOR with a longer period of influence during more prolonged head movements.

Evidence of VOR dysfunction can be readily elicited on examination. Spontaneous nystagmus is a hallmark of an uncompensated vestibular imbalance. This assessment can be enhanced by clinicians viewing the fundus with a direct ophthalmoscope while looking for repetitive shifts in the position of the optic nerve head. This test is first performed while the fellow eye is allowed to fixate on a target. Then, the effect of removing visual fixation (which is achieved simply by covering the fixating eye) is judged. An increase in nystagmus after removal of visual fixation, while the head and body are held in a stable position, suggests the presence of an uncompensated imbalance of the peripheral vestibular system. A drift of the optic disc to the patient's right (caused by drifting of the eyes to the left) reveals deficient vestibular input from the left vestibular end organ or nerve. (See Vestibular Nystagmus in Chapter 9.)

Horizontal head shaking for 10–15 seconds may induce a transient nystagmus after the head is held stable if there is an asymmetry (in the velocity storage signals) of the vestibular inputs. It is important to prevent the patient from visually fixating during the test, as fixation will suppress vestibular responses. This can be achieved by having the patient close his or her eyes in a dark environment or by using high-plus lenses (+20 D) on a trial frame or *Frenzel goggles* in front of both eyes. After the head shaking is completed, the eye movements should be examined in the still-darkened room with a light held to the side of 1 eye. Head-shaking nystagmus can result from either peripheral or central vestibular lesions.

The VOR *gain* (ie, the ratio of the amplitude of eye rotation to the amplitude of head rotation) can be assessed clinically with the head thrust maneuver or via ophthalmoscopy. The head thrust maneuver requires the clinician to briskly turn the patient's head (small amplitude) while the patient visually fixates on a target with his or her normal correction. The VOR system is the primary system dealing with this type of brief head movement. Normally, if the head is accelerated 10°, the eyes will move exactly 10° in the opposite direction to maintain foveation of a stationary target. Any imbalance in the vestibular gain results in the eyes being off target at the end of the head thrust, and a refixation saccade is required to recapture the target. A defective response is seen when the head is rotated toward the side of the lesion. Perhaps a more sensitive test of VOR gain can be performed by observing the fundus with a direct ophthalmoscope. When visual fixation is available, the pursuit system can maintain stable eye position at head movements up to only 2 Hz. At higher frequencies, as should be used with this testing strategy, the function of the VOR system can be isolated, and any abnormalities of that system will be revealed. A normal gain of 1 would allow the position of the optic nerve head to appear stationary as the head moves. Drifting of the optic nerve head to either the same or opposite side of the head movement reveals a hyper- or hypoactive VOR system, respectively.

Bilateral vestibular loss or hypofunction is easily assessed by measuring visual acuity during head rotations (dynamic visual acuity). While the patient reads the Snellen chart with the proper optical correction, relatively small horizontal head rotations at approximately 2 Hz are performed. Bilateral subnormal VOR gain will produce a mismatch between the amplitude of the eye and head movements, which will cause the intended target to fall off the fovea, and the acuity will fall by several lines (typically 4 or more) in bilateral vestibular loss.

Optokinetic Nystagmus

The OKN system maintains steady alignment of images on the retina during *sustained* rotation of the head (or environment). For approximately 30 seconds, the fluid dynamic properties allow the semicircular canals, via the VOR, to maintain neural output to compensate for head rotation (ie, the rotational-induced VOR will attenuate). Thereafter, the OKN provides a sustained output for eye position control that counters the effects of persistent rotations. Thus, the vestibular and OKN systems act synergistically to align the eyes properly during head rotations. However, the pursuit system, which is driven by visual attention to a target, is more influential in maintaining proper alignment during sustained rotations than the OKN system (which may be more important for this task in animals without foveae). Likewise, pursuit movements also contribute to ocular stability during brief head rotations that primarily activate the VOR.

The initial response of OKN is a pursuit movement, which thus employs the pathways for pursuit movements (described later in the chapter). Thereafter, a contraversive, corrective nystagmus is mediated by the same vestibular neurons that respond to vestibular stimulation, although, as stated earlier, that vestibular input wanes when the driving stimulus is head rotation. Thus, in instances of prolonged visual movement across the retina (eg, as occurs when one is running continuously), the OKN reflex is able to maintain adequate visual fixation even though any vestibular influence from head movement has waned. The integrity of the vestibular neurons can, therefore, be studied without using vestibular stimuli.

Proper OKN testing requires that the moving stimulus fill the complete visual environment and be associated with a brief period of *optokinetic after nystagmus* (OKAN) once the movement ceases; this type of testing can be done only in a specially equipped laboratory. Even then, however, the eye movement responses that are elicited do not "isolate" the OKN system but rather reflect the influence of both the pursuit and OKN systems (voluntary fixation on the moving target drives the pursuit system, whereas the involuntary eye movements induced by the moving stimuli are produced by the OKN system). The rotating drum of black and white stripes that clinicians use in the office, although quite practical, subtends only a portion of the visual field and, in reality, tests only the pursuit and saccade systems.

Saccadic System

The purpose of the saccadic system is to rapidly shift the fovea to targets of interest. Saccades are ballistic movements that generally cannot be altered once initiated. The speed of saccades is correlated with the extent of the eye movement—larger-amplitude saccades are faster than smaller-amplitude saccades, a relationship referred to as the *main sequence*. The velocity of saccades may exceed 500° per second, which allows the eyes to move from primary position to the farthest extent of the temporal visual field in only 0.2 second. Saccadic duration is generally less than 100 msec.

Volitional saccades are controlled by several areas of the cerebral cortex, including premotor zones that project to the *frontal eye fields* (FEFs) (see Chapter 1). The activation of these fields produces conjugate, contralateral saccades. The descending pathways from the FEFs primarily innervate the contralateral paramedian pontine reticular formation but also communicate with several intermediate structures, including the basal ganglia and superior colliculi, which also participate in eye movement control. Eventually, the outflow from the FEF via this network reaches the ocular motoneurons (CNs III, IV, VI), where the speed of eye movements is coded by the frequency of impulses and the amplitude of the eye movements is coded by the duration of the excitation. A consistent correlation exists between the speed and amplitude of saccadic eye movements. Each saccade reflects 2 components of the controlling neural signal—that is, a "pulse" signal followed by a "step" signal (Fig 7-1). The speed of the initial segment of the eye movements is produced by a relatively strong neural output called a *pulse*. The integration of horizontal eye movements to supply the required neural signal to control the eccentric positioning of the eyes (ie, the *step*) is performed by the medial vestibular nucleus and the accessory nucleus of CN XII (known commonly as the *nucleus prepositus hypoglossi*) in the medulla. The supranuclear brainstem center for control of conjugate vertical and torsional eye movements is the *rostral interstitial nucleus of the medial longitudinal fasciculus (riMLF)*, which is located in

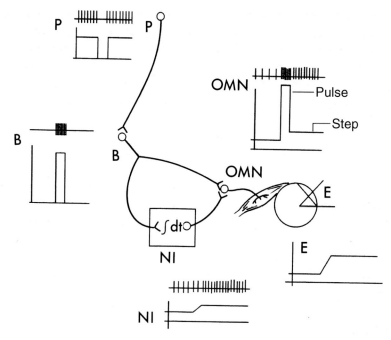

Figure 7-1 The combined influence of the pulse and step signal that contributes to the generation of a saccadic eye movement. This schematic shows the coordination among omnipause
cells *(P)*, burst cells *(B)*, and the cells of the neural integrator *(NI)* in the generation of a saccade. The NI performs an integration of the amount of neural activity required to execute an
eye movement over the duration of time *($\int dt$)*. The omnipause cells cease their discharge just
before the onset of a saccade. At the same time, the burst cells create the pulse that initiates
the saccade. This pulse is received by the NI, which determines the appropriate step needed
to maintain the eccentric position of the eyes. The pulse and step alter the firing of the ocular
motoneurons *(OMN)* that activate an extraocular muscle to execute an eye movement. The
lower right trace *(E)* represents the shift in eye position from baseline to a sustained eccentric
position. *Vertical lines* represent individual discharges of neurons. Underneath each schema-
tized neural (spike) discharge are plots of discharge rate versus time. *(Reproduced with permission
from Leigh RJ, Zee DS. The Neurology of Eye Movements. 3rd ed. Contemporary Neurology Series. New York: Oxford
University Press; 1999.)*

the midbrain. The integration of vertical eye movements to supply the step function that
controls the eccentric positioning of the eyes is performed at the nearby *interstitial nucleus
of Cajal (INC)*. (Note that this structure is the homologue to the accessory nucleus of CN
XII, which performs the integrative function for control of horizontal eye movements.)
Saccades and gaze holding are also strongly influenced by the cerebellum.

Saccades can be tested by having the patient rapidly shift gaze between 2 targets, such
as the extended index fingers of the examiner's outstretched hands, which are held to the
left and right of the patient. The *latency* (duration from stimulus to movement), *accuracy*
(arrival of the eyes on target), *velocity,* and *conjugacy* (degree to which the 2 eyes move
together) of the movements should be monitored. A *hypometric* saccade is one that falls
short of the intended target; 1–2 small catch-up saccades may be within normal limits. A
hypermetric saccade is one that overshoots the target.

Pursuit System

The pursuit system permits clear vision by maintaining foveation on a moving target and similarly provides foveal alignment when a person is moving through his or her environment. The neural substrate that controls pursuit movements at the cerebral level includes, among other areas, the FEF and the middle temporal area (area MT, where neurons preferentially respond to the speed and direction of moving stimuli), the medial superior temporal area (area MST), and the posterior parietal cortex. (Areas MT and MST are part of the *dorsal visual processing stream,* which plays an important role in detecting moving visual stimuli; see Chapter 1, Fig 1-26.) The descending pathways to the pons arise from an area at the confluence of the parietal, temporal, and occipital lobes and then pass through the posterior limb of the internal capsule. At the level of the brainstem, the pursuit system uses some of the same architecture described for saccades (the medial longitudinal fasciculus [MLF] and cranial nerve nuclei, in particular), with the addition of several other pontine nuclei. These nuclei project to the cerebellum, where the paraflocculus plays a role in sustaining pursuit movements.

Pursuit eye movements are tested by having the patient follow a predictably moving target horizontally and then vertically while the head and body are held in position. It is important that the target move relatively slowly, no faster than 30° per second (ie, one third the distance from primary position to the far extent of one's temporal visual field). The latency to initiate the eye movements and the accuracy of following the moving target can be assessed. The gain of the eye movements should be 1—that is, the eyes should accurately follow the slowly moving stimulus. A low gain causes the eyes to lag behind the stimulus, which typically generates a saccade that allows the eyes to catch up to the stimulus.

Vergence

Vergence eye movements drive the eyes in opposite directions to maintain the image of an object on the fovea of both eyes as the object moves toward or away from the observer. Vergence eye movements are driven primarily by a disparity in the relative location of images on the retinas. The cerebral structures that drive vergence movements in primates are not well understood. Binocularly driven cortical cells are selectively responsive to visual position disparity. Brainstem neurons that drive vergence movements are known to be located in the mesencephalic reticular formation, just dorsal to the third nerve nuclei. Convergence is tested with an accommodative target that has enough visual detail to require an effort to see it clearly (a penlight should *not* be used for ocular motor testing because the stimulus is diffuse). Apparent convergence deficiencies may be due to poor patient effort, which may limit clinical usefulness.

Clinical Disorders of the Ocular Motor Systems

Ocular Stability Dysfunction

The stability of ocular fixation may be disrupted by several types of abnormal eye movements known collectively as *saccadic intrusions* (see Chapter 9). These intrusions are of brief duration, quite rapid, and, in most cases, of small amplitude. The most common intrusions are *square-wave jerks (SWJs)*, which lead the eyes off and then back onto the target with symmetric movements (see the earlier discussion). Infrequent SWJs may be seen in normal individuals, especially during smooth pursuit movements and are often quite frequent or near-continuous in patients with PSP and certain diseases.

Square-wave jerks can be distinguished from other types of eye movement abnormalities such as nystagmus by simple clinical observation. They are composed only of fast phases, with no slow phases. Further, SWJs, which can vary in amplitude from 0.5° to >5° (the latter being known as *macrosquare-wave jerks*), are of much smaller amplitude than the eye movements of typical pendular nystagmus; the latter are more sustained and oscillate across a fixation point, whereas the former move the eye off to one side and then back onto fixation after a brief intersaccadic interval. See Chapter 9 for further discussion of saccadic intrusions.

Higher-order cognitive factors, like those evident in patients with dementing illnesses or attention deficit disorder, can confound the determination of whether a true ocular motor instability exists. Poor attention often leads to poor technical scores on automated perimetry, which requires long periods of cognitive focus and attention to a fixation target.

Vestibular Ocular Dysfunction

Eye movement abnormalities develop from either peripheral or central disruption of vestibular activity, although peripheral, end-organ disease of the semicircular canals is by far the most common cause (see Vestibular Ocular Reflex for bedside assessment of the VOR gain). Patients with vestibular disease often have nystagmus, the features of which are discussed in Chapter 9. Peripheral disease can also impair the otolithic organs, which, when disrupted unilaterally, may produce skew deviation or an *ocular tilt reaction* (ie, a combined head tilt, skew deviation, and cyclotorsional rotation of the eyes; Fig 7-2). With an ocular tilt reaction, both the head tilt and cyclotorsion (upper poles of both eyes) rotate away from the hypertropic eye, which is opposite to the normal compensatory rotation that is mediated by the VOR. Otolithic disturbance may also create a sense that the environment is tilted.

Vestibular imbalance is common with lesions of the caudal brainstem (lower pons and medulla) because of disruption to the vestibular nuclei or their interconnections. One of the better known stroke syndromes involving this area is the *lateral medullary syndrome of Wallenberg*. In general, damage to a lateral region of the brainstem disrupts the sensory pathways, and therefore the Wallenberg syndrome is one type of "stroke without paralysis" (see Chapter 2, Fig 2-5). Patients present with ipsilateral loss of pain and temperature sensation over the face (involvement of the descending tract of the fifth cranial nerve), contralateral loss of pain and temperature on the opposite side of the body (involvement of the lateral spinothalamic tract), ipsilateral cerebellar ataxia (damage to spinocerebellar tracts), ipsilateral first-order Horner syndrome, and sometimes the ocular tilt reaction. Patients may have dysarthria, dysphagia, vertigo, or persistent hiccups; there is no extremity weakness. Although the lateral medulla is in the distribution of the posterior

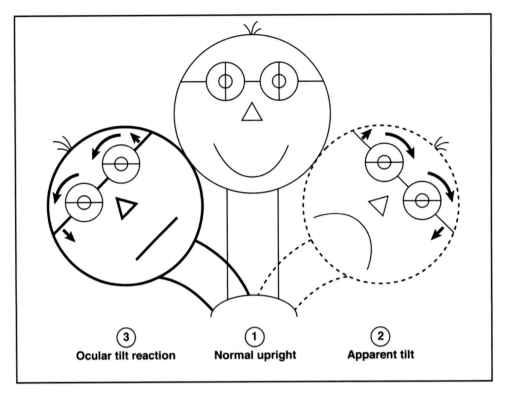

(3)
Ocular tilt reaction

(1)
Normal upright

(2)
Apparent tilt

Figure 7-2 Ocular tilt reaction. The apparent tilt of the environment (2) is compensated for (3) to achieve the appearance of normal upright orientation (1). With the ocular tilt reaction, the upper poles of each eye rotate toward the lower ear. *(Reproduced with permission from Kline L. Neuro-Ophthalmology Review Manual. 6th ed. Thorofare, NJ: Slack; 2008:71. Modified from Brandt T, Dieterich M. Pathological eye-hand coordination in roll: tonic ocular title reaction in mesencephalic and medullary lesions. Brain. 1987;110(Pt 3): 649–666.)*

inferior cerebellar artery, the syndrome usually results from occlusion of the more proximal vertebral artery. Patients with Wallenberg syndrome may experience *lateropulsion*, the sensation of being pulled to one side, which results from damage to the vestibular nuclei. Patients may also manifest *ocular lateropulsion*; this can be tested by examination of horizontal pursuit and saccadic movements, which will reveal a bias that produces hypermetric movements toward the side of the lesion and hypometric movements away from the side of the lesion. This directional bias also can be seen by noticing that the eyes turn toward the side of the lesion after visual fixation is removed for a couple of seconds (by, for instance, having a patient close his or her eyes).

Although an intact VOR is essential for clear viewing of a stationary object during head motion, there are situations when stable foveation depends on the ability to cancel or suppress the VOR. VOR suppression is important when viewing an object that moves with the head. The ability to suppress the VOR can be assessed at the bedside by having the patient fixate on a near card held in his or her outstretched hand while being rotated from side to side in a swivel chair (Fig 7-3). Normal VOR suppression allows the eyes to maintain fixation on the near card during rotation without requiring catch-up saccades;

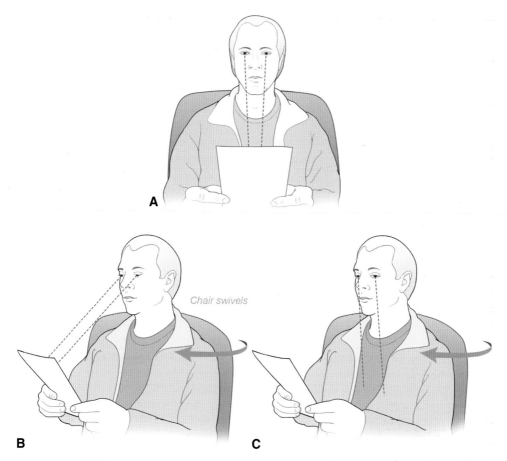

Figure 7-3 Clinical assessment of vestibular ocular reflex suppression. **A,** The patient is seated in a swivel chair, fixating on the letters of a near card held at arm's length. **B,** If VOR suppression is normal (intact), the eyes maintain fixation on the target as the chair, the patient's head and arms, and the card all rotate together as a unit. **C,** Conversely, if VOR suppression is abnormal, the eyes are dragged off the target during rotation due to an inability to cancel the VOR. In this example, the chair is rotated to the patient's right, and the VOR moves the eyes to the patient's left, prompting a rightward saccade to regain the target; this likely indicates right cerebellar system pathology. *(Illustration by Christine Gralapp.)*

impaired VOR suppression is evidenced by the eyes moving off the target during rotation. As directed by the VOR, rotation to the patient's right is met with conjugate eye movement to the patient's left, followed by a corrective saccade rightward, back to the target. Impaired VOR cancellation implies cerebellar disease and is particularly common in multiple sclerosis.

Optokinetic Nystagmus Dysfunction

Optokinetic nystagmus represents the combined response of the optokinetic and smooth pursuit systems. Separation of the optokinetic contribution from the smooth pursuit component of the response generally requires specialized experience or testing equipment. Abnormalities of the smooth pursuit or saccadic components, however, can be recognized by using an OKN drum. Asymmetry of the drum-induced responses can be found with a unilateral lesion of the cerebral pathways that descend from the ipsilateral parietal, middle temporal, or medial superior temporal areas to the brainstem ocular motor centers. An asymmetry of OKN responses produced by rotating the stripes toward the patient's right suggests a lesion in the right cerebrum. Typically, relatively large lesions of the parietal or parietal-occipital cortex are required to produce drum-induced asymmetries; these lesions are usually accompanied by a homonymous hemianopia. A lesion confined to the occipital lobe (eg, as usually occurs secondary to stroke within the distribution of the posterior cerebral artery) also produces a homonymous hemianopia but will not produce OKN asymmetry. Hence, OKN testing can provide clinical insight into the location and extent of a cerebral lesion that produces a homonymous hemianopia.

Saccadic Dysfunction

Saccadic disorders may produce abnormal latency to initiate eye movements, abnormal speed of eye movements (generally slow), or abnormal accuracy of eye movements (hypometria or hypermetria). The specific type of abnormality relates to the pattern of neural activity delivered to the ocular motoneurons. A pattern showing a subnormal peak of activity of the pulse produces slow saccades. A pattern with an inappropriate pulse amplitude produces inaccurate saccades. A drift off an eccentric target is produced by having an insufficient step for a given pulse amplitude. (See Gaze-Evoked Nystagmus in Chapter 9.) Saccadic dysfunction may also produce unwanted saccadic intrusions because of faulty suppression mechanisms, which may disrupt ocular fixation (see Ocular Stability Dysfunction earlier in this chapter and Saccadic Intrusions in Chapter 9).

In some cases, a patient is unable to initiate saccades. Use of the doll's head maneuver can demonstrate if this inability is the result of a supranuclear or infranuclear lesion. In the case of a supranuclear lesion, the doll's head maneuver can excite the vestibular pathways to drive the eyes in a manner that could not be initiated volitionally via descending pathways from the FEFs to the ocular motor nuclei. In other cases, saccades are initiated only after a prolonged period (ie, prolonged latency). Assessment of saccadic latency must take into account the patient's age; a gradual increase in latency may be seen with advancing age. Patients with PSP have slow volitional saccades, especially in the vertical plane, but their *reflexive* saccades (those directed to an unanticipated target, like a ball thrown toward a patient or the fast phases of OKN) often are initially normal. Other central nervous system disorders that cause slow saccades include cerebellar degeneration, Huntington disease, Wilson disease, Whipple disease, and pontine disease.

Central lesions that alter saccadic speed usually produce slower-than-normal saccades; this can also be seen with a variety of peripheral lesions (including nuclear, infranuclear, neuromuscular, or restrictive abnormalities). Peripheral lesions almost always produce slowed movements that are hypometric. In contrast, slow saccades with normal amplitude are typical of central lesions, especially of the cerebral hemispheres or basal ganglia. Wherever the location of a central lesion, ultimately slowed saccades result from lack of activation of the burst neurons or lack of inhibition from the omnipause neurons, both of which are in the paramedian pontine reticular formation. Slowness of saccades confined to the horizontal plane suggests pontine disease. Slowness of saccades confined to the vertical plane suggests dysfunction of the midbrain. In all these cases, there is typically a prolonged latency to initiate the eye movements.

Hypometric saccades can be seen with peripheral or central lesions. Hypermetric saccades are usually the result of disease of the cerebellum or its interconnections. Myasthenia gravis may produce faster-than-normal ("lightning-like") saccades, although these occur only over a reduced range of amplitude.

The accuracy of saccadic eye movements can be difficult to assess in patients with significant bilateral visual loss. Patients with large visual field defects (eg, homonymous hemianopia and bitemporal hemianopia) typically have difficulty directing their eyes accurately toward the abnormal visual field region. In these cases, saccades are essentially always hypometric. Repeated attempts to localize targets often result in improved performance, and thus one must use caution in describing the presence of hypometric saccades in patients with significant visual loss.

The most common saccadic dysfunction is the conjugate limitation of upgaze that is part of normal aging, characterized by eye movements that have reduced range but normal velocity. Although abnormalities of saccadic function are relatively nonspecific with regard to etiology and site of the lesion, there are notable exceptions in which saccadic abnormalities provide important clues to the diagnosis. These include

- discovery of obviously slowed saccades in a patient with extrapyramidal (ie, Parkinson-like) disease syndrome with imbalance and impaired cognition, which suggests a diagnosis of PSP
- presence of hypermetric saccades, which usually indicates disease of the cerebellum or its outflow pathways
- presence of unidirectional hypermetric saccades, ocular lateropulsion, and hypermetric pursuit movements, which are generally seen as part of the lateral medullary syndrome of Wallenberg

Ocular motor apraxia

One of the most extreme instances of saccadic dysfunction is the complete inability to volitionally initiate saccades, which is termed *ocular motor apraxia.* (An *apraxia* is an inability to voluntarily initiate a movement that can be initiated by some other means, usually via a reflex, which reveals that a paralysis is not present.) Patients with *congenital ocular motor apraxia* characteristically use horizontal *head thrusts* past the point of interest, employing the VOR to move the eyes into extreme contraversion until foveation on the target is possible; this is followed by slower head rotation in the opposite direction to primary position while the eyes maintain fixation on the target. Nonvolitional saccades that occur as a reflex to a moving object or sound and vertical eye movements are normal. The location of the lesion that causes congenital ocular motor apraxia is not known but probably is above the brainstem centers that drive volitional saccades. Patients may have other neurologic abnormalities, including delayed development. Also, ocular motor apraxia is associated with several diseases, including ataxia telangectasia, Pelizaeus-Merzbacher disease, Niemann-Pick type C, Gaucher disease, Tay-Sachs disease, Joubert syndrome, abetalipoproteinemia (vitamin E deficiency), and Wilson disease.

Acquired ocular motor apraxia results from bilateral lesions of the supranuclear gaze pathways of the frontal and parietal lobes, usually from bilateral strokes, often as part of an anoxic encephalopathy following cardiac arrest, or post–coronary artery bypass grafting. Patients often blink to break the fixation and then turn their head toward a new point of interest. Bilateral lesions at the parieto-occipital junction may impair the guidance of volitional saccades. Such inaccurate saccades, together with inaccurate arm pointing (ie, a patient may misdirect his or her hand when attempting to shake yours, despite being able to see your hand) and *simultanagnosia* (disordered visual attention that makes it difficult for a patient to perceive all the major features of a visual scene at once), are known as the *Balint syndrome;* this syndrome is often associated with cognitive dysfunction (see Chapter 6).

Cogan DG. Congenital ocular motor apraxia. *Can J Ophthalmol.* 1966;1(4):253–260.

Gaze palsy, gaze preference, and tonic deviations

Gaze palsy is a term used to indicate a symmetric limitation of the movements of both eyes in the same direction (ie, a conjugate ophthalmoplegia). With a cerebral lesion (supranuclear), the term *gaze preference* denotes an acute inability to produce gaze contralateral to the side of the lesion and is accompanied by a tendency for tonic deviation of the eyes toward the side of the lesion. In such cases, the doll's head maneuver generates a full range of horizontal eye movements because the infranuclear pathways are intact. Stroke is the most common etiology for this type of cerebral injury. The eye movement dysfunction is generally temporary, lasting only days or weeks. Presumably, alternative cerebral–bulbar pathways (perhaps from the parietal lobe) become increasingly capable of generating the saccades.

In contrast, brainstem lesions that produce a horizontal gaze palsy disrupt eye movements toward the side of the lesion (opposite to the pattern seen with lesions of the FEF) (Fig 7-4). With pontine lesions (nuclear and infranuclear), the final common site for supranuclear inputs (from volitional, reflex, and vestibular centers) is damaged, and thus the doll's head maneuver is ineffective in driving the paretic eyes. Bilateral pontine injury can abolish all horizontal eye movements. This devastating injury still allows vertical eye movements, which often occur spontaneously (ie, *ocular bobbing;* see Chapter 9).

Congenital horizontal gaze palsy can occur as part of the Möbius syndrome, in which aplasia of the sixth nerve nuclei is accompanied by bilateral facial paresis. A gaze palsy rather than just an ipsilateral limitation in abduction occurs because the sixth nerve nucleus also contains internuclear neurons destined for the contralateral oculomotor nucleus (CN III) via the MLF.

Vertical gaze palsies can manifest as selective limitation of upgaze or downgaze. In either case, the lesion is usually in the midbrain. Limitation of conjugate upgaze occurs with damage to the pretectum, an isthmus between the superior colliculi and the thalamus. Supranuclear fibers decussate through the pretectum as they pass to the riMLF, the midbrain structure that functions as the saccadic generator for vertical eye movements (and thus is the homologue for the paramedian pontine reticular formation for horizontal

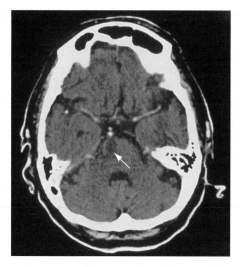

Figure 7-4 Cranial computed tomographic scan of an 82-year-old woman who developed an infarct on the right side of her pons. This infarct, which appears as a low-density lesion that extends to the midline *(arrow)*, damaged the paramedian pontine reticular formation and produced a conjugate gaze palsy to the right. The patient also had a hemiplegia on the left because the lesion extended to the ventral aspect of the pons and damaged the descending corticospinal tract, which decussates farther down the neuraxis. *(Courtesy of Eric Eggenberger, DO.)*

saccades). The *dorsal midbrain syndrome* (also known as the *pretectal* or *Parinaud syndrome;* Fig 7-5) includes

- conjugate limitation of vertical gaze (usually upgaze)
- co-contraction of extraocular muscles, which causes retraction and convergence of the globes (convergence retraction nystagmus)
- mid-dilated pupils with light–near dissociation
- retraction of the lids in primary position *(Collier sign)*
- skew deviation
- disruption of convergence (convergence spasm or convergence palsy)
- increased square-wave jerks

This syndrome often includes only a subset of these signs, although the limitation of conjugate upgaze is the most common feature. Common etiologies of the dorsal midbrain syndrome include mass lesions (especially pineal-based tumors), hydrocephalus, multiple sclerosis, and stroke.

The pretectum is the terminal structure supplied by the arteries of Percheron (small penetrating arteries that arise from the area around the top of the basilar artery; see Chapter 1). Stenosis at the origin of these vessels, disease of the more proximal basilar artery, and entrapment of emboli can all compromise flow through these vessels. Emboli that lodge at the top of the basilar artery can produce efferent and afferent neuro-ophthalmic problems.

Deviation of the eyes may occur with seizures involving any cerebral lobe. Most notably, a lesion of the FEF that causes excess neural activity, like a focal seizure, will drive the

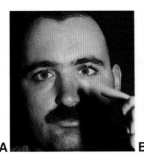 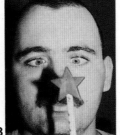 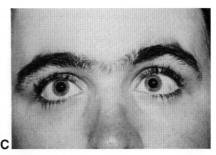

A B C

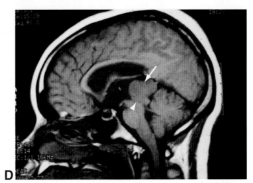

D

Figure 7-5 **A,** A patient with a germinoma pressing on the pretectum shows a poor pupillary light reaction. **B,** The near reaction of the pupils is good. **C,** Attempted upgaze is poorly done. **D,** Magnetic resonance scan showing compression of the dorsal midbrain region *(arrowhead)* by a germinoma *(arrow)* arising from the pineal gland. *(Parts A–C used with permission from Albert DM, Jakobiec FA. Principles and Practice of Ophthalmology. Philadelphia: Saunders; 1994:2476. Part D courtesy of Eric Eggenberger, DO.)*

eyes contralaterally during the period of the seizure. The head also may turn contralateral to the seizure focus during the ictus. In the post-ictal state, when there may be lingering hypoactivity of the FEF neurons, the eyes may deviate ipsilateral to the side of the lesion because of a relative increase in input from the unaffected FEF on the opposite side of the brain.

Transient and conjugate downward or upward ocular deviation may occur in healthy newborns. In these cases, vertical doll's head maneuver can move the eyes out of their tonically held position. Tonic downgaze in premature newborns, however, can be associated with serious neurologic disease, especially when intraventricular hemorrhage expands the third ventricle and impacts on the pretectum. The tonic deviation of the eyes, combined with retraction of the eyelids, is known as the *setting sun sign*; it is primarily seen in children as part of dorsal midbrain syndrome (Parinaud syndrome). Conjugate paresis of upgaze is an associated finding, and in these cases, the doll's head maneuver cannot induce upward movements of the eyes.

Oculogyric crisis is a tonic upward deviation, sometimes directed toward the right or left, that does not disrupt a patient's ability to move the eyes within the involved area. Patients find it difficult to direct their eyes downward. This disorder primarily is seen as an idiosyncratic reaction to neuroleptic drugs, especially the higher-potency antipsychotic drugs like haloperidol and fluphenazine (Prolixin), which are strong dopaminergic-blocking agents. These drugs alter the supranuclear influences onto the ocular motoneurons and thus create a tonic deviation of the eyes. The crisis may persist for hours if not treated. In the early 1900s, patients with postencephalitis parkinsonism often developed oculogyric crisis, but this syndrome is no longer seen. Very occasionally, patients with Wilson disease may develop an oculogyric crisis. Anticholinergic drugs (such as prochlorperazine) promptly stop the eye deviation.

Benjamin S. Oculogyric crisis. In: Joseph AB, Young RR, eds. *Movement Disorders in Neurology and Neuropsychiatry.* 2nd ed. Malden, MA: Blackwell Science; 1999:chap 14.

Caplan LR. "Top of the basilar" syndrome. *Neurology.* 1980;30(1):72–79.

Keane JR. The pretectal syndrome: 206 patients. *Neurology.* 1990;40(4):684–690.

Pursuit Dysfunction

Two main types of pursuit abnormalities occur: low gain and poor initiation. The former is more common because it is commonly seen in older patients without any definable neurologic problem or secondary to a wide range of medications. The subnormal gain results in eye movements that trail behind the target (ie, the motor output is not commensurate with the speed of the moving target), which prompts catch-up saccades to maintain visual fixation. (This combination of too-slow pursuit movements with interposed saccades is often referred to as *cogwheel,* or *saccadic, pursuit.*) Subnormal gain of pursuit eye movements is also common in patients with Parkinson disease and PSP. Deficient ability to initiate smooth pursuit eye movements is seen with relatively large lateralizing lesions of the posterior hemisphere or frontal lobes, or their underlying white matter. In such cases, the pursuit deficit is to the side of the lesion (this can be observed with the OKN drum). Pursuit movements are often poor or absent when made into a blind hemifield. Smooth pursuit deficits are usually found in both horizontal and vertical planes, although the vertical plane may be selectively involved in patients who have bilateral *internuclear ophthalmoplegia* or PSP. Generation of normal smooth pursuit eye movements depends on an adequate effort by the patient and sometimes will improve if more time is taken to assess this capability (ie, if the patient can quickly learn to match the eye movements to a particular speed of a moving target, such as an outstretched finger). The smoothness of pursuit eye movements declines with age (especially over age 60).

Vergence Disorders

Convergence disorders are common; however, bedside examination can be challenging because convergence depends heavily on patient effort. These disorders most commonly are classified as convergence insufficiency, convergence spasm, or divergence insufficiency.

Convergence insufficiency

Many neurologic conditions are associated with impaired convergence, most notably extrapyramidal disorders such as Parkinson disease and PSP. Lesions of the pretectal area may also be associated with convergence insufficiency; however, such lesions are typically accompanied by other features of the dorsal midbrain syndrome. Lesions of the midbrain (within the mesencephalic reticular formation and just dorsal to the third nerve nuclei) may cause convergence insufficiency with normal third nerve function. Closed-head trauma may also nonspecifically produce convergence insufficiency.

Convergence spasm

An excess of convergence tone is most typically seen in younger patients who have an inborn abnormality of convergence (that is, a high accommodative convergence to accommodation [AC/A] ratio, which produces an excessive amount of convergence for a given amount of accommodation) that manifests as an early-onset esotropia (see BCSC Section 6, *Pediatric Ophthalmology and Strabismus*). Isolated bouts of *convergence spasm* are usually not related to organic disease. However, convergence spasm associated with other abnormalities, especially convergence retraction nystagmus and reduced conjugate upgaze (as in the dorsal midbrain syndrome), indicates organic neurologic impairment. Acquired convergence spasm also can be seen in patients with lesions at the junction of the diencephalon and mesencephalon (eg, *thalamic esotropia* due to thalamic hemorrhage) and lower brainstem and cerebellar disorders in association with other signs and symptoms related to lesion location (eg, Wernicke encephalopathy, Arnold-Chiari malformation, multiple sclerosis).

Divergence insufficiency

Divergence insufficiency is an acquired disorder that produces comitant esodeviation that is greater at distance than at near. This disorder is usually benign, but it can be confused with bilateral sixth nerve palsy, although the latter is associated with abnormal speed and amplitude of abducting saccades. Divergence paralysis also may occur as an incipient manifestation of a unilateral sixth nerve palsy or appear in the resolving phase of a sixth nerve palsy; it has also been reported in association with altered intracranial pressure, midbrain tumors, craniocervical junction lesions, or spinocerebellar ataxia. Therefore, divergence paralysis should prompt the same evaluation as for a bilateral or chronic unilateral sixth nerve palsy, including neuroimaging.

CHAPTER 8

The Patient With Diplopia

Diplopia is one of the most common reasons why patients seek ophthalmic care. Substantial insight into the nature of diplopia can be gained from a series of important questions:

- Does the double vision resolve when 1 eye is covered (monocular vs binocular diplopia)?
- Is the double vision the same in all fields of gaze *(comitant)* or does it vary with gaze direction *(incomitant)?*
- Is the double vision horizontal, vertical, or oblique?
- To what extent is diplopia constant, intermittent, or variable?

History

Patients who develop an ocular misalignment may report double vision or may simply report "blurred vision." The cause of blurred vision can often be inferred to result from ocular misalignment (ie, diplopia) if closing 1 eye eliminates the visual disturbance ("binocular blur"). In contrast, monocular diplopia is usually optical but can occasionally be confused with metamorphopsia secondary to a maculopathy.

It is often helpful to determine if double vision is more bothersome at distance or at near or in a particular position of gaze. A history of head or eye pain, numbness, eye or eyelid swelling or redness, or other neurologic symptoms provides clues about possible orbital, cavernous sinus, or central nervous system causes for diplopia. A history of trauma, thyroid disease, or generalized weakness is also helpful in considering a differential diagnosis for diplopia.

Physical Examination

The ability to maintain alignment of the visual axes depends on the coordination of movement of both eyes. External examination may reveal obvious clues of the etiology, especially if proptosis or ocular redness is present. The movement of the eyes should be assessed individually *(ductions)* and together *(versions)*. Eye movement should also be assessed in all positions of gaze, with a comparison made at each point between near and far fixation.

One goal of the physical examination is to establish whether ocular misalignment is comitant or incomitant. The former is a feature often present in congenital strabismus,

215

whereas the latter is evidence of an acquired disorder. Assessment of an ocular misalignment is made by a sequential screening strategy. Abnormal ductions can often be recognized by gross observation, but in most cases, the *alternating cross-cover test* (including measurement of the amount of misalignment), performed at all 9 cardinal positions of gaze, is used to define whether an ocular misalignment is comitant or incomitant.

With a cooperative patient, subtle cases of strabismus may be revealed by using a *red Maddox rod,* which contains a series of parallel cylinders. When viewing a light source through the Maddox rod, a patient sees a line that is perpendicular to the orientation of the cylinders. Traditionally, a red Maddox rod is placed in front of the right eye, producing a red line, while the left eye views the fixation light. Viewing such disparate images often makes it easier for patients to appreciate the misalignment of the visual axes. A red glass can also be used, but this produces a large and somewhat diffuse red light, which frequently makes it more difficult for the patient to perceive misalignment of the images. Because these tests dissociate the 2 eyes, patients who have a phoria may report misalignment of the visual axes. It is therefore often useful to combine the subjective results of Maddox rod testing with the more objective results of the alternating cross-cover test, paying attention to the pattern of misalignment in all 9 positions of gaze. Nevertheless, Maddox rod testing is a sensitive method of obtaining quantitative information about the degree and pattern of ocular misalignment (Fig 8-1).

The double Maddox rod test helps quantify the degree of torsional misalignment. Usually, a red Maddox rod is placed in front of the right eye and a white Maddox rod in front of the left. When both rods are aligned vertically, the patient perceives 2 horizontal lines of light (red line, right eye; white line, left eye) and can judge if the lines are parallel or if 1 line is tilted with respect to the other. In the latter case, the Maddox rod is then rotated in the appropriate direction to quantify the amount of torsional misalignment (Fig 8-2). Discovery of a torsional component to diplopia is not uncommon with

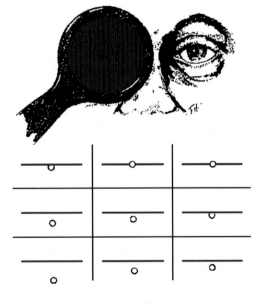

Figure 8-1 Maddox rod with the ridges held vertically causes the patient to see a horizontal line. In this particular case, the light seen by the left eye is under the line, indicating a left hyperdeviation increasing on down right gaze. This finding is compatible with a left superior oblique dysfunction or left fourth nerve palsy.

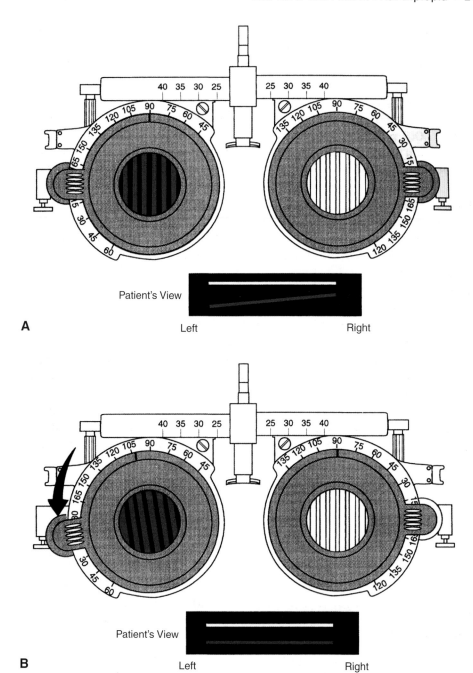

Figure 8-2 **A,** Double Maddox rod test for excyclotorsion. A red Maddox rod *(left)* is placed in front of the right eye and a white Maddox rod in front of the left. A patient with vertical diplopia sees the red line below the white line, indicating a right hypertropia. **B,** With cyclotorsion, the 2 lines are not parallel. The red Maddox rod is then rotated until the 2 lines appear parallel. The degree of rotation required (in this case about 12°) to make the lines parallel quantitates the amount of excyclotorsion. *(Used with permission from Kline LB, Bajandas FJ.* Neuro-Ophthalmology Review Manual. *Rev. 5th ed. Thorofare, NJ: Slack; 2004. Originally modified from Van Noorden GK.* Atlas of Strabismus. *4th ed. St Louis: Mosby; 1983.)*

dysfunction of the vertically acting extraocular muscles, particularly the superior oblique with a fourth nerve palsy.

A qualitative method for detecting relative cyclotropia uses a metal pointer or other straight line. A vertical prism is placed over 1 eye to dissociate the pointer such that 2 vertically displaced lines are visible; then the patient is asked if the 2 lines are parallel ("like railroad tracks") or if they converge to 1 side. A fourth nerve palsy is typically associated with convergence of the lines toward the side of the palsy.

Clues to the presence of ocular deviation may be provided by a consistent head tilt or head turn on examination. Evidence regarding chronicity may exist in old photographs (like that found on a driver's license).

Monocular Diplopia

Monocular optical aberrations may be described as producing distorted or double vision. Monocular diplopia usually results from abnormalities of the refractive media (high astigmatism; corneal irregularity, including keratoconus; and lens opacities) and typically resolves with a pinhole. Less commonly, monocular diplopia results from retinal pathology (eg, maculopathy with distortion of the retina because of fluid, hemorrhage, or fibrosis); cerebral diplopia or polyopia is extremely rare. In contrast to monocular diplopia, binocular diplopia can be relieved by closing either eye, because the diplopia results from misalignment of the visual axes. Occasionally, both monocular and binocular causes of diplopia may be present in the same patient. The demonstration of monocular diplopia effectively obviates the need for a neurologic workup to explain the cause of the diplopia.

Differentiating Paretic From Restrictive Etiologies of Diplopia

Restriction of eye movements should be strongly considered in patients with a history of orbital trauma, eye surgery, or evidence of orbital pathology such as enophthalmos or proptosis. Thyroid eye disease and orbital trauma are the most common causes of restrictive disease; these patients typically have associated orbital signs and symptoms. Patients may have both neural and restrictive components, especially following trauma.

Paretic and restrictive syndromes can be distinguished by the *forced duction test* (Fig 8-3). A restrictive process produces a mechanical limitation of the range of eye movements that can often be felt by an examiner when forceps or a cotton swab is used to advance the limited eye movement. Chronic neural lesions may also, rarely, cause mechanical limitation. This occurs, for example, with a sixth nerve palsy that has been present for many years and is associated with a large-angle esodeviation; over time, the medial rectus may become "tight" (ie, restricted) and limit abduction of the eye.

Ocular restriction, particularly from thyroid eye disease, can also be judged by measuring intraocular pressure in primary position and in eccentric gaze. An increase of ≥5 mm Hg of intraocular pressure in upgaze raises the possibility that this eye movement is being mechanically restricted by a "tight" inferior rectus muscle.

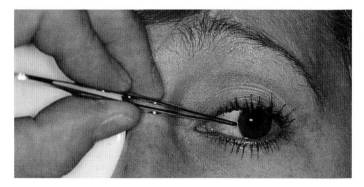

Figure 8-3 Forced duction testing. Before the eye is grasped with forceps, topical proparacaine drops are applied to the eye and held over the limbal region with a cotton tip for 1–2 minutes. This patient has a left esotropia and limited abduction. The conjunctiva is grasped with toothed forceps and the globe passively rotated in the direction of limited abduction to assess for restriction of the eye movement. *(Used with permission from Yanoff M, Duker JS, eds.* Ophthalmology. *2nd ed. St Louis: Mosby; 2004:569, fig 70-12.)*

Comitant and Incomitant Deviations

Comitant misalignment is characteristically found in patients with congenital or early-onset strabismus. These patients typically do not report diplopia because of *suppression,* an adaptation that reduces the responsiveness of the visual neurons in the occipital cortex to the input from 1 eye. Suppression is often associated with amblyopia but may occur in patients with normal acuity in both eyes, especially in patients with an alternating exodeviation. Patients with a history of childhood strabismus may develop diplopia later in life, when the degree of ocular misalignment changes. Patients with a long-standing exophoria, for example, may develop horizontal diplopia in their fifth decade of life when accommodation and convergence capacities wane.

Conversely, a long-standing incomitant deviation may become comitant with the passage of time. This "spread of comitance" is related to a gradual resetting of the innervation to yoke muscles of each eye. This apparent violation of Hering's law, which is probably mediated at a cerebellar level, produces an adjustment of the gain of the neural input signal to individual extraocular muscles. Spread of comitance may occur with either a restrictive or paretic incomitant deviation, especially with a fourth nerve palsy.

Incomitant strabismus is most frequently acquired and usually causes diplopia (Fig 8-4). If the deviation is very small, fusional amplitudes may eliminate the diplopia. Relatively small misalignments may produce blurred vision rather than an obvious perception of 2 images. Patients with subnormal acuity may not recognize diplopia or may have difficulty providing details of how the visual precept changes in various positions of gaze. Incomitant deviations that are congenital, such as overaction of the inferior oblique muscles, typically do not cause diplopia, even when the strabismus is quite obvious. One generally cannot distinguish with confidence by gross observation alone whether subnormal ductions are secondary to a neural or to a restrictive process.

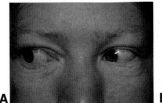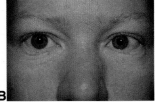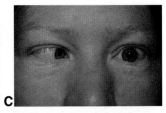

Figure 8-4 Left sixth cranial nerve palsy. **A,** In right gaze, the eyes are aligned. **B,** In straight-ahead gaze, the left eye is inwardly deviated. **C,** In left gaze, the left eye does not abduct, causing a marked misalignment of the eyes. *(Used with permission from Trobe JD.* The Physician's Guide to Eye Care. *3rd ed. San Francisco: American Academy of Ophthalmology; 2006:118. Image courtesy of W. K. Kellogg Eye Center, University of Michigan.)*

Localization

The clinician should attempt to localize the site of neural damage that produces an eye movement disorder. This localization will dictate patient evaluation, including imaging modality and differential diagnosis. Initially, conceptualize the anatomical pathway of the cranial nerve or nerves that are assumed to be involved (Fig 8-5). This "wiring diagram" concept takes into account supranuclear, internuclear, nuclear, and ocular motor nerve fascicles within the brainstem, which then traverse the subarachnoid space, cavernous sinus, superior orbital fissure, and orbit, ending in the neuromuscular junction of the extraocular muscle. In general, a lesion that involves the ocular motor cranial nerves within the brainstem typically damages other structures, such as a "long tract" (eg, the corticospinal and spinothalamic pathways), which produces deficits other than ophthalmoparesis. Current neuroimaging has revealed cases of clinically isolated (ie, no other clinically evident problems can be detected) sixth or third nerve palsy produced by a central lesion, such as a small stroke or a demyelinating plaque. In general, however, such isolated cranial neuropathies are the exception and not the rule for central lesions.

Methods for localizing lesions when the "wiring diagram" approach is not applicable include "common denominators" (structures the involved cranial nerves have in common, such as dura in meningeal-based diseases) and "pattern recognition" (eg, the Wernicke triad of ophthalmoplegia, ataxia, and mental status change is often more useful than anatomical localization of periaqueductal anatomy). In general, the more specific patterns of ocular misalignment concern nuclear, infranuclear, and internuclear dysfunction, but the clinician should always keep in mind potential mimics, including restrictive/myopathic and neuromuscular junction dysfunction (eg, myasthenia gravis).

Supranuclear Causes of Diplopia

The supranuclear pathway for eye movement control includes any afferent input to the ocular motor nerves (CNs III, IV, VI). The most important supranuclear pathways are those that drive volitional eye movement—that is, the corticobulbar pathways that are used, for

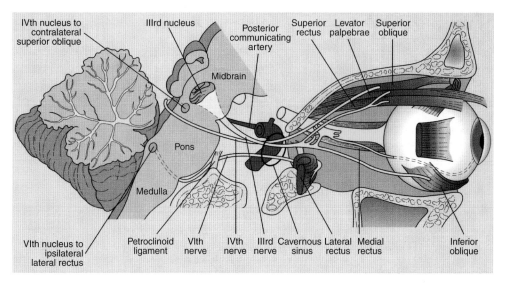

Figure 8-5 Anatomical substrate for localizing lesions of the infranuclear ocular motor pathways. This is a lateral view of CNs III, IV, and VI from the brainstem nuclei to the orbit. A sequential consideration of these pathways could begin either within the brainstem or within the orbit. The cranial nerve segments within the brainstem are often referred to as being "intramedullary." The subarachnoid space lies between the brainstem and cavernous sinus. The third nerve exits the midbrain anteriorly, crosses near the junction of the internal carotid and posterior communicating artery in the subarachnoid space, and enters the cavernous sinus, where it runs in the lateral wall. The fourth nerve exits the midbrain posteriorly and crosses to the opposite side; it then courses through the subarachnoid space and into the cavernous sinus. The sixth nerve exits the pons anteriorly, ascends along the clivus, crosses the petrous apex, and passes below the petroclinoid ligament to enter the cavernous sinus, where it runs between the lateral wall and the carotid artery. *(Used with permission from Yanoff M, Duker JS, eds.* Ophthalmology. *2nd ed. St Louis: Mosby; 2004:1324, fig 199-1.)*

example, to follow the command "Look to the right"—and the vestibular input to adjust the relative position of the eyes within the head. The vestibular input not only alters eye movements with respect to movements of the body but also changes the eye movements depending on the position of the head when the eye movement is initiated. For instance, if you were to initiate saccades to look at someone who was 45° to your right, the distance your eyes would have to move would depend on whether you were looking straight ahead or in some other direction. The distance of the horizontal eye movement is controlled by the selection of particular populations of neurons in the paramedian pontine reticular formation (PPRF). The vestibular system analyzes the relative position of your head and the direction of the intended visual target and makes the correct choice of which neurons to activate to drive the saccadic eye movements.

Typically, disruption of supranuclear pathways symmetrically limits the movements of both eyes. Hence, patients usually do not experience diplopia. An example of a supranuclear disruption of eye movements is seen in patients with dorsal midbrain syndrome in which neither eye is able to look upward (conjugate limitation of upgaze). However, certain supranuclear lesions can also produce misalignment and diplopia (Table 8-1).

Table 8-1 Supranuclear Ocular Motor Lesions That Produce Strabismus and Diplopia

Skew deviation
Alternating skew deviation
Ocular tilt reaction
Thalamic esodeviation
Convergence insufficiency or spasm
Divergence insufficiency

Skew Deviation

Skew deviation is an acquired vertical misalignment of the eyes resulting from asymmetric disruption of supranuclear input from the otolithic organs (the utricle and saccule of the inner ear, both of which contain otoliths, which are tiny calcium carbonate crystals). These organs sense linear motion and static tilt of the head via gravity and transmit information to the vertically acting ocular motoneurons, as well as to the *interstitial nucleus of Cajal (INC)*, all of which are in the midbrain.

Both peripheral and central lesions can produce skew deviation. Central causes of skew deviation are more common and can occur anywhere within the posterior fossa (brainstem and cerebellum). Skew deviation can be comitant or incomitant, and torsional abnormalities may be present. At times it may be difficult to distinguish some presentations of skew deviation from a fourth nerve palsy, and proper use of the Parks-Bielschowsky 3-step test (discussed later in the chapter) is essential. Skew deviation often produces diplopia and is an important exception to the general rule that supranuclear lesions do not produce double vision.

An *alternating skew deviation on lateral gaze* usually manifests as hypertropia of the abducting eye (ie, right hypertropia on right gaze) that switches when gaze is directed to the opposite side (ie, becomes left hypertropia on left gaze). Responsible lesions are located in the cerebellum, cervicomedullary junction, or dorsal midbrain. This disorder must be distinguished from bilateral fourth nerve palsies, which differ in that they produce a hyperdeviation that increases on gaze to the opposite side (eg, right hypertropia is larger on gaze to the left), in addition to excyclotropia.

Ocular tilt reaction is a combination of a head tilt, skew deviation, and cyclotorsional abnormalities of both eyes that can occur in tonic or, rarely, in paroxysmal fashion. This syndrome typically develops because of loss of otolithic input to the INC from a central lesion, which may be in the medulla, pons, or midbrain. Such a lesion can alter one's sense of true vertical, which in turn drives the head and rotates the eyes toward the same side in a compensatory response to correct to true vertical (see Chapter 7, Fig 7-1).

With an ocular tilt reaction, if the head is tilted to the left, the right eye is hypertropic, and the upper poles of both eyes rotate toward the lower ear. The opposite response of the eyes is present if the head tilt is to the right. The changes in head and eye position of an ocular tilt reaction should be distinguished from those of a normal response of head tilting as well as from those of a fourth nerve palsy; the normal ocular reflexes induced by tilting the head cause both eyes to rotate toward the higher ear (counterrolling), whereas the ocular tilt reaction causes the opposite response. With a fourth nerve palsy, the compensatory head tilt is typically contralateral to the side of the hypertropia (similar to ocular tilt reaction), but the higher eye is extorted—opposite the pattern of an ocular tilt reaction. Thus, in establishing the diagnosis of ocular tilt reaction, one must attend to both head position and ocular cyclotorsion.

Periodic alternating skew is a rare disorder producing alternating hypertropia, typically with a 30–60 second periodicity, indicative of a midbrain lesion.

Donahue SP, Lavin PJ, Hamed LM. Tonic ocular tilt reaction simulating a superior oblique palsy: diagnostic confusion with the 3-step test. *Arch Ophthalmol*. 1999;117(3):347–352.

Thalamic Esodeviation

Thalamic esodeviation is an acquired horizontal strabismus that may be seen in patients with lesions near the junction of the diencephalon and midbrain, most often thalamic hemorrhage. The esodeviation may develop insidiously or acutely and, in the case of expanding tumors, may be progressive. It is especially important to consider the possibility of a central nervous system lesion in children who are being evaluated for strabismus surgery.

Vergence Dysfunction

See Vergence Disorders in Chapter 7.

Nuclear Causes of Diplopia

The third nerve nucleus is actually a nuclear complex that contains subnuclei for 4 extraocular muscles (superior, inferior, and medial recti, and inferior oblique), a single subnucleus for the levator palpebrae muscles (central caudal nucleus), and paired subnuclei for the pupillary constrictor muscles (Edinger-Westphal nuclei) (see Chapter 1). Because the single central caudal nucleus controls both levator palpebrae muscles, and the superior rectus fascicles decussate just after emerging from their subnuclei, lesions of the third nerve nuclear complex affect (ptosis) or spare the eyelids and may bilaterally affect the superior rectus muscles. Injury to the third nerve nuclear complex is uncommon but may occur secondary to reduced perfusion through a small, paramedian-penetrating blood vessel, causing unilateral damage to 1 nuclear complex; such lesions are often asymmetric and affect the oculomotor nerve fascicle on one side in addition to the nucleus.

Intraparenchymal lesions of the fourth cranial nerve (either nuclear or intra-axial) are rare, given the relatively short course of this nerve within the brainstem. A lesion of the trochlear nucleus is clinically identical to a fascicular lesion. Microvascular or inflammatory lesions may nonetheless involve the central course of the fourth nerve. On occasion, a fourth nerve palsy may be accompanied by a contralateral Horner syndrome (first-order neuron lesion) because of the proximity of the descending sympathetic pathway. A selective lesion of the sixth nerve nucleus causes a horizontal gaze palsy and not an isolated abduction paresis in 1 eye, and thus patients may not experience diplopia. This situation arises because the sixth nerve nucleus contains 2 populations of neurons: those that innervate (1) the ipsilateral lateral rectus muscle and (2) the internuclear motoneurons, which travel via the medial longitudinal fasciculus to innervate the contralateral medial rectus subnucleus of the oculomotor nuclear complex.

Internuclear Causes of Diplopia

In the context of eye movement control, an "internuclear" lesion is one that disrupts the *medial longitudinal fasciculus (MLF)*, a bundle of fibers that connect the sixth nerve nucleus on one side of the pons to the medial rectus subnucleus (of the third nerve) on the contralateral side of the midbrain (see Chapter 1, Fig 1-29). This type of lesion produces an *internuclear ophthalmoplegia (INO)*.

The cardinal feature of a unilateral INO is slowed adducting saccadic velocity in 1 eye. This limitation is usually associated with nystagmus of the abducting eye. The eye with the slowed adduction may have limited or a full range of adducting movement (Fig 8-6). Convergence may be spared or disrupted. A skew deviation, often with a hyperdeviation ipsilateral to the lesion, may be present. By convention, the INO is named for the side of limited adduction. That is, a right INO is one that limits adduction of the right eye secondary to a lesion of the MLF on the right side of the brainstem. Although patients with INO may report horizontal diplopia, they may also experience vertical-oblique diplopia due to an associated skew deviation, episodic diplopia related to head–eye movements if the lesion is partial, or difficulty tracking fast-moving objects (especially, for instance, when playing tennis) because of the mismatch in saccadic velocity between the eyes.

A bilateral INO produces bilateral adduction lag, bilateral abducting nystagmus, and *vertical, gaze-evoked nystagmus* that is best appreciated in upgaze. This nystagmus is due

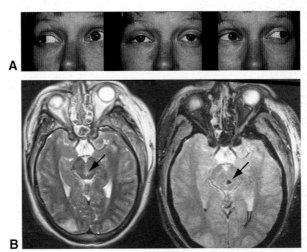

Figure 8-6 Left internuclear ophthalmoplegia. **A,** This 35-year-old woman had slowed adduction of the left eye and an increasing exodeviation on gaze right. **B,** T2-weighted *(left)* and T2*-weighted *(right)* axial MRIs demonstrate signal abnormality *(arrows)* in the left MLF within the midbrain. *(Part A courtesy of Steven A. Newman, MD; part B courtesy of Joel Curé, MD.)*

to disruption of vertical vestibular pursuit and gaze-holding commands, which ascend from the vestibular nuclei through the MLF. A large-angle exodeviation may occur in bilateral INO (ie, the "wall-eyed" bilateral INO, or *WEBINO,* syndrome) and is often caused by a midbrain lesion near the third nerve nuclei; Fig 8-7).

Davis SL, Frohman TC, Crandall CG, et al. Modeling Uhthoff's phenomenon in MS patients with internuclear ophthalmoparesis. *Neurology.* 2008;70(13 pt 2):1098–1106.

McGettrick P, Eustace P. The W.E.B.I.N.O. syndrome. *Neuro-Ophthalmology.* 1985;5(2): 109–115.

Mills DA, Frohman TC, Davis SL, et al. Break in binocular fusion during head turning in MS patients with INO. *Neurology.* 2008;71(6):458–460.

The two most common causes of INO are demyelination and stroke. In adolescents and younger adults, INO is typically caused by demyelination. In older adults, microvascular disease is the most common cause. Myasthenia gravis can produce pseudo-INO; this scenario usually lacks the vertical gaze-evoked nystagmus of a true INO and is often accompanied by myasthenic eyelid signs. The adduction paresis of myasthenic pseudo-INO may transiently resolve following IV edrophonium (Tensilon test) and typically responds to appropriate systemic therapy.

One-and-a-Half Syndrome

The *one-and-a-half syndrome* shares the features of a unilateral INO, plus it shows ipsilateral horizontal gaze palsy to the same side as the lesion (Fig 8-8). This syndrome is caused by a pontine abnormality that is large enough to involve the MLF and the PPRF (or the

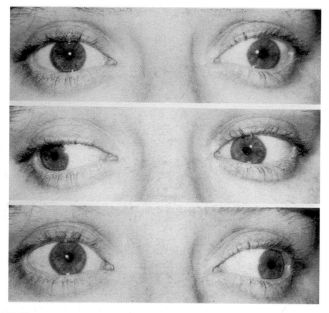

Figure 8-7 WEBINO syndrome. Exotropia in primary position *(top)* associated with impaired adduction of both the left *(middle)* and right *(bottom)* eyes. *(Courtesy of Lanning B. Kline, MD.)*

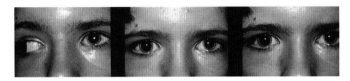

Figure 8-8 One-and-a-half syndrome. This 15-year-old patient had a brainstem glioma that caused a gaze palsy to the left *(right photograph)* and a left internuclear ophthalmoplegia (evident here as incomplete adduction of the left eye on gaze to the right; *left photograph*). The only horizontal eye movement was abduction of the right eye. *(Courtesy of Steven A. Newman, MD.)*

sixth nerve nucleus) on the same side of the brainstem. The only remaining horizontal eye movement is abduction of the eye contralateral to the lesion (horizontal eye movements are lost in 1 eye, whereas they are "half" lost in the fellow eye, hence the name); vertical gaze is preserved. A lesion producing the one-and-a-half syndrome but also involving the intra-axial portion of the facial nerve is termed the *eight-and-a-half syndrome* (7 + 1.5 = 8.5); familiarity with brainstem anatomy allows accurate localization of the various syndromic combinations. Stroke is the most common cause of this disorder.

Espinosa PS. Teaching NeuroImage: one-and-a-half syndrome. *Neurology.* 2008;70(5):e20.

Frohman TC, Galetta S, Fox R, et al. Pearls & Oy-sters: the medial longitudinal fasciculus in ocular motor physiology. *Neurology.* 2008;70(17):e57–e67.

Wall M, Wray SH. The one-and-a-half syndrome—a unilateral disorder of the pontine tegmentum: a study of 20 cases and review of the literature. *Neurology.* 1983;33(8):971–980.

Infranuclear Causes of Diplopia

Intra-axial *(fascicular)* ocular motor nerve palsies are due to lesions of the nerve distal to its nucleus but within the confines of the brainstem. Brainstem lesions tend to impact many structures and therefore produce multiple deficits, which allows accurate topographic localization of the lesion. At the level of the midbrain, intra-axial lesions can damage either the third or fourth nerve. Intra-axial involvement of the fascicle of the third nerve can produce 1 of 4 syndromes, each of which causes an ipsilateral third nerve palsy. Damage to the ventral midbrain can damage the cerebral peduncle and cause a contralateral hemiparesis *(Weber syndrome)*. Involvement of the red nucleus and substantia nigra may produce contralateral ataxia and/or tremor *(Benedikt syndrome)*. Damage to the dorsal midbrain may involve the superior cerebellar peduncle and produce contralateral ataxia *(Claude syndrome)*. A dorsal lesion with a slightly different configuration can produce the same type of ataxia plus a third nerve nuclear lesion and features of supranuclear eye movement dysfunction *(Nothnagel syndrome)*. The localization and direct anatomical correlation of these lesions is more important than the eponym, especially because use and definitions of these eponyms have varied in the literature.

Liu GT, Crenner CW, Logigian EL, Charness ME, Samuels MA. Midbrain syndromes of Benedikt, Claude, and Nothnagel: setting the record straight. *Neurology.* 1992;42(9):1820–1822.

As mentioned earlier, involvement of the fourth cranial nerve within the brainstem is uncommon. Pineal tumors may compromise the proximal course of both fourth nerves by compressing the tectum of the midbrain. Such lesions may also obstruct the Sylvian aqueduct, leading to elevated intracranial pressure and hydrocephalus (often producing the dorsal midbrain syndrome).

Intra-axial lesions of the sixth cranial nerve that involve its nucleus may also injure the seventh cranial nerve, whose fibers swing around the sixth nerve nucleus at the *facial genu*. Intra-axial lesions that involve the fascicle of the sixth nerve may also damage the fascicle of the seventh nerve, the tractus solitarius, and the descending tract of the trigeminal nerve, which produces an ipsilateral abduction palsy, facial weakness, loss of taste over the anterior two thirds of the tongue, and facial hypoesthesia, respectively *(Foville syndrome)*. Lesions of the ventral pons can damage the sixth and seventh nerves along with the corticospinal tract, which produces contralateral hemiplegia and ipsilateral facial nerve palsy and abduction deficit *(Millard-Gubler syndrome)*.

Gates P. The rule of 4 of the brainstem: a simplified method for understanding brainstem anatomy and brainstem vascular syndromes for the non-neurologist. *Intern Med J.* 2005; 35(4):263–266.

Wolf JK, ed. *The Classical Brainstem Syndromes.* Springfield, IL: Charles C Thomas; 1971.

The subarachnoid segment of the ocular motor nerves extends from the brainstem to the cavernous sinus, where the nerves exit the dura, and it is within this section that most ischemic cranial nerve palsies are thought to occur. The diagnosis of ischemic (microvascular or diabetic) ocular motor nerve palsies is one of exclusion. Ischemic cranial mononeuropathies typically occur in isolation and with maximal deficit at presentation; however, occasionally the loss of function progresses over 7–10 days. Pain may or may not be present and, if present, may be quite severe in some patients; pain does not distinguish benign from more serious causes.

The oculomotor nerve is a special case of isolated cranial mononeuropathy due to its close anatomical proximity to the cerebral vasculature (especially the posterior communicating artery) and potential for aneurysmal compression (see later in the chapter). Ocular misalignment due to ischemic ocular motor palsy always improves, and diplopia usually resolves within 3 months.

Progression of ocular misalignment beyond 2 weeks or failure to improve within 3 months is inconsistent with this cause of cranial neuropathy and should prompt a thorough evaluation for another etiology. Risk factors include diabetes mellitus, hypertensive vascular disease, and elevated serum lipids. Hence, these patients require a medical evaluation for vasculopathic risk factors.

Myasthenia gravis may mimic any pattern of painless, pupil-sparing extraocular motor dysfunction and should be kept in the differential diagnosis of such cases.

Asbury AK, Aldredge H, Hershberg R, et al. Oculomotor palsy in diabetes mellitus: a clinico-pathological study. *Brain.* 1970;93(3):555–566.

Jacobson DM, McCanna TD, Layde PM. Risk factors for ischemic ocular motor palsies. *Arch Ophthalmol.* 1994;112(7):961–966.

Richards BW, Jones FR Jr, Younge BR. Causes and prognosis in 4,278 cases of paralysis of the oculomotor, trochlear, and abducens cranial nerves. *Am J Ophthalmol.* 1992;113(5): 489–496.

Third Nerve Palsy

Third nerve palsies can cause dysfunction of the somatic muscles (superior, inferior, and medial recti; inferior oblique; and levator palpebrae superioris) and the autonomic (pupillary sphincter and ciliary) muscles. Patients with a complete third nerve palsy present with complete ptosis, with the eye positioned downward and outward and unable to adduct, infraduct, or supraduct, and a dilated pupil that responds poorly to light (Fig 8-9). Partial third nerve palsies are more common and present with variable limitation of upward, downward, or adducting movements; ptosis; or pupillary dysfunction.

Most isolated unilateral third nerve palsies result from (presumed) microvascular injury in the subarachnoid space or cavernous sinus. Occasionally, isolated third nerve palsies may occur due to brainstem lesions such as microvascular infarct. Less common causes include aneurysmal compression, tumor, inflammation (sarcoidosis), vasculitis, infection (meningitis), infiltration (lymphoma, carcinoma), and trauma.

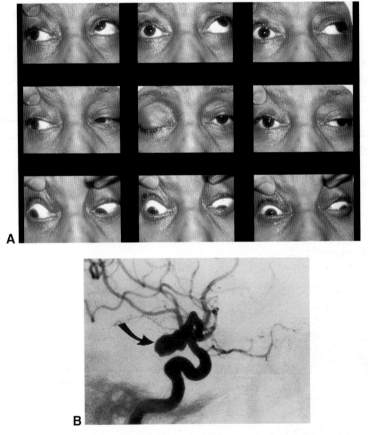

Figure 8-9 Complete third nerve palsy. This 62-year-old woman developed "the worst headache of my life." **A,** The examination revealed complete ptosis on the right; a nonreactive, dilated pupil; and severely limited extraocular movement except for abduction. **B,** Lateral view of a cerebral angiogram demonstrated a posterior communicating artery aneurysm *(arrow).*
(Part A courtesy of Steven A. Newman, MD; part B courtesy of Leo Hochhauser, MD.)

Pupil-involving third nerve palsy

Pupillary dysfunction with third nerve palsy results from loss of parasympathetic input, which produces a dilated pupil that responds poorly to light. Patients may present with a wide range of associated dysfunction, including dysfunction in the levator palpebrae and extraocular muscles. Aneurysms that arise at the junction of the posterior communicating and internal carotid arteries are juxtaposed to the third cranial nerve and are, therefore, in a position to produce a third nerve palsy with pupillary involvement as the initial manifestation of an expansion or rupture.

The pupillomotor fibers of the oculomotor nerve reside superficially in the medial aspect of the nerve adjacent to the posterior communicating artery, a common site for aneurysm formation. Thus, a nontraumatic third nerve palsy with pupillary involvement or evidence of progression to pupillary involvement must be assumed to be secondary to an aneurysm until proven otherwise. Such aneurysms are most commonly at the junction of the posterior communicating and internal carotid arteries, a location in close proximity to the third cranial nerve. Prompt neuro-ophthalmologic consultation and angiography (catheter angiography, MRA, or CTA, depending on clinical details) should be obtained (Fig 8-10). Almost all aneurysms at this location producing a third nerve palsy can be detected by these angiographic tests. CTA and MRA can reliably detect aneurysms as small as 2–3 mm in diameter under ideal circumstances. CTA is faster and provides slightly greater resolution and also may provide evidence of a subarachnoid hemorrhage. Lumbar puncture may yield evidence of a hemorrhage (xanthochromia of the spinal fluid) or detect an inflammatory or neoplastic cause when neuroimaging is normal. Aneurysms are uncommon before age 20 years, although, rarely, they may present as early as the first decade of life. Despite advances in noninvasive neuroimaging techniques, catheter angiography remains the "gold standard" in detecting intracranial aneurysms.

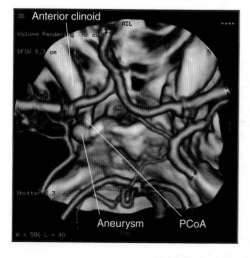

Figure 8-10 CTA demonstrating an aneurysm of the posterior communicating artery (PCoA). *(Courtesy of Michael Vaphiades, DO.)*

Pupil-sparing third nerve palsy

The term *pupil-sparing* should be reserved for situations in which there is normal pupillary function but complete loss of eyelid and ocular motor (somatic) functions of the third nerve. This is the typical finding of an ischemic cranial neuropathy, often associated with pain, which improves (and usually fully resolves) within 3 months.

A complete third nerve palsy with sparing of the pupil is almost always benign and secondary to microvascular disease, often associated with diabetes, hypertension, and/or hyperlipidemia. It is not uncommon, however, for the pupil to react normally and for there to be only minimal impairment of levator palpebrae and extraocular function (a partial third nerve palsy). Although the pupil is normal in this scenario, it should not be considered in the same category as pupil-sparing with otherwise complete oculomotor paresis, given that many other fibers within the third cranial nerve are also "spared." This distinction is crucial given that some proportion of partial third nerve palsies with normal pupillary function are related to compressive lesions and may later progress to involve the pupil. Management of a partial third nerve palsy without pupillary involvement must be individualized based on the demographics, historical features, and availability of accurate noninvasive imaging modalities. Some clinicians favor noninvasive imaging; others advocate close, frequent observation each day or so for 7–10 days. An aneurysm should be suspected even with a seemingly benign pupil-sparing third nerve palsy if the patient is within the high-risk age for developing an aneurysm (between 20 and 50 years) and does not have diabetes mellitus or other vascular risk factors.

Pupil dysfunction or a progressive loss of function does not always indicate the presence of an aneurysm or other serious problem. The vasculopathic form of oculomotor nerve palsy may produce some efferent pupillary defect in up to 20% of cases, although the pupillary involvement is generally mild (typically ≤ 1 mm anisocoria). Discovery of an elevation in fasting blood sugar, hemoglobin A_{1c}, serum lipids, or blood pressure would increase the probability that microvascular ischemia is the cause of the third nerve palsy, but patients with these risk factors may also harbor aneurysms. Thus, pupillary involvement or progression should prompt neuroimaging in search of an aneurysm.

Conversely, a patient who presents only with efferent pupillary dysfunction (ie, the pupil is dilated and responds poorly to light) and who has normal eyelid and extraocular muscle function almost always has a benign disorder. Such isolated pupillary involvement is not a form of third nerve palsy but rather represents either a tonic (Adie) pupil, a pharmacologically dilated pupil, or a pupil that is mechanically damaged (as may occur with posterior synechiae). The clinician must exclude minor degrees of incomitant strabismus (by careful alternate cover testing or by Maddox rod testing in all positions of gaze) to exclude subtle findings of a third nerve palsy before concluding that the problem is limited to the pupil. Tentorial herniation is not a plausible explanation for an isolated, fixed, and dilated pupil in the absence of an altered mental status or other neurologic abnormalities.

The presence of head and periorbital pain is not helpful in establishing the cause of the third nerve palsy. Although most third nerve palsies caused by aneurysms present with pain, many vasculopathic palsies also produce pain that, in some cases, may be intense. In older adults, vasculitis (eg, giant cell arteritis) must also be considered.

Jacobson DM. Relative pupil-sparing third nerve palsy: etiology and clinical variables predictive of a mass. *Neurology.* 2001;56(6):797–798.

O'Connor PS, Tredici TJ, Green RP. Pupil-sparing third nerve palsies caused by aneurysm. *Am J Ophthalmol.* 1983;95(3):395–397.

An acute, isolated, pupil-sparing but otherwise complete third nerve palsy in a patient over 50 years with appropriate vascular risk factors does not necessarily require neuroimaging but should prompt a general medical evaluation, with attention to serum glucose levels, systemic blood pressure, serum lipids, and a sedimentation rate. If and when progression occurs, if other cranial neuropathies develop, or if the expected recovery does not ensue within 3 months, then neuroimaging should be obtained to search for a mass or infiltrative lesion at the base of the skull or within the cavernous sinus. Occasionally, scans need to be repeated to discover a mass, especially if it is contained within the cavernous sinus. Lumbar puncture may be needed to detect carcinomatous meningitis, inflammation, or infection.

Jacobson DM, Broste SK. Early progression of ophthalmoplegia in patients with ischemic oculomotor nerve palsies. *Arch Ophthalmol.* 1995;113(12):1535–1537.

Trobe JD. Managing oculomotor nerve palsy. *Arch Ophthalmol.* 1998;116(6):798.

Divisional third nerve palsy

The third nerve divides into a superior and an inferior division at the superior orbital fissure or within the cavernous sinus. Isolated involvement of either division usually indicates a lesion of the anterior cavernous sinus or possibly the posterior orbit. The initial diagnostic study of choice is MRI. If neuroimaging is normal, then medical evaluation is warranted, including blood pressure determination, assessment of blood sugar level (glucose determination, hemoglobin A_{1c}), serum lipids, and Westergren sedimentation rate. Rarely, a divisional third nerve palsy may be secondary to brainstem disease, usually from small-vessel stroke (lacunae) or demyelination. Aneurysms are a much less common but potentially lethal cause of divisional third nerve palsy. Rare additional causes include tumors, inflammation (sarcoidosis, vasculitis), infection (meningitis), infiltration (carcinomatous meningitis or lymphoma), and trauma.

Bhatti MT, Eisenschenk S, Roper SN, Guy JR. Superior divisional third cranial nerve paresis: clinical and anatomical observations of 2 unique cases. *Arch Neurol.* 2006;63(5):771–776.

Third nerve palsies in younger patients

Children may have transient ophthalmoplegia following viral infection or vaccination. If an immediate workup is deferred, follow-up should be scheduled to monitor recovery. Aneurysms are rare in children. In adolescents and young adults, a pupil-involving third nerve palsy necessitates a workup to exclude an aneurysm or other structural etiology. *Ophthalmoplegic migraine,* with onset in childhood, can cause pain and third nerve dysfunction, but the 2 are not coincident. Curiously, the ophthalmoplegia develops days after the onset of head pain. Ophthalmoplegic migraine is a diagnosis of exclusion; all patients should undergo appropriate cranial neuroimaging as part of their initial evaluation. Although the pathophysiology of ophthalmoplegic migraine remains unknown, theories include recurrent demyelination with remyelination, or a benign ocular motor lesion such as schwannoma.

Carlow TJ. Oculomotor ophthalmoplegic migraine: Is it really migraine? *J Neuroophthalmol.* 2002;22(3):215–221.

Schumacher-Feero LA, Yoo SW, Solari FM, Biglan AW. Third cranial nerve palsy in children. *Am J Ophthalmol.* 1999;128(2):216–221.

Aberrant regeneration of the third nerve

Following damage to axons of the nerve, nerve fibers may regrow to innervate muscles other than those that they originally innervated (Fig 8-11). The misrouting of fibers produces several synkinetic phenomena (ie, co-contraction of muscles that normally are not activated at the same time). Classic findings include eyelid retraction with adduction or pupillary miosis with elevation, adduction, or depression.

Aberrant regeneration is common after trauma or compression by an aneurysm or tumor but does not occur with a third nerve palsy that is due to microvascular ischemia. Evidence of aberrant regeneration without a history of third nerve palsy—*primary aberrant regeneration*—is presumptive evidence of a slowly expanding parasellar lesion, most commonly a meningioma or carotid aneurysm within the cavernous sinus, and requires appropriate neuroimaging.

Grunwald L, Sund NJ, Volpe NJ. Pupillary sparing and aberrant regeneration in chronic third nerve palsy secondary to a posterior communicating artery aneurysm. *Br J Ophthalmol.* 2008;92(5):715–716.

Schatz NJ, Savino PJ, Corbett JJ. Primary aberrant oculomotor regeneration. A sign of intracavernous meningioma. *Arch Neurol.* 1977;34(1):29–32.

Fourth Nerve Palsy

A fourth nerve palsy typically causes diplopia that is worse in downgaze; hence, patients almost always report diplopia (or the tendency to close 1 eye) while reading. In some cases, examination of the affected eye reveals limited downgaze in the adducted position, but, in most cases, ocular motility appears grossly normal. Accordingly, it is essential to perform cover-uncover or Maddox rod testing to demonstrate a hypertropia that worsens on contralateral downgaze. Ipsilateral head tilting usually increases the vertical

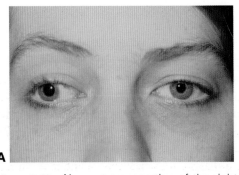 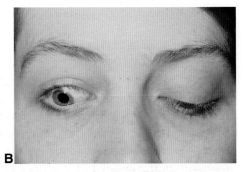

A   **B**

Figure 8-11 Aberrant regeneration of the right third nerve. **A,** In primary gaze, there is mild ptosis, pupillary mydriasis, and exotropia, all on the right. **B,** With attempted downward gaze, the right eyelid retracts as fibers of the right third nerve supplying the inferior rectus now also innervate the levator muscle. *(Courtesy of Rod Foroozan, MD.)*

strabismus, and, therefore, patients typically (subconsciously) tilt their head to the opposite side to avoid diplopia.

The *Parks-Bielschowsky 3-step test* is a time-honored algorithmic approach to identifying patterns of ocular motility that conform to dysfunction of specific vertically acting extraocular muscles. The 3 steps are

1. Find the side of the hypertropia.
2. Determine if the hypertropia is greater on left or right gaze.
3. Determine if the hypertropia is greater on left or right head tilt.

Beyond these 3 steps, it is also useful to determine if the vertical separation is greater in upgaze or downgaze (a fourth step) and check for relative cyclotropia.

The 3-step test is most helpful in determining whether a vertical strabismus conforms to the pattern of a fourth nerve palsy; for example, a right fourth nerve palsy shows right hyperdeviation that worsens on left gaze, right head tilt, and downgaze, with relative excyclotropia of the right eye. (More specific details on this testing are described in BCSC Section 6, *Pediatric Ophthalmology and Strabismus.*) Occasionally, a skew deviation mimics a fourth nerve palsy on the 3-step test but can distinguish itself by nonconformity to these rules. Practically speaking, the specific muscle(s) involved and the etiology of a vertical strabismus not due to a fourth nerve palsy is often not resolved by the 3-step plus fourth step test, because acquired vertical strabismus is often the result of the dysfunction of more than one muscle. In particular, thyroid eye disease, myasthenia gravis, or dysfunction of multiple ocular motor cranial nerves produces a wide variety of nonspecific patterns of ocular motility. The reliability of the 3-step test in identifying patterns of vertical strabismus lessens somewhat over time because of the phenomenon known as "spread of comitance" (see Chapter 7).

Bilateral fourth nerve palsy should always be considered whenever a unilateral palsy is diagnosed, especially after head trauma. Bilateral fourth nerve palsy presents with

- crossed hypertropia (ie, the right eye is higher on left gaze, and the left eye is higher on right gaze)
- excyclotorsion of 10° or greater (each eye rotates outwardly; best measured with double Maddox rod testing)
- a large (≥25 D) V pattern of strabismus

Brazis PW. Palsies of the trochlear nerve: diagnosis and localization—recent concepts. *Mayo Clin Proc.* 1993;68(5):501–509.

Fourth nerve palsies are often congenital. An anomalous superior oblique tendon, an anomalous site of its insertion, or a defect in the trochlea are now recognized as causes of some congenital fourth nerve palsies; similarly, some cases of presumed congenital fourth nerve palsy are secondary to a benign tumor (eg, schwannoma) of the fourth nerve. Patients are often asymptomatic until the fourth to sixth decades of life, when their vertical fusional amplitudes diminish and diplopia develops. Most patients maintain a chronic head tilt. The long-standing nature of the head tilt can often be confirmed by reviewing old photographs (Fig 8-12). Patients with a long-standing fourth nerve palsy have a relatively large vertical fusional range (>3 prism diopters).

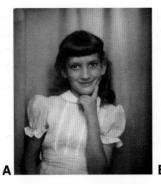 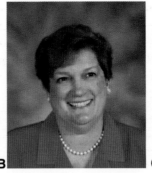 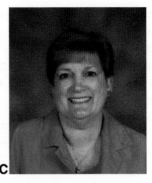

Figure 8-12 Congenital left fourth nerve palsy. **A,** Note the left hypertropia and right head tilt as a child. **B,** Forty years later, the right head tilt is still present, but the patient complains of more difficulty maintaining single, binocular vision. **C,** Following eye muscle surgery, the diplopia and head tilt have resolved. *(Courtesy of Lanning B. Kline, MD.)*

Helveston EM, Krach D, Plager DA, Ellis FD. A new classification of superior oblique palsy based on congenital variations in the tendon. *Ophthalmology.* 1992;99(10):1609–1615.

In patients older than 50 years, an isolated fourth nerve palsy is typically caused by microvascular ischemic disease, and function always improves and typically resolves within 3 months. The fourth nerve is particularly vulnerable to closed-head cranial trauma due to the unique dorsal midbrain crossing anatomy. In addition, the fourth nerve can be damaged by disease within the subarachnoid space or cavernous sinus.

Diagnostic evaluation for an isolated, nontraumatic fourth nerve palsy usually yields little information because most cases are congenital, ischemic, or idiopathic. In patients in the vasculopathic age group, a full medical evaluation looking for vascular risk factors, including diabetes, hyperlipidemia, and hypertension is appropriate. Older patients should be followed to ensure recovery. Lack of recovery after 3 months should prompt neuroimaging directed toward the base of the skull to search for a mass lesion. Other possible causes of an acquired vertical strabismus include orbital restrictive syndromes (eg, thyroid eye disease or previous trauma). Skew deviation, partial oculomotor nerve palsy, or myasthenia gravis should be considered in atypical cases.

Sixth Nerve Palsy

The sixth cranial nerve is the most frequent cause of an isolated ocular motor palsy; it typically presents as horizontal diplopia that worsens on ipsilateral gaze, especially viewing at distance. The abduction deficit is typically associated with an esodeviation that increases with gaze to the affected side (see Fig 8-4). As described earlier, a pattern of divergence paralysis may occur in the evolving or resolving phase of a sixth nerve palsy.

An ischemic mononeuropathy is the most common cause of an isolated sixth nerve palsy. Lesions of the *cerebellopontine angle* (especially acoustic neuroma or meningioma) may involve the sixth and other contiguous cranial nerves, causing decreased facial and corneal sensitivity (CN V), facial paralysis (CN VII), and decreased hearing with vestibular signs (CN VIII). Chronic inflammation of the petrous bone may cause an ipsilateral abducens palsy and facial pain *(Gradenigo syndrome)*, especially in children who have experienced recurrent infections of the middle ear. After exiting the pre–pontine space, the sixth nerve is vulnerable to meningeal or skull-based processes, such as meningioma, nasopharyngeal carcinoma, chordoma, or chondrosarcoma. In addition, the sixth nerve is susceptible to injury from shear forces of head trauma or elevated intracranial pressure. In such cases, injury occurs where the sixth nerve enters the cavernous sinus through the *Dorello canal* (the opening below the petroclinoid ligament).

Congenital sixth nerve palsies almost never occur in isolation. Abduction paresis present early in life usually manifests as a Duane syndrome (see Fig 8-15).

Isolated sixth nerve palsies in adults over the age of 50 are usually ischemic; ocular motility in these cases always improves and typically resolves within 3 months. In general, at the onset of an isolated sixth nerve palsy in a vasculopathic patient, neuroimaging is not required. As noted with other isolated ocular motor cranial nerve palsies, medical evaluation is appropriate. However, a cranial MRI is mandatory if obvious improvement has not occurred after 3 months. Other diagnostic studies that may be required include lumbar puncture, chest imaging, and hematologic studies to identify an underlying systemic process such as collagen vascular disease, sarcoidosis, or syphilis. Recovery does not necessarily indicate a benign cause. Occasionally, an ocular motor cranial nerve palsy will resolve spontaneously and then recur as a manifestation of an intracranial tumor.

Impaired abduction in patients under age 50 requires careful scrutiny, because few such cases are due to ischemic cranial neuropathy. Younger individuals should undergo appropriate neuroimaging. If negative, consideration should be given to neuromuscular junction disease, by obtaining acetylcholine antibodies or performing Tensilon testing; mechanical pathophysiologies, such as thyroid eye disease with medial rectus involvement; and meningeal-based disease, by obtaining a lumbar puncture. Leukemia or brainstem glioma are important considerations in children. In adolescents and young adults, demyelination may be the cause, in which case MRI with fluid-attenuated inversion recovery (FLAIR) imaging typically reveals T2 hyperintensities consistent with multiple sclerosis. (See Chapter 2 for a discussion of neuroimaging and Chapter 14 for a discussion of multiple sclerosis.)

Neuromyotonia

Neuromyotonia, a rare but important cause of episodic diplopia, is thought to be neurogenic in origin. Prior skull-base radiation therapy, typically for neoplasm (eg, meningioma), is the most common historical feature. Months to years postradiation, patients experience episodic diplopia lasting typically 30–60 seconds. Neuromyotonia may affect the oculomotor, trochlear, or abducens nerves. Diplopia is often triggered by activation of the offending nerve, during which overaction of the nerve produces ocular misalignment (eg, abducens nerve neuromyotonia episodes produce abduction of the involved eye and attendant exotropia). Often such patients undergo an extensive and largely unnecessary workup in the search for a recurrent neoplasm. The disorder generally responds quite well to medical therapy; carbamazepine and its derivatives are the first-line treatment.

Multiple Cranial Nerve Palsies

The guidelines for managing isolated cranial nerve palsies are based on the assumption that no other neurologic abnormalities are present. Benign, microvascular disease rarely causes simultaneous involvement of more than one ocular motor cranial nerve. Involvement of multiple contiguous nerves (CNs III, IV, V, VI, and sympathetic nerves) strongly suggests a lesion in the region of the cavernous sinus (see the following section). Bilateral involvement of the cranial nerves suggests a diffuse process such as infiltrative disease (eg, carcinoma, leukemia, or lymphoma), a midline mass lesion that extends bilaterally (eg, chordoma, chondrosarcoma, or nasopharyngeal carcinoma), a meningeal-based process, an inflammatory polyneuropathy (eg, Guillain-Barré syndrome or its variant, the Miller Fisher syndrome, or sarcoidosis), or myasthenia gravis.

A neurologic evaluation should be obtained if symptoms or signs indicate that more than one cranial nerve is involved. In this case, if neuroimaging is normal, a lumbar puncture should be considered with cytopathologic examination. Special testing for cancer-associated protein markers may be helpful in uncovering an elusive diagnosis. In suspected neoplastic meningeal involvement (meningeal carcinomatosis), a CT-PET scan is often the study of choice to demonstrate accessible biopsy sites. *Idiopathic multiple cranial neuropathy syndrome* should be considered only after neuroimaging, spinal fluid analysis, other tests, and observation over time have excluded a neoplastic, inflammatory, or infectious cause.

Cavernous Sinus and Superior Orbital Fissure Involvement

The hallmark of ophthalmoplegia secondary to a lesion of the cavernous sinus is multiple, ipsilateral ocular motor nerve dysfunction from some combination of third, fourth, fifth, and sixth cranial nerves and sympathetic fibers (see the illustrations in Chapter 1). Fifth nerve involvement with facial hypoesthesia or the presence of a third-order (postganglionic) Horner syndrome are helpful non–ocular motor clues to localize the lesion to the cavernous sinus. If only 1 ocular motor nerve is involved, it is usually the sixth nerve, which is the only ocular motor nerve not protected within the dural wall of the cavernous sinus. Aggressive lesions of the cavernous sinus, especially infectious or inflammatory processes, may compromise venous outflow and produce engorgement of ocular surface vessels, orbital venous congestion, increased intraocular pressure, and increased ocular pulse pressure.

It is often impossible to clinically distinguish cavernous sinus lesions from those involving the superior orbital fissure (the ocular motor nerves pass through this fissure from the cavernous sinus into the orbit), and lesions often cross this anatomical boundary. In recognition of this difficulty, the more general designation of *sphenocavernous,* or *parasellar, syndrome* may be used. The offending lesion may extend toward the optic foramen or into the orbital apex, in which case optic nerve function can be compromised. The designation *orbital apex syndrome* is then applied.

Tolosa-Hunt syndrome

Tolosa-Hunt syndrome is an idiopathic, sterile inflammation that primarily affects the cavernous sinus. Severe, "boring" pain is almost always present. Neuroimaging may show an enhancing mass within the cavernous sinus. The pain in patients with Tolosa-Hunt syndrome typically responds rapidly and dramatically to corticosteroid therapy, but a positive response may also occur with neoplastic mass lesions, especially lymphoma. Not infrequently, it is later discovered that the cause of the painful ophthalmoplegia in patients initially diagnosed with Tolosa-Hunt is neoplastic. Therefore, the Tolosa-Hunt syndrome is a diagnosis of exclusion. Other causes of cavernous sinus lesions include aneurysm, meningioma, lymphoma, schwannoma, pituitary adenoma (with or without apoplexy), carotid cavernous fistula, metastasis, sarcoidosis, and cavernous sinus thrombosis.

Kline LB, Hoyt WF. The Tolosa-Hunt syndrome. *J Neurol Neurosurg Psychiatry*. 2001;71(5): 577–582.

Carotid cavernous sinus fistula

Abnormal connections between the carotid artery (or its branches) and the cavernous sinus introduce high arterial pressures into the normally low-pressure venous contents of the cavernous sinus. This high-pressure connection may reverse blood flow within the superior ophthalmic vein and produce venous congestion within the orbit. Arterialization of conjunctival vessels is a classic sign of this fistula (Fig 8-13). Patients with this condition may have either direct, high-flow fistulous connections between the internal carotid artery and the cavernous sinus or indirect, "dural" low-flow connections mediated by small arterial feeders off the internal and/or external carotids. High-flow, direct fistulas most commonly occur after severe head trauma and produce a cranial bruit, whereas low-flow, indirect fistulas most often occur spontaneously, particularly in older women. The sequence of events leading to indirect fistula is not known. The clinical findings of the indirect fistulas are almost always less dramatic than those of a direct carotid cavernous fistula, although over time the low-flow state of the classic dural sinus fistula may become a greater flow as new arterial connections develop. Other than by the telltale symptom of a cranial bruit, differentiating high flow from low flow is best determined by angiographic studies.

Both direct and indirect fistulas often produce elevated intraocular pressure and proptosis but may also cause ocular motor neuropathy with diplopia, arterial or venous

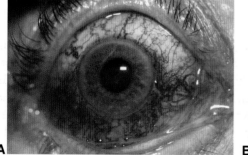 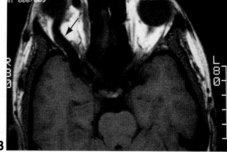

Figure 8-13 Right carotid cavernous sinus fistula. **A,** The elevated orbital venous pressure produces enlarged, corkscrew, arterialized conjunctival blood vessels that extend to the limbus. **B,** T1-weighted axial MRI reveals an enlarged, dilated superior ophthalmic vein *(arrow)*. *(Courtesy of Karl C. Golnik, MD.)*

compromise to the retina and eye, ischemic optic neuropathy, choroidal effusions (which can push the iris forward and produce angle-closure glaucoma), pain (which may partly result from ocular surface drying if proptosis is significant), and, in some patients, cerebral venous infarction. Some indirect fistulas remain stable or close spontaneously; however, both types of fistula may be successfully treated with interventional radiologic techniques or radiosurgery. Angiography is required to determine the location and configuration of the fistula, and then a variety of thrombogenic materials (eg, coils, beads, balloons) may be employed to eliminate the abnormal vascular flow.

Neuromuscular Junction Causes of Diplopia

Myasthenia gravis is the prototypical disease of the neuromuscular junction. It typically produces variable diplopia and ptosis with any pattern of pupil-sparing, painless ocular misalignment, and, conversely, it never produces sensory symptoms, pain, or autonomic or pupillary dysfunction. Accordingly, it belongs in the differential of any such cases of diplopia (see Chapter 14).

Myopathic, Restrictive, and Orbital Causes of Diplopia

Eye movements may be limited by mechanical factors that may be congenital or acquired. Congenitally deficient neural innervation to extraocular muscles can also be associated with limited eye movements, which sometimes also have a restrictive component.

Thyroid Eye Disease

The most common cause of restrictive strabismus in adults is *thyroid eye disease (TED)*. Any of the extraocular muscles may be involved, but the inferior and medial recti are most commonly affected. When the inferior rectus muscle is involved, there is typically an ipsilateral hypotropia in primary position that increases in upgaze—the restrictive process pulls the eye down and limits supraduction (see Chapter 14, Fig 14-3). When the medial rectus is the offending muscle, there is typically an esodeviation that increases on horizontal gaze to the same side (the enlarged, "tight" medial rectus restricts abduction). The diagnosis of TED is often straightforward if associated with proptosis, chemosis, eyelid retraction, and eyelid lag. Forced duction testing (see Fig 8-3) and measurement of intraocular pressure in different positions of gaze may provide information to support this diagnosis. Neuroimaging in TED typically reveals enlargement of the bellies of the extraocular muscles, with sparing of the tendons (see Chapter 4, Fig 4-23). For a more extensive discussion of TED, see Chapters 4 and 14 in this volume and BCSC Section 7, *Orbit, Eyelids, and Lacrimal System.*

Posttraumatic Restriction

Patients with blowout fractures of the orbit often develop diplopia. The most typical presentation involves fracture of the inferior orbital floor with entrapment of the inferior rectus muscle. This entrapment, best illustrated with coronal CT of the orbit, mimics the pattern of vertical strabismus often present in TED. Less commonly, the medial rectus muscle becomes entrapped (see Chapter 2, Fig 2-14). In some instances of orbital trauma, the orbital fascial scaffolds that are connected to the extraocular muscles fall into a bony fracture without actual muscle entrapment. In either case, there is usually diffuse swelling of the orbital tissue, which tends to resolve relatively quickly (within weeks), at times with resolution of diplopia. Hence, decisions about the need for surgery with orbital blowout fractures must be made judiciously. See also BCSC Section 7, *Orbit, Eyelids, and Lacrimal System.*

Post–Cataract Extraction Restriction

Injury or inflammation to the inferior rectus or other muscles secondary to retrobulbar injection for cataract or other ocular surgery can produce binocular diplopia. The onset of vertical diplopia just after surgery initially suggests nerve damage or possible myotoxicity from the local anesthetic. Over time, the initial paretic or myotoxic effect evolves into extraocular muscle fibrosis leading to restricted movement of the eye; concomitantly, the involved eye transitions from hypertropic status to hypotropic, with hypotropia increasing in upgaze.

Orbital Myositis

Idiopathic inflammation of one or more extraocular muscles typically produces ophthalmoplegia and pain, often with conjunctival hyperemia, chemosis, and sometimes proptosis. The pain may be quite intense and is accentuated by eye movements. If the inflammation is confined to the posterior orbit, the eye may appear at times to be white and quiet. Computed tomography or MRI typically shows enlargement of one or more of the extraocular muscles, with involvement of the tendon, and often the inflammation extends into the orbital fat. Orbital myositis–related pain usually responds promptly to systemic corticosteroid therapy, whereas diplopia may take longer to resolve. Orbital myositis is usually an isolated phenomenon but may be part of a systemic disease such as Wegener granulomatosis, systemic lupus erythematosus, or sarcoidosis (see also Chapter 14 of this volume and BCSC Section 7, *Orbit, Eyelids, and Lacrimal System*).

Neoplastic Involvement

Infiltration of the orbit by cancer, especially from the surrounding paranasal sinuses, can impair eye movements because of either extraocular muscle infiltration or involvement of the ocular motor cranial nerves. At times, extraocular muscles may be the site of a metastatic tumor.

Brown Syndrome

Brown syndrome is a restrictive ocular motor disorder that produces limited upgaze when the affected eye is in the adducted position (Fig 8-14). This pattern of motility is usually congenital but can be acquired. In congenital cases, the pathology is a short superior oblique tendon, which produces an ipsilateral hypodeviation that increases on upgaze to

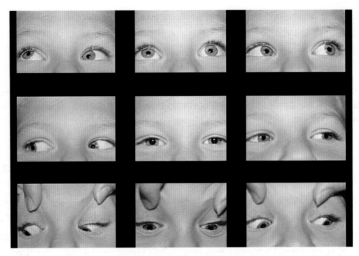

Figure 8-14 Brown syndrome. Selected gaze positions of a 7-year-old who was referred for a 2-year history of the left eye "moving funny." Visual acuity was 20/20 bilaterally. The patient's eyes were straight in primary position. The motility evaluation revealed a left hypotropia in upgaze to the right (see upper left photograph). This is the pattern of a congenitally short left superior oblique tendon that is characteristic of Brown syndrome. *(Courtesy of Steven A. Newman, MD.)*

the opposite side (impaired supraduction in adduction). The acquired cases result from damage or injury to the trochlea, which may cause a "click" that the patient can feel. Acquired disease is usually seen in patients with rheumatoid arthritis, idiopathic orbital inflammatory disease, or trauma but may, rarely, be a manifestation of a focal metastasis of a neoplasm to the superior oblique muscle.

Congenital Fibrosis Syndrome (Congenital Cranial Dysinnervation Syndrome, Agenesis Syndromes)

A group of congenital disorders that had been assumed to result from restrictive limitation of eye movements (hence the term *fibrosis*), in reality results from agenesis of ocular motoneurons in the brainstem. The prototype is *congenital fibrosis of the extraocular muscles type 1 (CFEOM1) syndrome,* which is an autosomal dominant disease, characterized by bilateral ptosis and external ophthalmoplegia. There is an agenesis of the superior division of the third cranial nerve with associated atrophy of the superior rectus and levator palpebrae muscles. Patients with this disorder have a characteristic extended neck posture as they attempt to look under their severely ptotic eyelids.

Other forms of nuclear agenesis also occur. *Duane retraction syndrome,* caused by failure of formation of the abducens nucleus and sixth nerve, produces a congenital abduction paresis. The involved lateral rectus muscle is innervated by an anomalous branch of the third nerve within the orbit. This unusual innervation pattern produces aberrant, co-contraction of the horizontal rectus muscles. This co-contraction can be observed as a retraction of the globe and narrowing of the eyelid fissure on attempted adduction, because activation of the third cranial nerve causes simultaneous contraction of both the

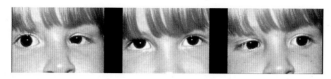

Figure 8-15 Bilateral Duane retraction syndrome. This 4-year-old was born with limited abduction of both eyes and narrowing of the palpebral fissure on attempted adduction in both eyes. *(Courtesy of Steven A. Newman, MD.)*

medial and lateral rectus muscles. Duane retraction syndrome usually is unilateral but may be bilateral (Fig 8-15).

Other variants of Duane syndrome include cases of limited adduction in 1 or both eyes, as well as cases with both limited adduction and abduction in 1 or both eyes (Table 8-2). In all instances, however, there is retraction of the globe on attempted adduction. Patients typically do not have diplopia with Duane syndrome and frequently develop a compensatory head position.

DeRespinis PA, Caputo AR, Wagner RS, Guo S. Duane's retraction syndrome. *Surv Ophthalmol.* 1993;38(3):257–288.

Miller NR, Kiel SM, Green WR, Clark AW. Unilateral Duane's retraction syndrome (type 1). *Arch Ophthalmol.* 1982;100(9):1468–1472.

Möbius syndrome occurs due to agenesis of the nuclei of the sixth and seventh cranial nerves bilaterally, which produces horizontal ophthalmoplegia and facial diplegia. Scoliosis, atrophy of the tongue, and deformities of the head may also be present. See also BCSC Section 6, *Pediatric Ophthalmology and Strabismus.*

Table 8-2 Duane Retraction Syndrome

Syndrome	Limitation*	Narrow Palpebral Fissure With Adduction
1	abDuction	Yes
2	aDDuction	Yes
3	aDD and abDuction	Yes

*Number of Ds equals the syndrome number.

CHAPTER 9

The Patient With Nystagmus or Spontaneous Eye Movement Disorders

Introduction

A variety of diseases, drugs, or other factors may disrupt the systems that provide ocular stability. Abnormal eye movements may occur because of inability to maintain fixation, loss of the normal inhibitory influences on the eye movement control system, or loss of the normally symmetric input from one of the vestibular pathways to the ocular motor nuclei. One form of excessive eye movements is known as *nystagmus,* a term that should be reserved for rhythmic, to-and-fro eye movements (horizontal, vertical, torsional, or a combination of these) that incorporate a slow phase. *Jerk nystagmus* has 2 phases: (1) a slow phase drift from the target of interest, followed by (2) a corrective saccade (fast phase) back to the target. *Pendular nystagmus* occurs when the back-and-forth slow-phase movements occur without a fast phase (Fig 9-1). Inappropriate saccadic movements may also affect the normal ability to fixate on a target. Collectively, these pathologic eye movements are known as *saccadic intrusions* or *saccadic oscillations;* because they have no slow phase, they do not conform to the definition of nystagmus.

Patients with acquired nystagmus often report a sensation of environmental movement termed *oscillopsia.* Oscillopsia is often absent in children with congenital nystagmus. Nystagmus in primary position may degrade visual acuity. Patients should be asked about any associated neurologic symptoms (eg, vertigo, ataxia, motor weakness, or sensory weakness) and any family history of abnormal eye movements.

Examination of ocular motility begins with assessing ocular stability with the eyes in primary gaze while fixating on a target. Eye movements in the 9 cardinal positions should then be examined to determine if

- the eye movement disorder is monocular or binocular
- the eyes behave similarly (conjugately)
- the abnormal eye movements are horizontal, vertical, torsional, or mixed
- the abnormal eye movements are continuous or are induced by particular eye position

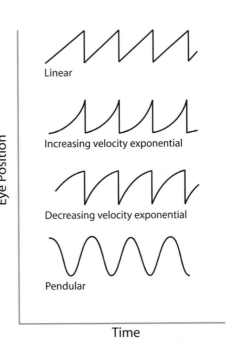

Figure 9-1 Nystagmus waveforms named for the velocity profile of the slow phase. Linear is typical of vestibular nystagmus; increasing velocity exponential, of congenital nystagmus; decreasing velocity exponential, of gaze-evoked nystagmus; and pendular may be seen with congenital or acquired nystagmus. *(Modified from Kline LB.* Neuro-Ophthalmology Review Manual. *6th ed. Thorofare, NJ: Slack; 2008.)*

- only slow phases (pendular nystagmus), fast and slow phases (jerk nystagmus), or only fast phases (saccadic intrusion) are seen
- there is a point at which the nystagmus is less evident (ie, a null point)

By convention, the direction of jerk nystagmus is reported as the direction of the fast-phase component; however, it is the slow phase that indicates the pathology. When the size of oscillations differs in each eye, it is referred to as *dissociated nystagmus*. When the direction of the oscillations differs between the 2 eyes, the term *disconjugate,* or *disjunctive,* is applied.

The amplitude of nystagmus often changes with gaze position. A few beats of nystagmus are normally present in the extremes of horizontal gaze (beyond 45°), especially in older patients. This should not be considered pathologic unless the nystagmus is persistent, asymmetric (present to the left but not the right, for instance), or accompanied by other features. Assessment for nystagmus can be complemented by strategies that search for subtler, smaller-amplitude eye movements. Illuminated Frenzel (high-magnification) goggles are extremely useful in detecting eye movements, but a 20 D lens, slit lamp, or direct ophthalmoscope can also be useful to block the patient's fixation and magnify abnormal eye movements. Ocular motor recordings (electro- or video-oculography, infrared tracking, or electromagnetic coil technique) provide an objective and highly sensitive measure of eye movements but are rarely needed in standard clinical practice. The characteristics of eye movements can be easily recorded and effectively communicated with videotape and drawing.

Leigh RJ, Zee DS. *The Neurology of Eye Movements.* 4th ed. Contemporary Neurology Series. New York: Oxford University Press; 2006.

Serra A, Leigh RJ. Diagnostic value of nystagmus: spontaneous and induced ocular oscillations. *J Neurol Neurosurg Psychiatry.* 2002;73(6):615–618.

Early-Onset (Childhood) Nystagmus

Congenital Nystagmus

Congenital nystagmus (CN, or *infantile nystagmus syndrome)* is usually recognized in the first few months of life; there may be a family history of the disorder. Patients with CN usually do not have oscillopsia. Congenital nystagmus may occur in the presence of poor vision or good acuity. Reduced acuity may be due to the nystagmus itself or related to an afferent visual pathway disorder. Therefore, the ophthalmologist must determine if there is evidence of damage to the visual pathways. In young children, it is important to detect any impairment of visual tracking (ie, determine that the eyes cannot follow visual stimuli equally) or optic atrophy. The presence of such abnormalities should prompt neuroimaging. Congenital nystagmus often occurs with such conditions as ocular albinism, achromatopsia, Leber congenital amaurosis, and aniridia. Frequently, electrophysiologic testing (ERG, VEP) is warranted.

Congenital nystagmus is almost always conjugate and horizontal, features that are maintained even in upgaze and downgaze. The nystagmus may be continuous or intermittent and can appear as jerk or pendular movements in different positions of gaze. There is frequently a null point, the field of gaze in which nystagmus intensity is minimal. If the null point is not in primary position, patients often adopt a head turn or other posture to improve vision by placing the eyes in the null position. Visual attention and fixation usually amplify CN (unlike the case with peripheral vestibular nystagmus, discussed later in the chapter), whereas convergence on a near target damps the amplitude of the nystagmus. Two characteristic signs of CN are

1. reversal of the normal pattern of optokinetic nystagmus characterized by the slow phase of eye movements moving in the direction opposite that of a rotating optokinetic drum
2. a unique pattern in which the velocity of the slow-phase movement increases exponentially with distance from fixation; this requires eye movement recordings (see Fig 9-1)

To summarize, the features of CN include

- jerk and/or pendular pattern
- presence with or without normal acuity
- conjugate horizontal eye movements that remain horizontal in up- and downgaze
- presence of a null point
- no oscillopsia
- increasing velocity of slow phase
- accentuation by distant fixation; diminishment by convergence
- 15% of patients with strabismus
- abolished in sleep

Abadi RV, Bjerre A. Motor and sensory characteristics of infantile nystagmus. *Br J Ophthalmol.* 2002;86(10):1152–1160.

Gelbart SS, Hoyt CS. Congenital nystagmus: a clinical perspective in infancy. *Graefes Arch Clin Exp Ophthalmol.* 1988;226(2):178–180.

Hertle RW, Dell'Osso LF. Clinical and ocular motor analysis of congenital nystagmus in infancy. *J AAPOS.* 1999;3(2):70–79.

Latent Nystagmus

Another form of nystagmus that appears very early in life is *latent nystagmus (LN)*, or *fusional development nystagmus syndrome*, which is a horizontal jerk nystagmus that is accentuated or appears only with monocular viewing conditions. Eyes with LN are stable until 1 eye is occluded, thus eliminating binocular fixation. The fast phase beats toward the viewing eye and away from the occluded eye (the slow phase of the viewing eye is toward the nose). Hence, the fast phase reverses direction each time the eyes are alternately covered. Use of an occluder when measuring visual acuity requires special care in patients with LN, because the onset of the nystagmus degrades acuity. Partial optical blurring of 1 eye (with a plus lens or filter) may permit better acuity measurements in the fellow eye without inducing nystagmus. Latent nystagmus is almost always associated with esotropia and, frequently, with dissociated vertical deviation.

Clinical characteristics of LN include

- conjugate jerk nystagmus
- beginning or accentuation when binocular fusion is disrupted
- direction changing with monocular occlusion: fast phase beats toward viewing eye; slow phase, toward the nose
- congenital esotropia usually present
- subnormal stereopsis
- may be seen with CN in the same patient

Nystagmus with characteristics of LN that is present when both eyes are open is known as *manifest latent nystagmus (MLN).* Because most patients with LN have esotropia (which may be a subtle microtropia), MLN is initiated when the esotropic eye is physiologically suppressed. In other words, the nystagmus spontaneously and intermittently develops whenever suppression occurs (ie, the examiner may not need to occlude 1 eye to induce this form of nystagmus). Both LN and MLN are benign entities. When studied with eye movement recordings, LN usually has a constant-velocity slow phase, in contrast with the increasing exponential waveform of CN.

Dell'Osso LF, Schmidt D, Daroff RB. Latent, manifest latent, and congenital nystagmus. *Arch Ophthalmol.* 1979;97(10):1877–1885.

Monocular Nystagmus of Childhood

Monocular nystagmus of childhood is a rare but important form of nystagmus that manifests early in life; causes range from the benign to the sight- and life-threatening. The eye movements are usually in 1 eye, vertical or elliptical, and of small amplitude. Monocular nystagmus in an eye with poor vision is often referred to as the Heimann-Bielschowsky phenomenon; it may occur with a variety of underlying pathophysiologies, including optic neuropathy and amblyopia. Monocular vertical nystagmus in an infant, often found in concert with an afferent pupillary defect and optic atrophy, is suggestive of an optic nerve/chiasmal tumor (glioma), and therefore neuroimaging is warranted.

Spasmus Nutans

Spasmus nutans is a disorder that often develops in the first year of life, manifesting as intermittent, binocular, very small amplitude, high-frequency, horizontal, pendular nystagmus. The nystagmus may be dissociated, even monocular, and the relationship of amplitude and phase of the eye movements may frequently vary between the eyes.

Small-amplitude vertical nystagmus may be present as well. This nystagmus is accompanied by head nodding, which is often subtle. Many patients have an abnormal head posture, or *torticollis*. There is an association between spasmus nutans and African-American ethnicity, Hispanic ethnicity, and low socioeconomic status.

In general, spasmus nutans is distinguished from congenital nystagmus (infantile nystagmus syndrome) by abnormal head movements and head posture, the intermittent and variable nature of the nystagmus, and the relatively high frequency of eye movements in spasmus nutans. However, the nystagmus of spasmus nutans is sometimes monocular and thus virtually impossible to distinguish from the more ominous conditions of monocular nystagmus of childhood (such as the Heimann-Bielschowsky phenomenon, discussed in the preceding section). Therefore, patients with presumed spasmus nutans should undergo neuroimaging to exclude a glioma of the anterior visual pathway.

Similarly, some authors have reported the association of a spasmus nutans–like syndrome with retinal dystrophies (eg, congenital stationary night blindness), and consideration should be given to electroretinography in such cases. Lack of the expected resolution of spasmus nutans or development of any other neurologic problems should likewise prompt appropriate evaluation, including neuroimaging.

Spasmus nutans is typically a benign disorder and patients generally have no other neurologic abnormalities, except perhaps strabismus and amblyopia. Typically, the abnormal eye and head movements disappear after several years (usually by the end of the first decade of life).

Newman SA, Hedges TR, Wall M, Sedwick LA. Spasmus nutans—or is it? *Surv Ophthalmol.* 1990;34(6):453–456.

Smith DE, Fitzgerald K, Stass-Isern M, Cibis GW. Electroretinography is necessary for spasmus nutans diagnosis. *Pediatr Neurol.* 2000;23(1):33–36.

Gaze-Evoked Nystagmus

Gaze-evoked nystagmus develops because of an inability to maintain fixation in eccentric gaze. The eyes drift back to the midline due to the elastic properties of the orbit, and a corrective saccade is generated to reposition the eyes on the eccentric target. Hence, the fast phase is always in the direction of gaze. The amplitude of the nystagmus increases as the eyes are moved in the direction of the fast phase. This pattern is in accordance with Alexander's law, which states that nystagmus increases in intensity (amplitude and frequency) as the eyes are moved in the direction of the fast phase.

Gaze-evoked nystagmus is caused by dysfunction of the neural integrator (see Chapter 1). For horizontal gaze, the neural integrator includes the nucleus prepositus hypoglossi and the medial vestibular nuclei. For vertical gaze, the interstitial nucleus of Cajal serves as the neural integrator. The flocculus and nodulus of the cerebellum also play a role in maintaining an eccentric position of gaze. The neural integrator receives a velocity signal (the "pulse") from the appropriate gaze center and, through the mathematical process of integration, generates a "step" signal to maintain the eccentric position of the eyes (see Chapter 7, Fig 7-1). That is, the neural integrator ensures a level of neural activity adequate to maintain the eyes in an eccentric position of gaze against the elastic forces of the orbit. If the neural integrator fails to function properly (becomes "leaky"), eccentric eye position cannot be maintained.

A few beats of symmetric jerk nystagmus at the extremes of far horizontal gaze without other features (eg, rebound nystagmus, saccadic dysmetria) is physiologic and of no clinical significance. However, sustained or asymmetric gaze-evoked nystagmus should prompt further evaluation. Metabolic and toxic etiologies include ethanol and a variety of medications, including anticonvulsants, sedatives, and hypnotics. Whenever gaze-evoked nystagmus is asymmetric, it can be presumed that an ipsilateral lesion of the brainstem or cerebellum—typically stroke, demyelination, or tumor—is present. This finding should prompt appropriate patient evaluation, including neuroimaging. End-organ disease such as extraocular myopathies and myasthenia can also cause gaze-evoked nystagmus, with a pattern similar to that seen with lesions of the central nervous system.

Rebound Nystagmus

Prolonged eccentric viewing may induce *rebound nystagmus*. Such eccentric viewing may produce a directional bias in ocular motor control in an attempt to counteract the centripetal tendency of the eyes to return to primary position (primarily due to elastic forces within the orbit). This induced bias becomes evident when the eyes return to primary position and then show a tendency to return to the prior eccentric direction of gaze. The bias induces corrective saccadic movement in the direction opposite to the initial eccentric position of gaze. Rebound nystagmus is often a manifestation of cerebellar disease.

Vestibular Nystagmus

Peripheral Vestibular Nystagmus

Patients with *peripheral vestibular nystagmus* typically present with a sudden, sometimes dramatic, onset of dysequilibrium with vertigo, nausea, and vomiting (Table 9-1). Patients often recognize that their symptoms are worsened by particular head movements or postures. Oscillopsia, tinnitus, and hearing loss may also occur. After the acute phase of peripheral vestibular loss, which typically lasts days, patients experience a slow period

Table 9-1 Clinical Characteristics of Peripheral and Central Vestibular Nystagmus

Symptom or Sign	Peripheral Dysfunction	Central Dysfunction
Vertigo	Severe	Milder
Duration of symptoms	Days to weeks, improving over time (may be recurrent)	May be more chronic
Tinnitus or hearing loss	Common	Typically absent
Horizontal nystagmus with torsion	Typical	Not typical
Horizontal nystagmus without torsion	Rare	May be present
Pure vertical or torsional nystagmus	Almost never	Diagnostic
Visual fixation	Dampens nystagmus	No effect
Common causes	Labyrinthitis; Ménière disease; trauma; toxicity	Demyelination; stroke; drugs

(weeks to months) of gradually waning symptoms. Even patients who become asymptomatic may experience discomfort months to years later, when their vestibular system is challenged, as when riding in a fast-moving car or boat.

Peripheral vestibular nystagmus occurs in patients with dysfunction of the end organ (semicircular canals, otolithic structures, vestibular nerve). End-organ damage, which is usually unilateral or at least asymmetric (except in cases of toxicity), disrupts the otherwise symmetric vestibular afferent inputs to the neural integrator, which stabilizes eye position in eccentric locations. The output of the neural integrator is routed to the contralateral paramedian pontine reticular formation. This loss of tonic symmetry produces a directional bias in eye position. A reduction in input from a left-sided vestibular lesion, for instance, produces a leftward bias, which then induces a corrective saccade away from the side of the lesion. Thus, a left-sided lesion would produce leftward slow phases and right jerk nystagmus.

Peripheral vestibular nystagmus related to vestibular neuropathy typically disrupts output from all 3 semicircular canals and the otolithic organs, producing a mixed horizontal-torsional pattern of nystagmus that changes depending on the direction of gaze. This follows Alexander's law: The nystagmus is more pronounced when gaze is directed toward the side of the fast-beating component. Depending on the severity of the lesion, the nystagmus may be evident in primary position. A skew deviation may also be present due to disruption of peripheral vestibular structures. Nystagmus that is purely vertical or torsional almost always signifies a central lesion (see the following section).

A characteristic feature of peripheral vestibular nystagmus is the ability of visual fixation to dampen the nystagmus. The effect of visual fixation on nystagmus can be evaluated during direct ophthalmoscopy by temporarily covering the contralateral fixing eye. Other methods for enhancing vestibular nystagmus include vigorous head shaking, hyperventilation, mastoid vibration, and the Valsalva maneuver.

Peripheral vestibular dysfunction, often accompanied by nystagmus, usually occurs in 1 of 4 clinical settings. The first is an acute, monophasic disorder that occurs secondary to a (presumed viral) vestibular neuronitis. The second is a recurrent form of vestibular dysfunction that is usually associated with auditory symptoms (tinnitus and hearing loss). This disorder, exemplified by *Ménière disease,* is usually progressive, although typically there are long symptom-free intervals. The third clinical setting is a paroxysmal dysfunction of the vestibular system that produces vertigo in response to certain postures of the head. This disorder, known as *benign, paroxysmal, positional vertigo (BPPV),* develops because of free movement of otoconia particles (calcium carbonate crystals normally contained within the utricle and saccule), which act as foreign debris within a semicircular canal. The Dix-Hallpike maneuver, during which the patient's head is turned 45° to the right or left and lowered below the horizontal plane of an examining table to induce symptoms, can be used to diagnose which side and semicircular canal are dysfunctional. Once that is determined, repositioning treatments such as the Epley maneuver can remove the otoconia from that semicircular canal. The Epley procedure for the right ear, for example, begins in the right Dix-Hallpike position, with the head 45° to the right and below the horizon; the head is then turned slowly (over minutes) 180° to the patient's left. These patients often enjoy a remission after a bout of BPPV, but it is not uncommon for patients to be intermittently plagued by this disorder. A fourth clinical setting for the occurrence of peripheral vestibular dysfunction is a toxic etiology, primarily the use of aminoglycosides (but also other medications such as chemotherapeutics). Systemic ototoxins typically produce head movement–related oscillopsia and decreased vestibular ocular reflex (VOR) gain bilaterally with little or no nystagmus (vestibular hypofunction without asymmetry).

Some patients with cerebellopontine angle tumors (usually acoustic neurinoma or meningioma) may experience *Bruns nystagmus,* which is a combination of gaze-evoked and peripheral vestibular nystagmus. Initially, as the vestibular nerve is affected, the eyes drift toward the side of the lesion, with a corrective fast phase in the opposite direction. As the lesion enlarges, the ipsilateral brainstem is compressed, causing problems in maintaining ipsilateral eccentric gaze; thus, as the patient looks to the side of the lesion, large-amplitude, lower-frequency gaze-evoked nystagmus is noted, whereas in contralateral gaze, small-amplitude, high-frequency vestibular nystagmus is seen.

Baloh RW. Clinical practice: vestibular neuritis. *N Engl J Med.* 2003;348(11):1027–1032.

Fife TD, Tusa RJ, Furman JM, et al. Assessment: vestibular testing techniques in adults and children. Report of the Therapeutics and Technology Assessment Subcommittee of the American Academy of Neurology. *Neurology.* 2000;55(10):1431–1441.

Hotson JR, Baloh RW. Acute vestibular syndrome. *N Engl J Med.* 1998;339(10):680–685.

Central Forms of Vestibular Nystagmus

There are extensive interconnections between the central vestibular structures of the brainstem and the phylogenetically older regions of the cerebellum (flocculus, nodulus, and vermis). Therefore, it can be difficult, if not impossible, to determine by clinical examination alone the precise location of some lesions that produce central nystagmus. Although some forms of central vestibular nystagmus do provide good localizing information (Table 9-2), it is often more appropriate to think of the central vestibular pathways as a single system and to obtain neuroimaging if more specific information about localization is desired. If

Table 9-2 Selected Nystagmus/Oscillatory Movements and Their Most Common Lesion Locations

Abnormal Eye Movement	Probable Location of Lesion
Downbeat nystagmus	Cervical-medullary junction
Upbeat nystagmus	Posterior fossa (medulla most common)
See-saw nystagmus	Parasellar/diencephalon
Monocular nystagmus of childhood	Optic nerve/chiasm/hypothalamus
Periodic alternating nystagmus	Cerebellar nodulus
Convergence-retraction nystagmus	Pretectum (dorsal midbrain)
Ocular bobbing	Pontine destructive lesion
Flutter/opsoclonus	Pons (pause cells); cerebellum (connections to pons)

central vestibular nystagmus is of small amplitude and only present outside of primary position, patients may have no visual complaints.

Downbeat nystagmus

Downbeat nystagmus is the most common form of central vestibular nystagmus and results from defective vertical gaze holding that allows for a pathologic upward drift of the eyes, which is then corrected with a downward saccade. Lesions that cause downbeat nystagmus compromise the vestibulocerebellum (nodulus, uvula, flocculus, and paraflocculus) and diminish the tonic output from the anterior semicircular canals to the ocular motoneurons (the vertical VOR is asymmetric for up and down movements, as distinct from the symmetric horizontal VOR). Downbeat nystagmus may be present in primary position, but in accordance with Alexander's law, the downbeating movements are usually accentuated in downgaze (especially downgaze to either side). Patients usually report oscillopsia, which can be debilitating.

A structural lesion may be associated with downbeat nystagmus, in which case the lesion is often located at the cervical-medullary junction. An Arnold-Chiari type I malformation, in which the cerebellar tonsils herniate through the foramen magnum and compress the brainstem and spinal cord, is the most common structural etiology (Fig 9-2). Lesions at the foramen magnum are best assessed with sagittal MRI. In some cases of unexplained downbeat nystagmus, antibodies to glutamic acid decarboxylase have been discovered in the blood of affected patients. These antibodies might produce downbeat nystagmus by interfering with the GABAergic neurons of the vestibular complex that normally inhibit the cells of the flocculus.

The differential diagnosis of downbeat nystagmus includes

- Arnold-Chiari type I malformation
- tumors (meningioma, cerebellar hemangioma) at the foramen magnum
- demyelination
- stroke
- cranial trauma
- drugs (alcohol, lithium, anticonvulsants)
- platybasia

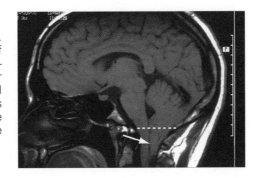

Figure 9-2 Arnold-Chiari type I malformation. This 26-year-old patient reported a sense of movement of his environment. Downbeat nystagmus was identified as the explanation for his oscillopsia. This sagittal, T1-weighted MRI scan shows herniation of the cerebellar tonsils *(arrow)* through the foramen magnum. (The level of the foramen magnum is shown by the *dotted line.*)

- basilar impression
- spinocerebellar degenerations
- syrinx of the brainstem or upper cervical spinal cord
- brainstem encephalitis
- paraneoplastic syndrome
- nutrition (Wernicke encephalopathy, parenteral feeding, magnesium deficiency)
- antibodies to glutamic acid decarboxylase
- idiopathic

Clonazepam, baclofen, gabapentin, base-out prisms (to induce convergence), memantine, and 3,4-diaminopyridine are common (off-label) treatments for downbeat nystagmus, but they are frequently only partially successful or unsuccessful.

Upbeat nystagmus

Upbeat nystagmus is caused by an inappropriate downward drift of the eyes, followed by corrective, upward saccades. Upbeat nystagmus may be caused by lesions in the brainstem (often medulla) or the anterior cerebellar vermis; hence, the lesions may exist at variable locations within the posterior fossa. Common causes of upbeat nystagmus include demyelination, stroke, cerebellar degeneration, and tobacco smoking.

Torsional nystagmus

In contrast to the mixed patterns of nystagmus seen with peripheral vestibular disease, nystagmus that is purely torsional is indicative of a central lesion. *Torsional nystagmus* is usually associated with a medullary lesion (syringobulbia, lateral medullary infarction) and may be part of an ocular tilt reaction.

Periodic alternating nystagmus

Periodic alternating nystagmus (PAN) is a strictly horizontal nystagmus that predictably oscillates in direction, amplitude, and frequency. For instance, a rightward beating nystagmus develops progressively larger amplitudes and higher frequencies up to a certain point, then wanes, eventually leading to a short period of downbeat or no nystagmus. Then, the nystagmus reverses direction, with a crescendo–decrescendo pattern that again leads to a short period without nystagmus, to complete the cycle. PAN may be congenital or acquired. The acquired form has a characteristic oscillation cycle of 2–4 minutes. A cursory examination may lead to the erroneous conclusion that the nystagmus is directed only to 1 side. For this reason, any presentation of nystagmus that is purely horizontal and is present in primary position should be observed for at least 2 minutes to be certain one is not dealing with PAN. A patient with PAN may also demonstrate periodic alternating head turn to minimize the nystagmus, according to Alexander's law.

PAN is typically associated with dysfunction of the cerebellar nodulus and uvula, which play a role in the time constant of rotational velocity storage. An oscillatory shifting of the null point results. Common causes include multiple sclerosis, cerebellar degeneration, Arnold-Chiari type I malformation, stroke, anticonvulsant therapy, and bilateral visual loss. If the last is reversible (eg, vitreous hemorrhage), PAN may be abolished. Baclofen (Lioresal) can be effective for the acquired form of this nystagmus.

Acquired Pendular Nystagmus

Acquired pendular nystagmus includes pendular, slow-phase eye movements in the horizontal, vertical, and torsional planes (often forming elliptical waveforms). (In contrast, the much rarer congenital pendular nystagmus usually manifests with only horizontal movements.) Pendular nystagmus with both vertical and horizontal components produces oblique nystagmus (if the components are in phase) or circular or elliptical nystagmus (if the components are out of phase). The eye movements may be conjugate or disconjugate and are often dissociated.

The localizing value of acquired pendular nystagmus is poor. It is most commonly seen in patients with multiple sclerosis, who may exhibit asymmetric or monocular forms. This form of nystagmus can also be seen following blindness secondary to optic nerve disease, including that due to multiple sclerosis. Assuming reduced vision in both eyes, the nystagmus is typically larger in the eye with poorer vision.

Oculopalatal Myoclonus or Tremor

Acquired pendular nystagmus may accompany *palatal myoclonus,* an acquired oscillation of the palate. The eye movements are continuous and rhythmic, approximately 1 Hz, and typically conjugate in the vertical plane, and they persist during sleep. This eye movement disorder may also be associated with synchronous movements of the facial muscles, pharynx, tongue, larynx, diaphragm, trunk, and extremities. The condition usually occurs several months (rarely ranging to years) following a lesion involving the Guillain-Mollaret triangle, which encompasses pathways from the deep cerebellar nuclei through the superior cerebellar peduncle, then through the central tegmental tract to the inferior olive in the medulla. Lesions within this pathway (most often within the central tegmental tract) can disrupt transmission between the cerebellum, specifically the flocculus, and the inferior olive. The lesion produces hypertrophy of the inferior olivary nucleus, which is easily visualized with MRI as a T2 hyperintensity within 1 or both inferior olives.

See-Saw Nystagmus

See-saw nystagmus is a form of disconjugate nystagmus in which 1 eye elevates and intorts while the other eye depresses and extorts, movement reminiscent of that of a see-saw. The eye movements are typically pendular, the frequency typically slow, and the amplitude similar between eyes. See-saw nystagmus may be congenital, but it is most commonly found in patients with large tumors in the parasellar region. Craniopharyngioma is one of the most frequent causes. Other parasellar–diencephalic tumors and trauma may also produce see-saw nystagmus; congenital achiasma is a rare cause. There may be associated visual loss, often bitemporal hemianopia. Asymmetric visual loss may influence the amplitude of the eye movements (ie, the amplitude may be larger in the poorer seeing eye).

Daroff RB. See-saw nystagmus. *Neurology.* 1965;15:874–877.

Dissociated Nystagmus

Nystagmus that is characterized by a difference in the size of the ocular oscillation is referred to as "dissociated." Perhaps the most common form of *dissociated nystagmus* is seen with lesions of the medial longitudinal fasciculus (MLF), which produces an internuclear ophthalmoplegia (INO; see Chapter 8). Isolated slowing of adduction of the eye ipsilateral to an MLF lesion is the primary feature required to establish a diagnosis of INO. In addition, there is often nystagmus of the abducting eye when gaze is directed to the side opposite the lesion. One explanation for this pattern of dissociated nystagmus is the development of increased neural pulsing in an attempt to overcome the adduction weakness. According to Hering's law, the increased neural signaling would also be delivered to the contralateral yoke muscle, which would create excessive saccadic movements in the contralateral lateral rectus muscle.

Saccadic Intrusions

Several forms of saccadic intrusions have been identified. Based on eye movement recordings, 2 classes may be distinguished by the presence or absence of an intersaccadic interval, which is defined as the temporal separation between sequential saccades extending 180–200 msec.

Saccadic Intrusions With Normal Intersaccadic Intervals

The most common saccadic intrusions are *square-wave jerks,* which have a normal intersaccadic interval (amplitude typically <2°; latency to refixation: 200 msec). *Macrosquare-wave jerks* are much less common but also include an intersaccadic interval (amplitude 5°–15°; latency to refixation: 70–150 msec; Fig 9-3). The smaller square-wave jerks may be seen in low frequencies in normal elderly people. Macrosquare-wave jerks tend to have a slightly higher frequency and are always pathologic. Lesions that disrupt the fastigial nucleus of the cerebellum or the superior colliculus, or their interconnecting fibers, may give rise to these inappropriate eye movements. The abnormal eye movements may be created by an alteration of the omnipause neurons of the pons, which would lower the typically high threshold for initiation of saccadic eye movements during attempted fixation. The larger-amplitude macrosquare-wave jerks are mostly seen in patients with cerebellar disease or multiple sclerosis.

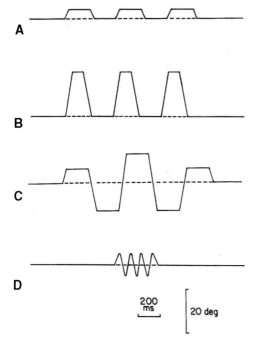

Figure 9-3 Schematic of saccadic intrusions and oscillations. **A,** Square-wave jerks: small, uncalled-for saccades away from and back to the position of the target. **B,** Macrosquare-wave jerks. **C,** Macrosaccadic oscillations: hypermetric saccades about the position of the target. **D,** Ocular flutter: back-to-back, to-and-fro saccades without an intersaccadic interval. *(Used and modified with permission from Leigh RJ, Zee DS.* The Neurology of Eye Movements. *3rd ed. Contemporary Neurology Series. New York: Oxford University Press; 1999.)*

Macrosaccadic oscillation is another type of saccadic intrusion that breaks fixation. These oscillations differ from the square-wave jerks in that the oscillations extend equally to 1 side and then the other side of the fixation. Relatively large movements that break fixation, like macrosquare-wave jerks, tend to occur in short bursts. This disorder develops because of a hypermetria that produces repetitive inaccuracies in attempts to fixate on a target. The hypermetria is a manifestation of cerebellar dysfunction.

Saccadic Intrusions Without Normal Intersaccadic Intervals

Two types of eye movement abnormalities lack the intersaccadic interval that is normally present between sequential saccades: ocular flutter and opsoclonus. Both conditions can be diagnosed with reasonable confidence by clinical examination alone, although a definitive demonstration of the lack of an intersaccadic interval requires eye movement recordings. The pathology for these eye movements is unknown but may relate to dysfunction of the omnipause neurons of the pons or to connections with these cells (see Chapter 7).

Ocular flutter typically presents as bursts of horizontal movements that have quite small amplitude but very high (10–15 Hz) frequency (Fig 9-3D). Whereas flutter is horizontal, multidirectional eye movements with a similarly high frequency but often larger amplitude are known as *opsoclonus* (or *saccadomania*). A patient may have both ocular flutter and opsoclonus, or the movements may change from 1 form to the other during the course of disease.

In evaluating patients with these types of eye movements, a paraneoplastic etiology must be excluded. In children, neuroblastoma (or other tumor of neural crest origin) is the primary consideration, whereas in adults, small cell carcinoma of the lung or cancer of the breast or ovaries is of prime concern. Abnormal antibodies directed against neuronal RNA are found in some patients with paraneoplastic-induced ocular flutter or opsoclonus. Serologic or CSF assay for the anti-Ri antibody (also known as ANNA-2) can help confirm the diagnosis in cases secondary to cancer of the breast or ovary, whereas anti-Hu antibodies (also known as ANNA-1) are present in some children with neuroblastoma. Multiple sclerosis is a common cause of ocular flutter in young adults. Ocular flutter and opsoclonus may occur following brainstem encephalitis. Other reported causes include drug intoxication, toxins, and hyperosmolar coma. Despite the generally dire implications, opsoclonus may be seen as a transient finding in normal infants and may occur, rarely, in some patients without explanation in the absence of associated neurologic or systemic abnormalities. Opsoclonus may coexist with myoclonus (opsoclonus-myoclonus syndrome).

Digre KB. Opsoclonus in adults. Report of three cases and review of the literature. *Arch Neurol.* 1986;43(11):1165–1175.

Lennon VA. Paraneoplastic autoantibodies: the case for a descriptive generic nomenclature. *Neurology.* 1994;44(12):2236–2240.

Voluntary Nystagmus

Voluntary "nystagmus" consists of rapidly oscillating eye movements (almost always horizontal) that can be induced volitionally. The movements, which are not a form of nystagmus (because they lack slow phases), appear as high-frequency, conjugate, back-to-back saccades without an intersaccadic interval associated with convergence and often with eyelid flutter and facial grimacing. At times, voluntary nystagmus can be difficult to distinguish from ocular flutter; however, ocular flutter is typically associated with other abnormal examination features and does not have the convergence and eyelid accompaniments of voluntary nystagmus (see Chapter 13).

Additional Eye Movement Abnormalities

Convergence-Retraction Nystagmus

Convergence-retraction nystagmus, which in reality does not meet the definition of nystagmus because it lacks slow phases, results from co-contraction of the extraocular muscles on attempted upgaze. The medial rectus muscles are the most powerful of the extraocular muscles, and their contraction produces convergent movements even when all other extraocular muscles are contracting. The co-contraction of all extraocular muscles produces retraction of the globe into the orbit. Convergence-retraction nystagmus localizes the disease process to the dorsal midbrain, and hence the "nystagmus" is often associated with paresis of upgaze, pupillary light–near dissociation, skew deviation, and bilateral lid retraction (Collier sign). Convergence-retraction nystagmus is best demonstrated by having the patient make an upward saccade or follow a downward-rotating OKN drum.

Superior Oblique Myokymia

Superior oblique myokymia is a disorder that produces paroxysmal, monocular, high-frequency bursts of contraction of the superior oblique muscle. These bursts typically last for seconds, occur numerous times per day, and usually produce vertical or torsional oscillopsia. The movements are of very small amplitude, and magnification (obtained, for instance, with a slit lamp or 20 D lens) is usually required. The abnormal movements may occur spontaneously or immediately following a downward eye movement. The contraction of the superior oblique muscle may also produce transient vertical diplopia, because a tonically contracting superior oblique muscle will depress the affected eye. Electromyographic recordings of some patients have demonstrated abnormal discharge from some muscle fibers, either spontaneously or following contraction of the muscle. The etiology of superior oblique myokymia is unknown. It is almost always benign, although there are rare reports of its association with multiple sclerosis or posterior fossa tumor. Some clinical and neuroimaging findings suggest this disorder may be due to neurovascular compression, similar to cases of hemifacial spasm and trigeminal neuralgia.

The clinical course of superior oblique myokymia is highly variable. Some patients enjoy spontaneous recovery or experience only brief spells of symptoms. Most patients, however, are chronically bothered by oscillopsia or intermittent diplopia. Carbamazepine, phenytoin, baclofen, gabapentin, or topical β-blockers may be helpful in some patients. In more severe cases, a combined superior oblique muscle tenotomy and recession of the ipsilateral inferior oblique muscle may effect a cure.

> Brazis PW, Miller NR, Henderer JD, Lee AG. The natural history and results of treatment of superior oblique myokymia. *Arch Ophthalmol.* 1994;112(8):1063–1067.

Oculomasticatory Myorhythmia

Vertical saccadic palsy may be an early neurologic finding in Whipple disease. In addition, patients may develop pendular, vergence oscillations that occur with contractions of the masticatory muscles. This combination of abnormal movements is known as *oculomasticatory myorhythmia.* Patients may have only the neurologic manifestations, but, more commonly, they also have unexplained fever, diarrhea, cognitive dysfunction, weight loss, and lymphadenopathy. Whipple disease can be diagnosed by duodenal biopsy (using PAS staining) to document infection with *Tropheryma whippelii* or by serologic polymerase chain reaction (PCR) testing. Whipple disease is a progressive and potentially life-threatening disease that is curable with antibiotic therapy.

> Lowsky R, Archer GL, Fyles G, et al. Brief report: diagnosis of Whipple's disease by molecular analysis of peripheral blood. *N Engl J Med.* 1994;331(20):1343–1346.
> Schwartz MA, Selhorst JB, Ochs AL, et al. Oculomasticatory myorhythmia: a unique movement disorder occurring in Whipple's disease. *Ann Neurol.* 1986;20(6):677–683.

Treatment of Nystagmus and Other Eye Movement Abnormalities

Nystagmus is generally difficult to treat, although successful forms of therapy have been reported for some forms. Several treatment options are described here, but readers should review the referenced publications to obtain a more in-depth overview.

Perhaps the most well-documented and successful therapy for nystagmus and related disorders is the use of baclofen (a $GABA_B$ agonist) for the acquired form of PAN and carbamazepine derivatives for superior oblique myokymia. Downbeat and other central vestibular forms of nystagmus can occasionally be helped by clonazepam, a $GABA_A$ agonist.

Memenatine or gabapentin (also GABAergic medication) may help some patients with the acquired form of pendular nystagmus.

Nonmedical treatment options are also available. Nystagmus associated with amblyopia can be improved with traditional amblyopia therapy. Base-out prisms to induce convergence may be helpful for some patients whose nystagmus diminishes with convergence. Use of contact lenses may improve visual acuity in patients with congenital nystagmus.

Unilateral, retrobulbar injection of botulinum toxin reduces the amplitude of nystagmus and may produce a visual benefit for patients who are willing to view monocularly. However, total cessation of eye movements has its own consequences; for example, some patients report blurred vision when walking because of the loss of the normal VOR that adjusts eye position as the head moves.

Some patients with congenital nystagmus can be helped by extraocular muscle surgery (Anderson-Kestenbaum procedure) to mechanically shift the null point to primary position. Clinicians have achieved variable reduction of the amplitude of eye movements and improved visual acuity in some adult patients with congenital nystagmus by performing horizontal rectus muscle tenotomy, with reattachment of the muscles to their original insertion site.

Leigh RJ, Averbuch-Heller L, Tomsak RL, Remler BF, Yaniglos SS, Dell'Osso LF. Treatment of abnormal eye movements that impair vision: strategies based on current concepts of physiology and pharmacology. *Ann Neurol.* 1994;36(2):129–141.

Straube A, Leigh RJ, Bronstein A, et al. EFNS task force—therapy of nystagmus and oscillopsia. *Eur J Neurol.* 2004;11(2):83–89.

Eye Movements in Comatose Patients

Coma is caused by *bilateral* lesions of the brainstem (typically structural) or cerebral hemispheres (structural or metabolic disturbances). Coma also can develop in patients who have a large, unilateral hemispheric stroke when the accompanying edema or hemorrhage produces a mass effect that is sufficient to cause midline shift or tentorial herniation and compression of the brainstem.

A variety of eye movement abnormalities may be seen in unconscious patients. Patients may have conjugate deviation of the eyes. In a gaze preference, the eyes deviate toward the side of a cerebral hemispheric lesion (and away from the side of the hemiparesis, if present) because the intact contralateral frontal eye field imposes a bias that drives the eyes to the opposite side. Intact horizontal eye movements are demonstrable with supranuclear activation such as the VOR. This type of ocular deviation typically persists for only a few days, after which compensatory adjustments are made by the brain to balance the tonic input that controls resting eye position. A pontine brainstem stroke that produces coma may also produce conjugate ocular deviation, although in this situation (gaze palsy) the eyes deviate away from the side of the lesion (remember, "Brainstem lesions are too terrible to look at"). Here, the intact, contralateral horizontal gaze center drives the eyes to the ipsilateral side. Ocular deviation from brainstem strokes usually persists for long periods of time.

Comatose patients may also manifest spontaneous, slow, roving horizontal eye movements. The conjugate nature of these eye movements indicates intact brainstem ocular motor pathways, as may occur in patients whose coma is due to metabolic derangement. Spontaneous eye movements of this type may also be somewhat disconjugate. In cases of coma caused by bilateral hemispheric lesions, spontaneous eye movements may be confined to the horizontal plane and rapidly alternate in gaze from 1 side to the other every few seconds ("Ping-Pong" gaze). Longer periods of alternating deviation lasting minutes are termed *periodic alternating gaze deviation* and may be seen in patients with metabolic coma.

Ocular Bobbing

Ocular bobbing is a rare sign of rapid downward movement of both eyes, followed by a slow return of the eyes to the midline position. The offending lesion is usually in the pons, secondary to infarction or hemorrhage. Ocular bobbing portends an extremely poor prognosis for neurologic recovery. Bilateral pontine lesions lead to loss of horizontal eye movements.

Similar vertical eye movements may have an initially slow downward movement followed by a fast return to primary position (*inverse bobbing*, or *ocular dipping*), or the deviation from primary position may be upward. An initially fast upward deviation followed by a slow return to primary position has been referred to as *reverse ocular bobbing;* a slow initial upward drift followed by a fast return to primary position has been termed *converse bobbing*, or *reverse ocular dipping*. Although ocular bobbing has valuable localization and prognostic information, inverse bobbing, reverse bobbing, and dipping are nonlocalizing (most often noted with hypoxic-ischemic encephalopathy).

CHAPTER 10

The Patient With Pupillary Abnormalities

Pupillary function is an important objective clinical sign in patients with visual loss and neurologic disease. In some patients, an abnormal pupillary response may be the only objective sign of organic visual dysfunction; in others, it may herald the presence of a life-threatening cerebral aneurysm or tumor. Fortunately, the presence of efferent and afferent pupillary defects can be determined quickly and easily in the clinic by evaluating the size and reaction of the pupils. Pupillary anatomy and innervation are discussed in Chapter 1, and the evaluation of relative afferent pupillary defect is described in Chapter 3. This chapter reviews the clinical approach to patients with pupillary disorders, including irregular pupils, anisocoria, and light–near dissociation.

History

Patients with pupillary disturbances, particularly anisocoria, may not be aware of any abnormality. This is especially true in persons with dark-colored irides. Frequently, a spouse, friend, or physician brings the abnormality to the patient's attention.

The patient's medical history may be helpful in assessing the significance of a disturbance in pupil size or shape. A history of previous infection (eg, herpes zoster), trauma, surgery (especially ocular), or migraine may suggest the etiology of the pupillary disturbance. The patient's occupation may also be important. A farmer or gardener may be exposed to plants or pesticides that can produce pupillary dilation or constriction by topical contamination. A physician, nurse, or other health professional may work with or have access to topical dilating or constricting substances that may produce changes in pupil size by design or chance.

Reports of symptoms in patients with pupillary disturbance are highly variable. Frequently, none are reported. When present, symptoms may include photophobia, difficulty focusing when going from dark to light or light to dark, and blurring of vision.

Pupillary Examination

Documenting the onset of the pupillary abnormality may be facilitated by careful inspection of patient photographs. The clinician can look at the patient's driver's license or other photographic identification card at the time of initial evaluation or can ask the patient to return with old photographs spanning several years ("biopsy of the family album").

A thorough clinical examination of the pupils requires only simple, inexpensive tools: a bright, even, handheld light source (such as a halogen transilluminator); a pupil-measuring gauge, preferably in half-millimeter increments; neutral density filters in 0.3, 0.6, and 0.9 log unit values to quantitate relative afferent pupillary defects; and an examination room in which background illumination is easily controlled. For measuring afferent pupillary defects, see Chapter 3.

In evaluating pupil size, the clinician shines a handheld light obliquely from below the nose for indirect illumination and a clear view of the pupils in both darkness and room light. To avoid accommodative miosis, the patient is instructed to fix on a distant target, and the examiner should be careful not to block the patient's fixation. The pupils are measured 5–10 seconds after changes in illumination to avoid pupillary fluctuations. It is important to remember that at any given moment, multiple factors may influence pupil size and reactivity; the pupil is in a state of constant physiologic unrest.

Shining a light in 1 eye of a normal subject causes both pupils to constrict equally. The pupillary reaction in the illuminated eye is called the *direct response,* and the reaction in the other eye is the *consensual response.* Because of the hemidecussation of afferent pupillomotor fibers in the chiasm, and because a second hemidecussation of the pupillomotor fibers takes place in the brainstem, direct and consensual responses are equal. If 1 eye is blind, all input to the pupillary centers in the brainstem comes from the other eye, but the double hemidecussation ensures equal pupillary motor innervation and prevents inequality of the pupils (anisocoria).

In addition, the near response should be examined. This should be carried out in moderate room light, such that the patient's pupils are midsize and the near object is clearly visible. The patient is given an accommodative target with fine detail to look at. The near response, although it is usually triggered by blurred or disparate imagery, has a large volitional component, and the patient may need encouragement. If the patient has not made sufficient effort, "practice runs" may be needed. Often, a good near response is obtained on the third or fourth try. Sometimes a better response is obtained if other sensory input is added to the stimulus, such as a ticking watch; or a proprioceptive target such as the patient's own thumbnail can be used. A lack of near response usually indicates that the patient (or the doctor) is not trying hard enough.

Slit-lamp examination of the anterior segment is also essential in defining a pupillary abnormality. For example, the finding of corneal injury or anterior chamber inflammation may explain a small pupil in the setting of ciliary spasm. Gonioscopy to assess the anterior chamber angle should be performed in a patient with a dilated pupil, particularly when there is a history of pain or redness in the eye. Assessment of the iris should include not only inspection of the integrity of the sphincter muscle but also transillumination of the iris to seek evidence of iris damage from previous trauma, infection, or inflammation. In addition, by placing a wide beam at an angle to the iris and turning the light off and on, the clinician can assess the light reflex for segmental defects such as those that occur in eyes with tonic pupils or aberrant regeneration of the oculomotor nerve.

Normally the pupil is black, but on occasion it may appear white. Leukocoria (white pupil) has several causes, one of which is a light-reflecting abnormality in the posterior segment of the eye. In small children, leukocoria may indicate the presence of a malignant tumor such as retinoblastoma. Other causes include persistent hyperplastic primary vitreous, retinopathy of prematurity, and cataract.

Pharmacologic agents can be used to evaluate pupillary reactivity and can confirm a clinical suspicion of Horner syndrome, tonic pupil, or pharmacologic mydriasis. It is important to remember, however, that pharmacologic pupil testing is not infallible, as false-positive and false-negative results can occur, and test results must be interpreted in the individual setting.

Baseline Pupil Size

The resting pupil size is influenced by several factors; most important are the amount of ambient light, the status of retinal adaptation, the level of arousal, and the patient's age. Pupils, in general, become smaller with age. Sleep results in decreased sympathetic activity and smaller pupils. Arousal, excitement, or startle increases pupil size. Elevated intraocular pressure may result in enlargement of the pupil, possibly by inducing ischemia in the iris. Pupils are often dilated following grand mal seizures.

Extremely small pupils usually suggest pontine hemorrhage, narcotic intoxication, or pilocarpine use. Extremely large pupils suggest parasympathetic pharmacologic blockade from either topical or systemic agents.

Pupil Irregularity

Any disorder that physically damages the mechanical compliance of the iris or iris musculature can result in an irregular pupil. *Blunt trauma* to the eye can cause focal tears in the sphincter muscle. An *iridodialysis* occurs when the outer edge of the iris is torn away from its ciliary attachment. *Intraocular inflammation* can damage the iris or cause it to adhere to the lens or cornea *(synechiae)*. *Neovascularization* can also distort the iris and impair pupillary reactivity. *Iris malformation* such as coloboma and aniridia will affect pupil size and function. The leading cause of a misshapen pupil in an adult is probably *cataract surgery,* but any operative procedure in the anterior segment may have similar results. To avert an extensive and unnecessary neurologic evaluation, it is essential to recognize these iris structural abnormalities as the cause of abnormal pupil size, shape, and reactivity.

The following 2 rare conditions may cause pupillary irregularity by means of alteration in iris innervation:

1. *Tadpole pupil.* This disorder is uniformly benign and occurs in healthy individuals, often with a history of migraine. The pupil undergoes sectoral dilation lasting for a few minutes before returning to normal. This phenomenon may occur multiple times for several days or a week and then disappears. It is thought to represent segmental spasm of the iris dilator muscle. (See: http:/library.med.utah.edu/NOVEL/.)

2. *Midbrain corectopia.* In rare cases, eccentric or oval pupils are seen in patients with rostral midbrain disease. This abnormality is presumably caused by incomplete damage of the pupillary fibers leading to selective inhibition of iris sphincter tone.

Selhorst JB, Hoyt WF, Feinsod M, Hosobuchi Y. Midbrain corectopia. *Arch Neurol.* 1976;33(3): 193–195.

Thompson HS, Zackon DH, Czarnecki JS. Tadpole-shaped pupils caused by segmental spasm of the iris dilator muscle. *Am J Ophthalmol.* 1983;96(4):467–477.

Anisocoria

Efferent disturbances of pupil size are usually unilateral, which produces inequality in the diameters of the 2 pupils. This condition is called *anisocoria*. Although it is important for the clinician to look for anisocoria when assessing the pupil, its presence does not necessarily represent an abnormality. The evaluation of a patient with isolated anisocoria is much easier with the systemic approach illustrated in the flowchart in Figure 10-1. In many individuals, anisocoria is physiologic.

Physiologic Anisocoria

Physiologic anisocoria (also known as *simple* or *essential anisocoria*) is the most common cause of a difference in pupil size of 0.4 mm or more. At any given moment, about 20% of individuals have noticeably asymmetric pupil diameters. Usually, the difference in pupil diameters is less than 1.0 mm. The amount of anisocoria in an individual can vary from day to day.

Physiologic anisocoria is sometimes more apparent in dim light than in bright light, simulating Horner syndrome. Congenital or acquired ptosis on the side of the smaller pupil can further create diagnostic confusion. When questions arise, pharmacologic testing with cocaine will demonstrate symmetric dilation of pupils in patients with physiologic anisocoria.

Lam BL, Thompson HS, Corbett JJ. The prevalence of simple anisocoria. *Am J Ophthalmol.* 1987;104(1):69–73.

Thompson BM, Corbett JJ, Kline LB, Thompson HS. Pseudo-Horner's syndrome. *Arch Neurol.* 1982;39(2):108–111.

Anisocoria Equal in Dim and Bright Light

Anisocoria that is equal in dim and bright light indicates no difference in the relative function of the pupillary sphincter and dilator muscles. It is consistent with physiologic anisocoria and the patient can be reassured.

Anisocoria Greater in Dim Light

With some conditions, such as those described in the following sections, anisocoria becomes more apparent in dim light.

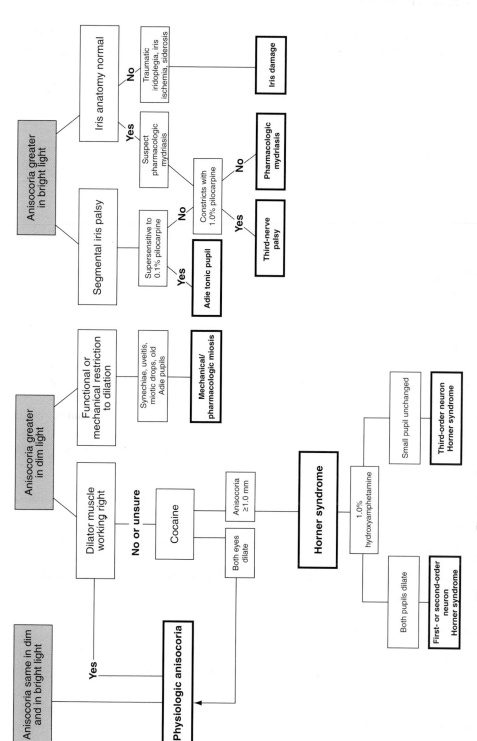

Figure 10-1 Flowchart for evaluation of anisocoria. *(Courtesy of Lanning B. Kline, MD.)*

Mechanical anisocoria

Occasionally, previous trauma (including surgery) or inflammation can lead to adhesions between the iris and the lens or intraocular lens. These adhesions may prevent dilation in conditions of dim illumination. Posterior synechiae should be visible with a magnifying lens or slit lamp.

Pharmacologic anisocoria

The use of pilocarpine may result in a small, poorly reactive pupil. Anisocoria will not be present if both eyes are treated, but the unilateral use of medication may cause confusion. This condition is seen less often today than formerly because of the wider range of choices in glaucoma medications.

Physiologic anisocoria

Physiologic anisocoria was discussed earlier in the chapter.

Horner syndrome

A lesion at any point along the oculosympathetic pathway results in Horner syndrome, which includes ptosis, miosis, and anhidrosis on the same side. With Horner syndrome, anisocoria is more apparent in dim illumination, and the affected pupil shows dilation lag when the room light is abruptly turned off. (See: http://library.med.utah.edu/NOVEL/.) Light and near pupillary reactions are intact, but the eyelid is ptotic due to paresis of Müller muscle. There is apparent enophthalmos because the lower eyelid may be elevated; however, exophthalmometry readings are equal. When the lesion is congenital, iris heterochromia develops (the affected iris appears lighter in color). The distribution of anhidrosis depends on the location of the lesion. Interruption of the central (first-order) or preganglionic (second-order) neuron causes anhidrosis of the ipsilateral face. Lesions at or distal to the superior cervical ganglion—that is, the postganglionic (third-order) neuron—result in anhidrosis limited to the ipsilateral forehead.

The oculosympathetic dysfunction can be confirmed pharmacologically with topical drops: either cocaine or apraclonidine. Cocaine blocks the re-uptake of norepinephrine released at neuromuscular junctions of the iris dilator muscle, thereby increasing the amount of norepinephrine available to stimulate the muscle. Following instillation of cocaine in a normal eye, the pupil will dilate; but in Horner syndrome, the pupil dilates poorly because little or no norepinephrine is being released into the synaptic cleft. The test is performed by instilling 2 drops of 4% or 10% cocaine in each eye and measuring the amount of anisocoria after 45 minutes. A postcocaine anisocoria of 1 mm or more is diagnostic of Horner syndrome on the side of the smaller pupil (see Fig 10-1). A false-positive test result is occasionally encountered in a patient with a mechanically restricted pupil. In such a case, the adhesions and synechiae responsible for keeping the pupil constricted and immobile are usually detectable at the slit lamp. Otherwise, 5% or 10% (full-strength) topical phenylephrine will distinguish between the 2 conditions: a mechanically restricted pupil remains small following phenylephrine, but the direct drug action on the dilator muscle easily dilates a Horner pupil.

Apraclonidine has weak α_1-agonist action, which, in most normal eyes, produces no significant effect on the pupil. In sympathetically denervated eyes, the iris dilator muscle develops adrenergic supersensitivity; thus, apraclonidine dilates a Horner pupil. Following instillation of 0.5% or 1% apraclonidine in each eye, a reversal of anisocoria is diagnostic of a Horner syndrome (Fig 10-2). If the apraclonidine test is negative in a patient suspected of having Horner syndrome, cocaine testing (still considered the gold standard pharmacologic test) should be performed on a separate day.

The lesion producing Horner syndrome can be further localized by use of hydroxamphetamine (see Fig 10-1), which acts by releasing norepinephrine from the presynaptic terminal. Hydroxyamphetamine in a normal eye will dilate the pupil; but with a *postganglionic* Horner syndrome, the nerve terminal has degenerated, and the pupil dilates poorly, if at all. In other words, if the amount of baseline anisocoria is increased following hydroxyamphetamine, then it is a postganglionic lesion. With a *preganglionic* Horner syndrome, the postganglionic neuron is intact, and hydroxyamphetamine dilates the Horner pupil as much as it does the normal pupil. Any pharmacologic test of pupillary function should not be done within 24 hours of instillation of other drops.

Localization of the lesion causing Horner syndrome is important. *First-order neuron lesions* are caused by central disorders of the nervous system, such as vascular occlusion, particularly in the lateral medulla (Wallenberg syndrome), as well as by tumors, cervical disc disease, and other disorders involving the upper cervical spinal cord. *Second-order neuron lesions* are caused by apical lung tumors (Pancoast syndrome), metastases, chest surgery, thoracic aortic aneurysms, or trauma to the brachial plexus (Fig 10-3). *Third-order neuron lesions* are caused most commonly by degenerative changes in the wall of the carotid artery or following vasospasm. Other causes include surgery on the carotid artery or structures nearby, internal carotid artery dissection (Fig 10-4), and extension of tumors such as nasopharyngeal carcinomas into the cavernous sinus.

In addition to testing with cocaine and hydroxyamphetamine drops, careful history taking and examination are also helpful in localizing Horner syndrome. Clues for the localization of first-order neuron lesions include accompanying neurologic symptoms and signs such as numbness, weakness, ataxia, and nystagmus. Second-order neuron lesions are associated with trauma and symptoms such as cough, hemoptysis, and swelling in the neck. Symptoms associated with third-order neuron lesions include numbness over the first as well as the second and/or third divisions of CN V, and double vision from sixth nerve palsy. Congenital Horner syndrome is usually caused by birth trauma to the brachial plexus. Horner syndrome acquired in early childhood indicates the possibility of neuroblastoma arising in the sympathetic chain of the chest. Analysis for catecholamine

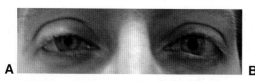 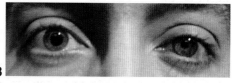

Figure 10-2 Apraclonidine test for Horner syndrome. **A,** A patient with suspected right oculosympathetic defect (ptosis and miosis). **B,** Following instillation of 1% apraclonidine, the anisocoria is reversed, confirming Horner syndrome on the right side. Note also the eyelid retraction on the right side. *(Courtesy of Aki Kawasaki, MD.)*

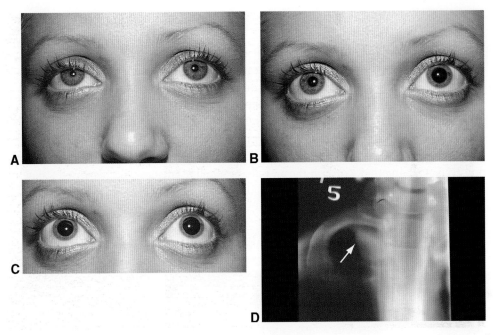

Figure 10-3 Second-order neuron Horner syndrome. **A,** This patient demonstrates right-sided ptosis and miosis in bright light. **B,** The anisocoria increases in the dark. **C,** Following instillation of hydroxyamphetamine 1% drops, both pupils dilate, indicating that the third-order neuron is intact. **D,** The patient's chest tomography demonstrates a right apical mass *(arrow)* that proved to be a schwannoma. *(Courtesy of Lanning B. Kline, MD.)*

excretion in the urine can be especially important, because catecholamines are often increased in neuroblastoma patients. Imaging of the neck, chest, and abdomen may also be warranted.

Isolated postganglionic Horner syndrome is often benign. If examination of old photographs verifies that the Horner syndrome has been present for several years, further investigations will probably be unrewarding. However, Horner syndrome associated with pain deserves extra attention.

Painful postganglionic Horner syndrome is a distinct clinical entity associated with several causes, most importantly carotid artery dissection. Patients with spontaneous dissection of the internal carotid artery commonly present with a Horner syndrome and ipsilateral headache, usually located around the temple, orbit, or throat. Such patients may also have amaurosis fugax and altered taste (dysgeusia). This condition must be recognized, because, in the acute stage, stroke is a possible complication. MRI typically shows an intramural hemorrhage, and, in rare cases, MRA or cerebral arteriography is needed to provide definitive evidence of dissection. Patients with typical cluster headaches may develop Horner syndrome on the ipsilateral side during an acute attack. (See: http://library.med.utah.edu/NOVEL/.) The Horner syndrome often resolves, but it may become permanent after repeated attacks. Some patients, usually middle-aged men, have Horner syndrome and daily unilateral headaches not characteristic of cluster; no underlying pathology can be identified. The term *Raeder paratrigeminal syndrome* has been used to describe this condition. This condition mandates careful patient evaluation, diagnosed

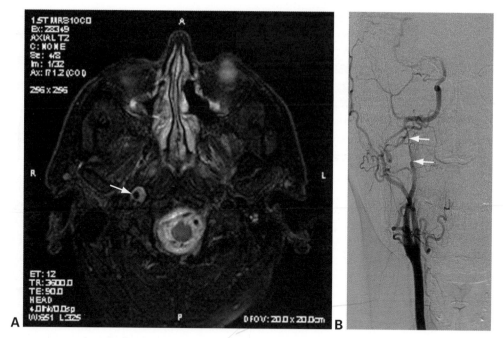

Figure 10-4 **A,** Internal carotid artery dissection. Axial MRI showing blood *(arrow)* in the wall of the right internal carotid artery ("crescent moon sign"). **B,** Catheter angiogram demonstrates "string sign" *(arrows)*, confirming internal carotid artery dissection. *(Part A courtesy of Karl C. Golnik, MD; part B courtesy of Lanning B. Kline, MD.)*

only after exclusion of possible underlying lesions, particularly pathology in the parasellar and cavernous sinus regions.

Cremer SA, Thompson HS, Digre KB, Kardon RH. Hydroxyamphetamine mydriasis in Horner's syndrome. *Am J Ophthalmol.* 1990;110(1):71–76.

Kardon RH, Denison CE, Brown CK, Thompson HS. Critical evaluation of the cocaine test in the diagnosis of Horner's syndrome. *Arch Ophthalmol.* 1990;108(12):384–387.

Mahoney NR, Liu GT, Menacker SJ, Wilson MC, Hogarty MD, Maris JM. Pediatric Horner syndrome: etiologies and roles of imaging and urine studies to detect neuroblastoma and other responsible mass lesions. *Am J Ophthalmol.* 2006;142(4):651–659.

Maloney WF, Younge BR, Moyer NJ. Evaluation of the causes and accuracy of pharmacologic localization of Horner's syndrome. *Am J Ophthalmol.* 1980;90(3):394–402.

Morales J, Brown SM, Abdul-Ralim AS, Crosson CE. Ocular effects of apraclonidine in Horner syndrome. *Arch Ophthalmol.* 2000;118(7):951–954.

Anisocoria Greater in Bright Light

With the conditions described in the following sections, anisocoria is greater in bright light.

Iris damage

Blunt trauma to the eye can cause mydriasis by damaging the pupillary sphincter. The pupil may be relatively miotic after injury, but it soon becomes midsized and poorly responsive to bright light in dim illumination. Notches can be seen in the pupillary margin, and the iris may transilluminate near the sphincter muscle. Iris injury occurs frequently in patients with head trauma, and the dilated pupil may be mistakenly identified as a sign of third nerve palsy due to uncal herniation.

Because of direct iris sphincter damage, instillation of pilocarpine 1% may not lead to pupillary constriction. Thus, diagnostic eyedrop testing in patients with traumatic mydriasis sometimes mimics the findings of pharmacologic mydriasis.

Prolonged or recurrent angle closure can also impair a pupil's function. Iris function is frequently abnormal following intraocular surgery, and interruption of pupillary responses in this setting must be approached with caution.

Pharmacologic pupil

When mydriatic medications are instilled in the eye accidentally or intentionally, the pupil becomes dilated and reacts poorly to light and near stimulation. The sphincter muscle should be examined at the slit lamp. Drug-induced dilation causes paralysis of the *entire* sphincter, in contrast to an Adie pupil, which causes segmental sphincter contraction. Pilocarpine may be used to test for drug-induced mydriasis. Pilocarpine 1% causes constriction of the pupil in a normal eye or one with an Adie pupil or third nerve palsy but not in a pharmacologically dilated pupil.

With adrenergic mydriasis, the pupil is large, the palpebral fissure is widened, and the conjunctiva may be blanched. Accommodation is not impaired.

Pharmacologic agents such as those used to treat glaucoma may cause anisocoria if they are administered in only 1 eye or if absorption is asymmetric. The anisocoria can be pronounced if a patient inadvertently injures the surface of 1 cornea while instilling drops or if 1 cornea is exposed, for example, from a Bell's palsy.

Adie tonic pupil

Diagnostic features of tonic pupils include sluggish, segmental pupillary responses to light and better response to near effort followed by slow redilation. A tonic pupil is caused by postganglionic parasympathetic pupillomotor damage. Seventy percent of patients are female. Tonic pupils are unilateral in 80% of cases, although the second pupil may later become involved (4% per year). *Holmes-Adie syndrome* includes other features, notably diminished deep tendon reflexes and orthostatic hypotension.

In the initial stages, a tonic pupil is dilated and poorly reactive. The examiner at the slit lamp can usually see segments of the sphincter constrict. The iris crypts stream toward the area of normal sphincter function, bunching up along the pupillary border in areas of normal function and thinning in the areas of paralysis (Fig 10-5). After a few weeks, a tonic pupil constricts to near effort with a slow, tonic movement and redilates just as slowly, whereas a normal pupil redilates promptly (Fig 10-6). This may account for symptomatic complaints of difficulty refocusing for distance.

The denervated iris sphincter is supersensitive to topical parasympathomimetic solutions. Pilocarpine drops (0.1%) can be used to demonstrate this, as the normal pupil will constrict slightly, if at all. (This strength of pilocarpine can be obtained by diluting commercial 1% solution with sterile saline for injection.) After 60 minutes, the pupils are reexamined, and if Adie is present, the affected pupil (dilated pupil) will constrict more than

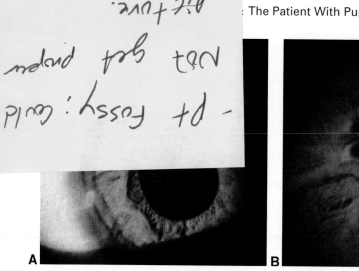
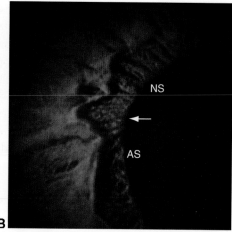

Figure 10-5 Adie tonic pupil. **A,** The pupil is not round; the sphincter contracts from the 11 o'clock to 1 o'clock areas, with puckering of the iris stroma. Where the sphincter is paralyzed, the regions of iris stroma are relatively flat. **B,** Same patient as in part A. The *arrow* indicates the junction of the normal sphincter *(NS)* and the atonic sphincter *(AS)*. *(Reprinted with permission from Thompson HS. Segmental palsy of the iris sphincter in Adie's syndrome. Arch Ophthalmol. 1978;96(9):1615–1620. Copyright 1978, American Medical Association.)*

the normal pupil (Fig 10-7). About 80% of patients with a tonic pupil show cholinergic denervation supersensitivity.

Patients with tonic pupils may have accommodative symptoms or photophobia, but just as often they have no symptoms and report that anisocoria was first noticed by a friend or relative. Accommodative symptoms are difficult to treat. Fortunately, they usually resolve spontaneously within a few months of onset. When photophobia from a dilated pupil is a problem, topical dilute pilocarpine (0.1%) may be helpful. With time (months to years), an Adie tonic pupil gets smaller. Histopathologic examination of the ciliary ganglion in patients with Adie tonic pupil has shown a reduction in the number of ganglion cells.

Systemic conditions associated with tonic pupils only rarely include varicella-zoster, giant cell arteritis, syphilis, and orbital trauma. Bilateral tonic pupils may be seen in patients with diabetes, alcoholism, syphilis, cancer-associated dysautonomia, and amyloidosis.

Kardon RH, Corbett JJ, Thompson HS. Segmental denervation and reinnervation of the iris sphincter as shown by infrared videographic transillumination. *Ophthalmology.* 1998;105(2): 313–321.

Thompson HS. Segmental palsy of the iris sphincter in Adie's syndrome. *Arch Ophthalmol.* 1978;96(9):1615–1620.

Third nerve palsy

For additional discussion of third nerve palsy, see Chapter 8.

Pupillary involvement in third nerve palsy is almost always accompanied by ptosis and limited ocular motility. At times, the motility disturbance may be subtle, requiring careful quantitation with alternate cover testing. Pupillary dysfunction is an important

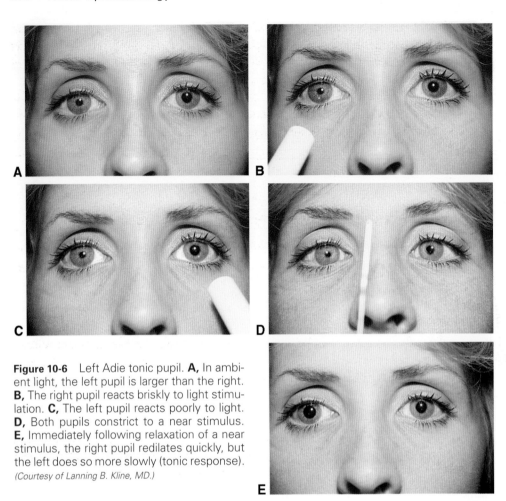

Figure 10-6 Left Adie tonic pupil. **A,** In ambient light, the left pupil is larger than the right. **B,** The right pupil reacts briskly to light stimulation. **C,** The left pupil reacts poorly to light. **D,** Both pupils constrict to a near stimulus. **E,** Immediately following relaxation of a near stimulus, the right pupil redilates quickly, but the left does so more slowly (tonic response). *(Courtesy of Lanning B. Kline, MD.)*

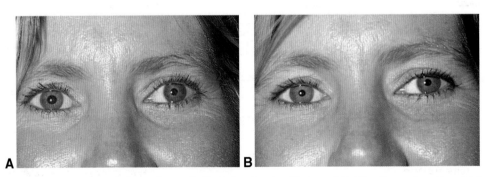

Figure 10-7 **A,** Right Adie tonic pupil. **B,** Following instillation of 0.1% pilocarpine, the right pupil becomes miotic, demonstrating supersensitivity. *(Courtesy of Lanning B. Kline, MD.)*

factor in evaluating an acute third nerve palsy. When the pupil is involved, an aneurysm at the junction of the internal carotid and posterior communicating arteries must be excluded (see Chapter 2, Fig 2-10). If the pupil is spared and all other functions of the third nerve are completely paretic, an aneurysm can likely be ruled out.

Aberrant regeneration of the oculomotor nerve may cause mydriasis and a synkinetic pupillary reaction. (See: http:/library.med.utah.edu/NOVEL/.) Portions of the pupillary sphincter contract with attempted movement of the eye, especially medially.

Czarnecki JS, Thompson HS. The iris sphincter in aberrant regeneration of the third nerve. *Arch Ophthalmol.* 1978;96(9):1606–1610.

Disorders of Pupillary Reactivity: Light–Near Dissociation

At times, the near response exceeds the best pupillary constriction that bright light can produce. This clinical observation of light–near dissociation may arise in a variety of settings (Table 10-1).

Afferent Visual Pathway

Because the pathways subserving light reflex (more dorsal) and near reflex (more ventral) are separated in their approach to the Edinger-Westphal nuclei in the midbrain, patients with anterior visual pathway disease still have intact, brisk pupillary responses to near stimuli.

Midbrain

Dorsal midbrain damage causes midposition pupils with poor light response and preserved near response (see Chapter 7, Fig 7-5). Associated findings may include bilateral eyelid retraction (Collier sign), vertical gaze palsy, accommodative paresis, and convergence-

Table 10-1 Causes of Light–Near Dissociation of the Pupil

Cause	Location	Mechanism
Severe loss of afferent light input to both eyes	Anterior visual pathway (retina, optic nerves, chiasm)	Damage to the retina or optic nerve pathways
Loss of pretectal light input to Edinger-Westphal nucleus	Tectum of the midbrain	Infection (Argyll Robertson pupils) or compression
Adie syndrome	Ciliary ganglion	Aberrant reinnervation of iris sphincter by accommodative neurons
Panretinal photocoagulation, retinal cryotherapy, orbital surgery	Short, posterior ciliary nerves	Aberrant reinnervation following damage to short, posterior ciliary nerves
Third nerve aberrant reinnervation	Course of CN III	Aberrant reinnervation of iris sphincter by accommodative neurons or extraocular muscle neurons
Peripheral neuropathy	Short, posterior ciliary nerves/ciliary ganglion	Axonal loss

retraction nystagmus. Typically, midbrain damage causes midposition pupils that are poorly reactive to both light and near stimuli.

The *Argyll Robertson pupil* occurs in patients with tertiary syphilis involving the central nervous system. Affected patients have small pupils (<2 mm) that are often irregular. The pupils do not react to light, but the near response and subsequent redilation are normal and *brisk*. This feature distinguishes Argyll Robertson pupils from bilateral chronic tonic pupils. In addition, iris atrophy frequently occurs, portions of the iris transilluminate, and dilation is poor after instillation of mydriatics.

Argyll Robertson–like pupils are seen in widespread autonomic neuropathies such as bilateral tonic pupils (chronic), diabetes, and chronic alcoholism, as well as in encephalitis and following panretinal photocoagulation. Bilateral tonic pupils have been reported in neurosyphilis. Serologic tests for syphilis, such as serum FTA-ABS and TPHA, should be considered in the evaluation of patients with bilateral pupillary light–near dissociation with miosis.

Aberrant Regeneration

Light–near dissociation can also occur from aberrant regeneration of damaged nerves, which restores the near reflex but not the light reflex. In tonic pupil syndrome, the injured short ciliary nerves resprout and accommodative fibers mistakenly reinnervate the iris sphincter. Similar misdirection can follow traumatic injury or chronic compression of the oculomotor nerve. In both situations, the pupil near response is restored, but the pupil light reflex remains absent or dysfunctional. Sometimes aberrant regeneration involves the medial rectus fibers. In such a case, a pupillary contraction occurs during attempted adduction, including gaze deviation. This synkinetic pupil movement can be mistaken for a restored near response.

Other Pupillary Disorders

Benign Episodic Pupillary Mydriasis

Also known as *springing pupil, benign episodic pupillary mydriasis* typically occurs in young, healthy individuals who frequently have a history of headache. Episodic mydriasis may last from minutes to hours and may be accompanied by mild blurring of vision, periocular discomfort, and headache. Each episode is self-limited, and the condition has not been associated with any systemic or neurologic disease.

Jacobson DM. Benign episodic unilateral mydriasis: clinical characteristics. *Ophthalmology.* 1995;102(11):1623–1627.

Paradoxical Pupillary Reactions

In rare cases, paradoxical pupillary constriction in dim illumination after exposure to light can be observed in patients with congenital stationary night blindness, congenital achromatopsia, or dominant optic atrophy.

Frank JW, Kushner BJ, France TD. Paradoxic pupillary phenomena. A review of patients with pupillary constriction to darkness. *Arch Ophthalmol.* 1988;106(11):1564–1566.

CHAPTER 11

The Patient With Eyelid or Facial Abnormalities

Patients with disorders of the eyelids or facial movement often present to the ophthalmologist. Some may complain of visual difficulties (eg, visual loss from ptosis) or pain (eg, exposure keratopathy from facial palsy), but most patients are aware of an abnormality in the position of the lid. Occasionally, patients will attribute the problem to the wrong eye, for example, mistaking ptosis for contralateral lid retraction or widening of the palpebral fissure for contralateral ptosis. Many of these eyelid and facial problems are neurologic in origin. In evaluating these disorders, the clinician should ask about onset and duration of symptoms, as well as associated symptoms. These latter include variability, fatigability, and systemic symptoms such as weakness, dysarthria, or difficulty swallowing. Congenital ptosis can often be confirmed by a review of old photographs of the patient. Patients should be asked about diabetes, thyroid disease, hypertension, sarcoidosis, and focal motor weakness. Before discussing these entities, the clinician must carefully examine eyelid function and facial movement. Diagnosis and management of eyelid disorders are discussed at greater length in BCSC Section 7, *Orbit, Eyelids, and Lacrimal System*.

Examination Techniques

An examination of the eyelids begins with observation of the eyelids' general shape and appearance (an S shape may indicate neurofibromatosis [Fig 11-1; see also Chapter 14] or pathology affecting the lacrimal gland), blink rate (low in Parkinson disease and high in blepharospasm), and abnormal movements (synkinesis with other facial muscles). The opening of the palpebral fissure should be measured in primary position (adult normal is 9–10 mm, with the upper eyelid covering 1 mm of the limbus and the lower eyelid just touching it) (Fig 11-2). If the ptosis is unilateral, the examiner should verify that it is not an artifact of vertical strabismus (hypotropia) (Fig 11-3) or contralateral lid retraction. The eyelids should be everted to rule out a local cause of ptosis, such as retained contact lens or giant papillary conjunctivitis. If the ptosis is asymmetric—and especially if the higher eyelid appears retracted—the clinician should manually raise the ptotic eyelid to see if the higher eyelid drops to a new position (Fig 11-4).

To evaluate levator function, the examiner measures the total excursion of the eyelid margin, from downgaze to upgaze, while firmly pressing on the patient's eyebrow to

275

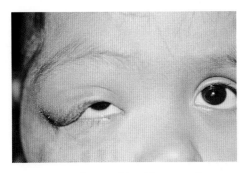

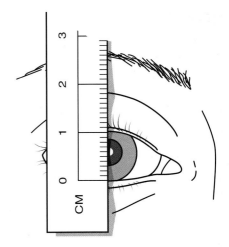

Figure 11-1 2-year-old with neurofibromatosis has ptosis on the right; the S-shaped eyelid margin results from the presence of a plexiform neurofibroma. *(Courtesy of Steven A. Newman, MD.)*

Figure 11-2 The upper lid normally crosses approximately 1 mm below the limbus. Fissure height can be measured by placing a ruler between the borders of the upper and lower eyelids.

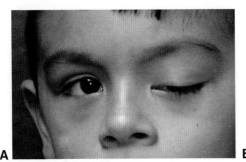

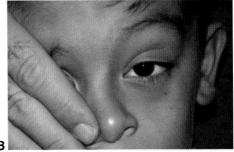

A　　　　　　　　　　　　　　　　**B**

Figure 11-3 **A,** Patient with pseudoptosis from a large left hypotropia. **B,** Occlusion of the right eye revealed that the left upper eyelid is in a normal position. *(Courtesy of Tariq Bhatti, MD.)*

prevent frontalis action. Normal upper eyelid excursion is 12–16 mm (Fig 11-5). In addition, the upper eyelid margin–corneal reflex distance (Fig 11-6) and the upper eyelid margin–upper eyelid crease distance are measured (Fig 11-7).

The movement of the eyelid during target pursuit from upgaze to downgaze should be observed. Normally, this motion is smoothly accomplished, but there may be eyelid lag in patients with thyroid eye disease (Fig 11-8; see also Chapter 14) or as a result of aberrant regeneration of the third cranial nerve (CN III) (see also Chapter 8 on diplopia).

In cases of suspected fatigable ptosis caused by myasthenia gravis, the patient fixates on the examiner's hand, which is elevated to provoke extreme upgaze. The clinician watches for progressive ptosis as the patient attempts to hold this position. A patient without myasthenia gravis can maintain the position without developing ptosis. The Cogan lid-twitch sign is identified by having the patient fixate in downgaze for a few seconds and

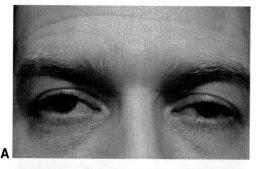

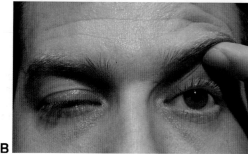

Figure 11-4 **A,** Patient with ptosis on the left from myasthenia gravis that is greater than that on the right. **B,** Manual opening of the left eyelid results in greater right-sided ptosis (enhanced ptosis). This sign, although often present with myasthenia gravis, is not specific. It may be seen with other disorders producing asymmetric ptosis and is a manifestation of Hering's law of equal innervation. *(Courtesy of Rod Foroozan, MD.)*

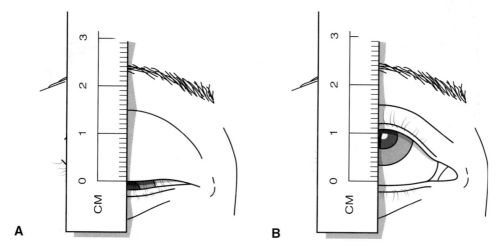

Figure 11-5 Upper eyelid excursion can be measured by splinting the frontalis while asking the patient to look down at the floor **(A)** and up to the ceiling **(B)**.

then rapidly refixate straight ahead. The sign appears as an overshoot upward of the eyelid and fluttering as the lid settles into position.

Evaluation of facial motor function includes assessing the strength of the orbicularis oculi and other facial muscles. Eyelid closure should be assessed to determine if it is incomplete (lagophthalmos). Reinnervation phenomena such as synkinesis with eyelid closure and facial tics may be signs of a previous seventh nerve injury (see Fig 11-11). The clinician should note the presence of exophthalmos (thyroid eye disease, discussed

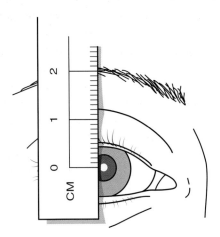

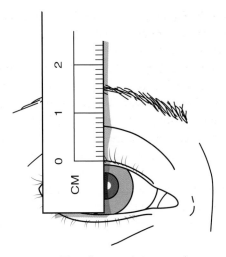

Figure 11-6 The marginal reflex distance can be measured from the first Purkinje image in the visual axis to the upper eyelid position. This is normally approximately 4–5 mm.

Figure 11-7 The distance between the upper eyelid margin and the primary eyelid crease can be measured with a ruler.

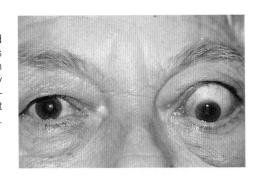

Figure 11-8 Eyelid retraction from thyroid eye disease (Graves ophthalmopathy). This 73-year-old woman presented with a 6-month history of foreign-body sensation (previously treated as "dry eye syndrome"). Eyelid retraction on the left side is enhanced by severe left inferior rectus restriction. See also Chapter 14. *(Courtesy of Steven A. Newman, MD.)*

in Chapter 14) or enophthalmos. Enophthalmos may result in apparent ptosis and narrowing of the palpebral fissure because the eyelid follows the contour of the globe as the eye retracts into the orbit. Anisocoria (discussed in Chapter 10) may suggest sympathetic or parasympathetic nervous system involvement, either of which will alter lid position. Finally, "neighboring" cranial nerves should be assessed. If ptosis is caused by third nerve weakness, the function of CNs IV, V, and VI should also be evaluated. Ocular motility should be checked for subtle weakness. Similarly, if seventh nerve dysfunction is found, facial sensation and hearing should be evaluated.

Ptosis

Congenital Ptosis

The most common form of congenital ptosis is thought to result from dystrophic development of the levator muscle without associated innervational abnormalities. Congenital ptosis (Fig 11-9) may be unilateral or bilateral and may be associated with other congenital ocular or orbital abnormalities, including blepharophimosis syndrome, congenital fibrosis of the extraocular muscles, superior rectus weakness, and Marcus Gunn jaw-winking syndrome (Fig 11-10). This last phenomenon is a synkinetic movement of the eyelid associated with jaw movement. In the external pterygoid–levator form of the syndrome, the eyelid elevates with movement of the mandible to the opposite side, jaw protrusion, or wide opening of the mouth. With the internal pterygoid–levator form, the eyelid elevates when the teeth are clenched. In some patients with Marcus Gunn jaw-winking, ptosis may worsen with movement of the jaw, although this is not common. Congenital tumors, such as hemangiomas and neurofibromas, may also lead to congenital ptosis. These tumors are typically associated with a palpable mass. Whatever the origin of a child's congenital ptosis, the ophthalmologist must be aware of the potential for amblyopia as a result of occlusion or anisometropia.

Acquired Ptosis

Table 11-1 summarizes the most common causes of acquired ptosis. *Neurogenic* ptosis requires careful attention to associated abnormalities in pupillary size and extraocular

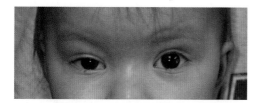

Figure 11-9 Congenital ptosis of the right upper eyelid in a 2-year-old child. *(Courtesy of Rod Foroozan, MD.)*

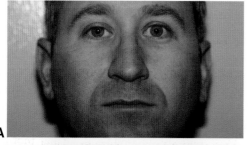

A

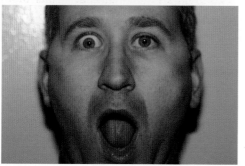

B

Figure 11-10 Marcus Gunn jaw-winking syndrome. **A,** This 25-year-old has mild right upper eyelid ptosis. **B,** Opening the mouth results in eyelid retraction. This pattern indicates synkinesis between the fifth nerve and the third nerve. *(Reprinted with permission from Levin LA, Arnold AC, eds. Neuro-Ophthalmology: The Practical Guide. New York: Thieme; 2005.)*

Table 11-1 Causes of Acquired Ptosis

Neurogenic
Third nerve palsy
Horner syndrome
Ophthalmoplegic migraine
Apraxia of lid opening
Miller Fisher syndrome

Myogenic
Progressive external ophthalmoplegia
Steroid eyedrops
Myotonic dystrophy

Neuromuscular
Myasthenia gravis
Botulism

Aponeurotic
Disinsertion
Attenuation

Traumatic
Eyelid laceration
Postsurgical ptosis
Foreign body

Mechanical
Chalazion
Cicatricial

movements. *Cerebral* ptosis refers to ptosis in association with a lesion of the cerebral (typically right) hemisphere. The ptosis may be bilateral or unilateral, and in the majority of cases it is transient.

Averbuch-Heller L, Leigh RJ, Mermelstein V, Zagalsky L, Streifler JY. Ptosis in patients with hemispheric strokes. *Neurology.* 2002;58:620–624.

Suspicion of systemic disorders such as *myasthenia gravis, progressive external ophthalmoplegia,* and *myotonic dystrophy* (discussed in Chapter 14) requires questions regarding the patient's general strength, fatigability, and family history. *Botulism poisoning* leads to bilateral ptosis associated with poorly reactive pupils and ophthalmoplegia. Patients also have associated facial paralysis and generalized proximal muscle weakness. Areflexia, ataxia, and ophthalmoplegia characterize *Miller Fisher syndrome,* a variant of Guillain-Barré syndrome (discussed later in the chapter). In addition to bilateral ptosis, these patients may also have facial diplegia, as well as respiratory and swallowing difficulties. Chronic use of steroid eyedrops is thought to lead to ptosis as a localized steroid-induced myopathy of the levator muscle.

Levator aponeurotic defects are the most frequent cause of acquired ptosis, replacing the former concept of "senile" ptosis. The ptosis is caused by stretching, dehiscence, or disinsertion of the levator aponeurosis. Because the levator muscle itself is healthy, levator function is usually normal. Patients with aponeurotic defects usually have a high eyelid crease.

Traumatic and *mechanical* causes of acquired ptosis are generally evident from inspection of the eyelids and require appropriate medical or surgical therapy.

Pseudoptosis

Pseudoptosis encompasses conditions such as brow ptosis and laxity and dermatochalasis that mimic true ptosis. Pseudoptosis can also be caused by microphthalmos or by phthisis bulbi, conditions resulting in the eyelids not being adequately supported by the globe. Hypotropia also causes pseudoptosis, because the perception of eyelid position is related to the position of the eye (see Fig 11-3). Contralateral lid retraction may also give rise to pseudoptosis.

Apraxia of Eyelid Opening

Apraxia of the eyelid opening is a rare disorder causing unilateral or bilateral ptosis. Thought to be supranuclear in origin, it is characterized by inability to voluntarily open the eyelids, associated with frontalis contraction and facial grimacing. It is often associated with extrapyramidal disease such as Parkinson disease, Shy-Drager syndrome, Huntington disease, Wilson disease, and progressive supranuclear palsy. It has also been seen following bilateral frontal lobe infarcts. Apraxia of the eyelid opening may be seen in patients with essential blepharospasm.

Tozlovanu V, Forget R, Iancu A, Boghen D. Prolonged orbicularis oculi activity: a major factor in apraxia of lid opening. *Neurology.* 2001;57(6):1013–1018.

Eyelid Retraction

Eyelid retraction is considered to be present if, with the eyes in primary position, the sclera is visible above the superior corneal limbus. It is usually acquired but may be present at birth. Preterm infants occasionally have a benign transient conjugate downgaze associated with upper eyelid retraction. This finding is thought to be caused by immature myelination of the vertical eye movement system and immaturity or dysfunction of the extrageniculocalcarine visual pathways. Many normal infants (80% of children 14–18 weeks of age) have an eye-popping reflex when ambient lighting levels are reduced.

Causes of eyelid retraction are listed in Table 11-2. The most common cause of eyelid retraction in adults is thyroid eye disease (see Fig 11-8). The eyelid retraction *(Collier sign)* in *dorsal midbrain syndrome* (see Chapter 7, Fig 7-5) is a less common cause. Unilateral eyelid retraction as a result of contralateral ptosis may occur in patients with levator aponeurotic defects; this phenomenon results from Hering's law of equal innervation. Bilateral eyelid retraction can be associated with thyroid eye disease, familial periodic paralysis, Cushing syndrome, and midbrain disease, or hydrocephalus with vertical nystagmus. Unilateral eyelid retraction is caused chiefly by thyroid eye disease but may also occur from aberrant regeneration of the third nerve (see Chapter 8, on diplopia), Marcus Gunn jaw-winking syndrome (see Fig 11-10), and idiopathic levator fibrosis. Subconjunctival

Table 11-2 Causes of Acquired Lid Retraction

Neurogenic
Dorsal midbrain syndrome
Progressive supranuclear palsy
Aberrant regeneration of third nerve
Marcus Gunn jaw-winking
Sympathomimetic eyedrops (eg, phenylephrine hydrochloride, apraclonidine)

Myogenic
Thyroid eye disease
Myasthenia gravis
Postsurgical (ptosis repair, orbicularis myectomy)

Mechanical
High axial myopia
Buphthalmos
Orbital fracture with entrapment
Proptosis secondary to orbital mass

injections of botulinum toxin and several surgical procedures have been used to reduce the degree of eyelid retraction in patients with thyroid eye disease.

Chang EL, Rubin PA. Upper and lower eyelid retraction. *Int Ophthalmol Clin.* 2002;42(2):45–59.

Abnormalities of Facial Movement

Facial (seventh) nerve weakness is a frequent clinical problem that the ophthalmologist may be asked to evaluate. Assessment of the facial nerve includes testing not only motor function but also sensory and autonomic functions. Motor function can be readily assessed by observation. With the patient at rest, any asymmetry of facial expression or eyelid blink is noted. The palpebral fissure on the side of seventh nerve paresis will be wider as a result of the relaxed tone of the orbicularis oculi muscles. The clinician can test the various muscle groups by asking the patient to smile, to forcibly close the eyes, and to wrinkle the forehead. The degree to which the eyelashes become buried on each side can reveal subtle orbicularis oculi weakness. The corneal blink reflex provides an assessment of both seventh and fifth nerve function. The clinician can whisper or use a quiet watch to test hearing and assess possible involvement of the eighth nerve as a result of cerebellopontine angle tumors.

Testing autonomic functions such as salivation, lacrimation, and sensation can help to localize seventh nerve lesions. Sugar or vinegar placed on the anterior two thirds of the tongue can be used to test taste. Cutaneous sensation can be tested along the posterior aspect of the external auditory canal and tympanic membrane. Lesions of the seventh nerve from the cerebellopontine angle to the geniculate ganglion typically impair all functions of the nerve, whereas lesions distal to the geniculate ganglion affect only certain functions, depending on their location, as shown in Figure 11-11. A dissociation of motor, sensory, and autonomic functions is also possible with pontine lesions proximal to the joining of the motor portion of the seventh nerve with the intermediary nerve. Testing should

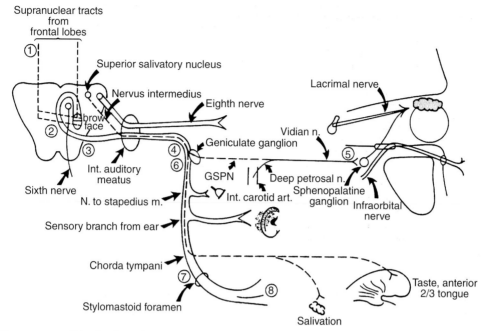

Figure 11-11 Distribution of seventh nerve and topical diagnosis of lesions.

1. *Supranuclear facial palsy:* contralateral weakness of lower two thirds of the face with some weakness of the orbicularis oculi; retained expression
2. *Nuclear facial palsy:* facial monoplegia (congenital) plus sixth nerve nucleus involvement (ipsilateral gaze palsy) and frequent ataxia, occasional Horner syndrome

   Peripheral lesions result in facial monoplegia including the orbicularis oculi and frontalis muscles, *plus:*

3. *Cerebellopontine angle:* decreased tearing, dysgeusia, loss of salivary secretion, loss of taste from anterior two thirds of tongue, hearing impairment, nystagmus, vertigo, ataxia, and adjacent cranial nerve findings (V, VI)
4. *Geniculate ganglionitis* (Ramsay Hunt syndrome, zoster oticus): same findings except without involvement of brainstem and other cranial nerves
5. *Isolated ipsilateral tear deficiency* due to involvement of vidian nerve or sphenopalatine ganglion (accompanying sixth nerve palsy with cavernous sinus involvement)
6. *Fallopian canal:* involvement of nerve to stapedius muscle, dysacusis, involvement of chorda tympani, loss of taste to anterior two thirds of tongue, impaired salivary secretion
7. *Distal to chorda tympani:* isolated paralysis of facial muscles
8. *Distal to branching of seventh nerve after it leaves stylomastoid foramen:* only certain branches of seventh nerve are affected (localized facial; in addition, bilateral seventh nerve palsy may result from weakness)

   In addition, bilateral seventh nerve palsy may result from congenital conditions (Möbius syndrome), sarcoidosis, Guillain-Barré syndrome, or neurofibromatosis type 2 (bilateral acoustic neuromas). *(Adapted with permission from Kline LB, Bajandas FJ. Neuro-Ophthalmology Review Manual. 5th ed. Thorofare, New Jersey: Slack; 2000.)*

include functions of the fifth, sixth, and eighth nerves, which, if abnormal, may help localize the cause of a seventh nerve palsy.

Any aberrant facial movements at rest or during volitional movement should be noted (Fig 11-12). Following any facial neuropathy, but most commonly as a result of Bell's palsy,

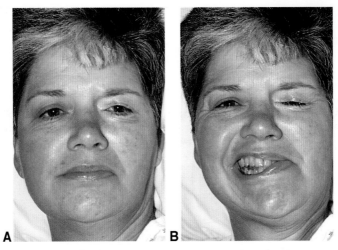

Figure 11-12 Facial nerve synkinesis. Misdirection may occur with recovery of seventh nerve function following trauma or surgery. **A,** In this 54-year-old patient, aberrant regeneration of the left seventh nerve following resection of a cerebellopontine angle meningioma caused eyelid closure when she attempted to smile **(B).** *(Courtesy of Steven A. Newman, MD.)*

regenerating axons may reinnervate muscles different from those originally served; such aberrant regeneration can cause synkinetic movements. In this situation, the involved facial muscles may remain weak. When axons originally destined for the orbicularis oculi reinnervate the lower facial muscles, each blink may cause a twitch of the corner of the mouth or a dimpling of the chin. Conversely, movements of the lower face—such as pursing the lips, smiling, or chewing with the mouth closed—may produce involuntary lid closure.

Other disorders of aberrant facial innervation include lacrimation caused by chewing *(crocodile tears)*, in which fibers originally supplying mandibular and sublingual glands reinnervate the lacrimal gland by way of the greater superficial petrosal nerve. This syndrome usually follows severe proximal seventh nerve injury and may be accompanied by decreased reflex tearing and decreased taste from the anterior two thirds of the tongue. Marcus Gunn jaw-winking syndrome is caused by anomalous communication between the trigeminal (pterygoid) and oculomotor (levator) nerves.

Seventh Nerve Disorders

Disorders of Underactivity of the Seventh Nerve

Facial weakness or paralysis may occur with supranuclear, nuclear, or infranuclear lesions (Table 11-3).

Supranuclear lesions

A lesion in the facial portion of the precentral gyrus results in a contralateral paralysis of volitional facial movement, which involves the lower face more severely than the upper face (upper motor neuron lesion). Emotional and reflex facial movements such as smiling

Table 11-3 Etiologies of Facial Paralysis

Idiopathic Bell's palsy

Infections
Herpes zoster
Lyme disease
Acute or chronic otitis media
Other: syphilis, meningitis, infectious mononucleosis, varicella, enterovirus, rubella, mumps,
 leprosy, tuberculosis, mucormycosis, tetanus, diphtheria, human immunodeficiency virus

Pontine infarct or hemorrhage

Pontine demyelination

Neoplasms
Pontine glioma
Cerebellopontine angle
Intratemporal bone
Parotid gland
Other: sarcoma, hemangioma, histiocytosis X, leukemia, lymphoma, epidermoids

Trauma

Miscellaneous
Congenital facial paralysis
Guillain-Barré syndrome
Sarcoidosis
Diabetes mellitus
Vasculitis
 Polyarteritis nodosa
 Wegener granulomatosis
Melkersson-Rosenthal syndrome

and spontaneous blinking are usually preserved because they are controlled through extrapyramidal pathways.

With extrapyramidal disorders, such as parkinsonism or progressive supranuclear palsy, spontaneous facial expression is minimal, and the spontaneous blink rate is usually reduced. Volitional facial movements generally remain intact.

Brainstem lesions

Ipsilateral facial weakness involving both the upper and lower face may occur with a pontine disorder. Vascular lesions and intraparenchymal tumors are the most common causes. Other evidence of a pontine disturbance is to be expected, such as ipsilateral corneal and facial anesthesia, sixth nerve palsy, lateral gaze palsy, cerebellar ataxia, and contralateral hemiparesis. A dissociation between the autonomic, sensory, and motor functions of the seventh nerve may be present. Large lesions of the pons may produce facial diplegia, which is also seen in Möbius syndrome, a congenital disorder involving bilateral sixth nerve palsies.

Peripheral lesions

Peripheral or lower motor neuron lesions result in ipsilateral facial weakness and may have a multitude of causes. Testing of the sensory and autonomic functions of the seventh nerve helps to pinpoint the responsible lesion. Concomitant impairment of the fifth, sixth, or eighth cranial nerve or cerebellar signs may indicate tumors in the cerebellopontine angle.

Bell's palsy, which typically occurs in adults, represents the most common type of facial neuropathy, but it must remain a diagnosis of exclusion. Bell's palsy is characterized by the sudden onset of facial paresis. Pain may either precede the palsy or occur concurrently. Facial numbness may be reported, although cutaneous sensation is usually intact. Decreased tearing, diminished taste, and dysacusis also may be noted.

Although the etiology of Bell's palsy is unknown, the palsy may be caused by autoimmune or viral-induced inflammatory or ischemic injury with swelling of the peripheral nerve. The external auditory canal and ear should be examined for vesicles caused by herpes zoster (Ramsay Hunt syndrome). The incidence of Bell's palsy is higher in pregnant women and in patients with diabetes mellitus or a family history of Bell's palsy. If the facial weakness progresses over a period of more than 3 weeks, a neoplastic etiology must be ruled out.

Approximately 85% of patients with Bell's palsy experience a satisfactory spontaneous recovery, although subtle signs of aberrant regeneration are commonly found. In these patients, recovery typically begins within 3 weeks of onset of the deficit and is complete by 2–3 months. In the remaining patients, recovery is incomplete, and aberrant regeneration is common. Complete facial palsy at the time of presentation, impairment of lacrimation, dysacusis, and advanced age are all poor prognostic signs. Electrical stimulation testing provides an assessment of the degree of nerve degeneration and has been reported to be helpful in predicting recovery.

Corticosteroids are commonly used to treat Bell's palsy, and evidence from meta-analyses and randomized trials supports their efficacy. It is postulated that edema of the nerve within a tight fallopian canal contributes to nerve damage, and a 7–10-day course of oral corticosteroids is recommended for patients without specific systemic contraindications who are seen within the first 72 hours. Several experimental and clinical reports have suggested that a combination of antiviral agents (acyclovir, famciclovir) and corticosteroids may provide additional benefit over the use of corticosteroids alone in the treatment of Bell's palsy. However, a large randomized trial found that, although corticosteroids improved the chances of recovery at 3 and 9 months, the addition of acyclovir, either alone or in combination with corticosteroids, conferred no benefit.

Grogan PM, Gronseth GS. Practice parameter: steroids, acyclovir, and surgery for Bell's palsy (an evidence-based review): Report of the Quality Standards Subcommittee of the American Academy of Neurology. *Neurology.* 2001;56(7):830–836.

Magaldi JA. Bell's palsy. *N Engl J Med.* 2005;352(4):416–418.

Sullivan FM, Swan IR, Donnan PT, et al. Early treatment with prednisolone or acyclovir in Bell's palsy. *N Engl J Med.* 2007;357(16):1598–1607.

Neoplasms may involve the seventh nerve in the cerebellopontine angle (acoustic neuroma [Fig 11-13], meningioma), within the fallopian canal, or in the parotid gland. Such lesions can compress the seventh nerve, resulting in facial synkinesis. Most of these lesions are histologically benign and slow growing. When small, they may be missed on CT; MRI with intravenous contrast is recommended. Infections may spread to involve the seventh nerve from otitis media.

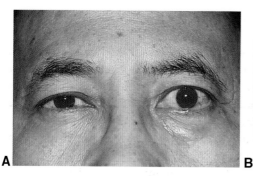 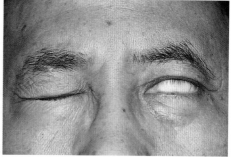

Figure 11-13 Facial nerve palsy. This 60-year-old patient had complaints of ocular irritation on the left side following excision of a left acoustic neuroma. **A,** The left eye will not close due to weakness of the left orbicularis oculi. **B,** Fortunately, corneal sensation remains intact, and the patient demonstrates an excellent Bell's phenomenon. *(Photographs courtesy of Steven A. Newman, MD.)*

Various infectious agents can cause seventh nerve pathology. The nerve may be impaired from meningitis. Lyme disease, caused by infection with the tick-borne spirochete *Borrelia burgdorferi,* can cause unilateral or bilateral facial palsies. Classic manifestations include a characteristic rash, arthritis, and meningopolyneuritis (see Chapter 14). The prognosis for seventh nerve recovery is excellent. Herpes zoster involving the seventh nerve is called *Ramsay Hunt syndrome.* It is diagnosed by the identification of vesicles along the posterior aspect of the external auditory canal, over the tympanic membrane, or on the pinna. Pain is often severe, and postherpetic neuralgia may result. The prognosis for recovery is less promising than with Bell's palsy. An isolated seventh nerve palsy, as well as other isolated or multiple cranial nerve palsies, may be the first sign of human immunodeficiency virus (HIV) seroconversion.

The seventh nerve is the cranial nerve most commonly involved in sarcoidosis. The site of involvement is usually the parotid gland, which develops noncaseating granulomatous inflammation. Seventh nerve involvement is frequently bilateral yet asymmetric.

Facial diplegia may occur in *Guillain-Barré syndrome,* especially in the variant known as *Miller Fisher syndrome,* when ophthalmoplegia and ataxia are also present. Cerebrospinal fluid analysis reveals an elevated protein level with a normal cell count, and deep tendon reflexes should be absent. A high percentage of patients with Miller Fisher syndrome have GQ1b IgG autoantibodies in their serum. Recovery is generally complete, and the serology improves with clinical improvement.

A seventh nerve palsy may occur with head trauma. The *Battle sign* (ecchymosis over the mastoid) may be present, and fractures of the temporal bone should be suspected. A congenital facial palsy is frequently related to birth trauma from forceps and tends to resolve.

In *Melkersson-Rosenthal syndrome,* recurrent unilateral or bilateral facial paralysis is accompanied by chronic facial swelling and lingua plicata (furrowing of the tongue). The etiology of this disorder, which usually begins in childhood or adolescence, is unknown. The facial swelling is frequently marked and may be bilateral, even when facial paresis is only unilateral.

Given the large differential diagnosis of seventh nerve weakness, etiologic considerations in specific clinical settings deserve emphasis. *Bilateral* seventh nerve palsies are most frequently due to sarcoidosis, basilar meningitis (bacterial, viral, spirochetal), and Guillain-Barré syndrome. *Recurrent unilateral* seventh nerve involvement is often caused by diabetes mellitus, Lyme disease, and Melkersson-Rosenthal syndrome. *Progressive* seventh nerve palsy is highly suggestive of a neoplastic etiology, with tumor invasion (brainstem, cerebellopontine, parotid gland) or diffuse infiltration (meningeal carcinomatosis). Further, accompanying cranial nerve palsies will aid in topographic localization of the lesion.

Treatment

In cases of orbicularis oculi involvement, treatment of corneal exposure may be necessary. Artificial tear preparations (preferably preservative free) and lubricants are sufficient in mild cases. Taping the eyelid shut with lubricating ointment in the eye for sleep may be necessary. Moisture chambers have been used at night. Patients should be advised to avoid a dusty or windy environment. Breakdown of corneal epithelium indicates the need for punctual plugs, tarsorrhaphy, or the injection of botulinum toxin type A (Botox) to induce ptosis.

In the setting of a facial nerve palsy, the most critical question is the status of the trigeminal nerve. Loss of corneal sensation combined with a facial nerve palsy is a particularly difficult clinical problem. The risk of neurotrophic combined with neuroparalytic keratitis demands an aggressive approach that possibly includes early tarsorrhaphy or gold weight implant.

Surgical treatment may include attempts at reinnervation with hypoglossal to facial anastomosis or transfacial cable grafts. Unfortunately, these procedures, even when successful, tend to protect the cornea poorly. Silicone bands (Arion sling) tend to be unpredictable, and implanted springs have a high incidence of extrusion. The simplest and most successful surgical treatment for corneal problems associated with chronic facial nerve palsies is the use of gold eyelid weights. Because there is a tendency to implant too small a weight, preoperative evaluation should include trials of various weights taped to the eyelid surface. The heaviest weight that can be lifted clear of the visual axis should be chosen. Although the weight is more visible when implanted low over the tarsus, this position is more predictable than placement over the septum. The weight can be removed later if facial nerve function recovers.

Dresner SC. Ophthalmic management of facial nerve paralysis. *Focal Points: Clinical Modules for Ophthalmologists.* San Francisco: American Academy of Ophthalmology; 2000, module 4.

Rahman I, Sadiq SA. Ophthalmic management of facial nerve palsy: a review. *Surv Ophthalmol.* 2007;52(2):121–144.

Disorders of Overactivity of the Seventh Nerve

Disorders of the seventh nerve, its nucleus, or the pyramidal or extrapyramidal pathways may produce hyperexcitable states. Essential blepharospasm, hemifacial spasm, and facial myokymia are the 3 most common disorders of overactivity (Table 11-4).

Table 11-4 Comparison of the Common Causes of Seventh Nerve Overactivity

	Laterality	Site of Dysfunction*	Etiology	Treatment
Essential blepharospasm	Bilateral	Basal ganglia	Unknown	Botulinum toxin (preferred treatment) *Medical:* Haloperidol, clonazepam, other drugs *Surgical:* extirpation of eyelid protractors, selective seventh nerve section
Hemifacial spasm	Unilateral	Facial root in cerebellopontine angle	Nerve compression by blood vessel or tumor	Botulinum toxin (preferred treatment) *Medical:* Carbamazepine, baclofen, other drugs *Surgical:* microsurgical decompression of facial root
Facial myokymia	Unilateral	Facial nucleus or fascicle in pons	Glioma, multiple sclerosis	Treatment of the underlying cause
Eyelid myokymia	Unilateral	Unknown	Unknown	Reassurance, botulinum toxin

*Presumed

Essential blepharospasm

This bilateral condition consists of episodic contraction of the orbicularis oculi. Onset usually occurs between ages 40 and 60. Initially, the spasms are mild and infrequent, but they may progress to the point that the patient's daily activities are severely disrupted. In advanced cases, the patient's eyelids cannot be pried open during an episode of spasm. Facial grimacing and other movements may be associated with blepharospasm (*Meige syndrome*) (Fig 11-14), and cogwheeling in the neck and extremities or other extrapyramidal signs may be noted. *Tardive dyskinesia* secondary to neuroleptic and antipsychotic drugs can produce spasms that involve the mouth. Extrapyramidal disorders such as parkinsonism, Huntington disease, and basal ganglia infarction may be accompanied by some degree of blepharospasm.

The exact cause of benign essential blepharospasm is unknown, but increasing evidence using functional neuroimaging suggests that it is caused by basal ganglia dysfunction. The clinician evaluating a patient with blepharospasm should exclude causes

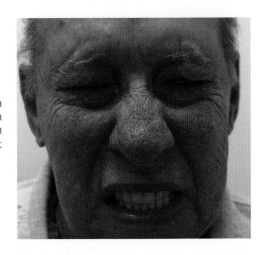

Figure 11-14 Essential blepharospasm with Meige syndrome. This patient has contraction of the orbicularis oculi muscles in association with facial grimacing. *(Courtesy of Eric Eggenberger, DO.)*

of reflex blepharospasm, in particular severely dry eyes, intraocular inflammation, and meningeal irritation. Stress may exacerbate the condition. Neuroradiologic studies are generally unrevealing.

The efficacy of medical therapy, including neuroleptics and benzodiazepines, for blepharospasm is generally limited. Currently, the treatment of choice for essential blepharospasm is injection of botulinum toxin into the orbicularis oculi muscle.

Dutton JJ, Fowler AM. Botulinum toxin in ophthalmology. *Surv Ophthalmol.* 2007;52(1): 13–31.

Although there are several types of botulinum toxin, only type A has been used extensively in clinical practice. The effect of the toxin is temporary, lasting only a few months, so that repeated injections are necessary. The efficacy of the drug relates to its ability to cause muscle weakness. Complications such as ptosis, exposure of the cornea, diplopia, and local ecchymosis are usually mild and transient. The dosage varies from 2.5 to 5 units per injection site and 4 to 8 sites per eye. The central portion of the pretarsal orbicularis should be avoided to minimize the chance of inducing ptosis.

Occasionally, when medical treatment fails, surgical therapy consisting of the meticulous extirpation of the eyelid protractors may be indicated. Selective ablation of the seventh nerve is an alternative procedure that carries the risk of greater complications and has a lower success rate. See also BCSC Section 7, *Orbit, Eyelids, and Lacrimal System.*

Essential blepharospasm may cause psychological distress, with some patients withdrawing socially as the symptoms worsen. Thus, counseling may be as valuable as the medical and surgical management of the condition. The Benign Essential Blepharospasm Research Foundation (BEBRF) (http://www.blepharospasm.org) has provided education and support to blepharospasm sufferers and aided research efforts since 1981.

Ben Simon GJ, McCann JD. Benign essential blepharospasm. *Int Ophthalmol Clin.* 2005;45(3): 49–75.

Patel BCK, Anderson RL. Essential blepharospasm and related diseases. *Focal Points: Clinical Modules for Ophthalmologists.* San Francisco: American Academy of Ophthalmology; 2000, module 5.

Hemifacial spasm

Hemifacial spasm is characterized by unilateral episodic spasm that involves the facial musculature and typically lasts from a few seconds to minutes. The disorder frequently begins as intermittent twitching of the orbicularis oculi muscle but, over the course of several years, spreads to involve all the facial muscles on 1 side (Fig 11-15). Episodes may increase in frequency for weeks to months and then abate for months at a time. Seventh nerve function is usually intact, although over time subtle ipsilateral facial weakness may develop.

The pathogenesis of hemifacial spasm is most commonly compression of the seventh nerve root exit zone by an aberrant vessel. Abnormal firing in the motor nucleus or ephaptic transmission of nerve impulses causes innervation directed toward 1 muscle group to excite adjacent nerve fibers directed to another muscle group. Less commonly (perhaps 1% of hemifacial spasm), tumors within the cerebellopontine angle or previous seventh nerve injury may lead to the spasms; therefore an MRI of the brain, including the course of the facial nerve, is typically performed to exclude a compressive lesion.

Botulinum toxin type A injection into the facial muscles has proven very effective and is the treatment of choice for hemifacial spasm in most patients. Reinjection is required at intervals of several months. Hemifacial spasm responds to lower doses of botulinum toxin than does blepharospasm. Side effects are similar to those seen in patients with blepharospasm treated with botulinum toxin.

Carbamazepine, clonazepam, or baclofen may provide improvement in some patients. Facial myectomy and neurectomy have been shown to give patients with hemifacial spasm limited relief. Suboccipital craniotomy with placement of a sponge between the seventh nerve and the offending blood vessel (*microvascular decompression*) may be considered in advanced cases.

Spastic paretic facial contracture

Spastic paretic facial contracture is a rare disorder characterized by unilateral facial contracture with associated facial weakness. Typically, it begins with myokymia of the orbicularis oculi muscle, which gradually spreads to most of the ipsilateral facial muscles. At the same time, tonic contracture of the affected muscles becomes evident. Over weeks to months, ipsilateral facial weakness develops, and voluntary facial movements of the

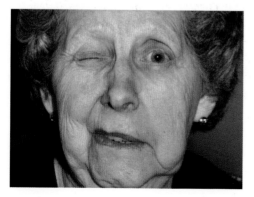

Figure 11-15 Hemifacial spasm. This 73-year-old woman has intermittent twitching involving the entire right side of the face. *(Courtesy of Rod Foroozan, MD.)*

affected side diminish. Spastic paretic facial contracture is a sign of pontine dysfunction in the region of the seventh nerve nucleus, often caused by a pontine neoplasm. Damage to the nucleus causes facial weakness, and involvement of supranuclear connections leads to facial spasticity.

Facial myokymia

Facial myokymia is characterized by continuous unilateral fibrillary or undulating contraction of facial muscle bundles. When confined to the eyelid, it is most commonly a self-limited, benign condition. Occasionally, these rippling movements begin within a portion of the orbicularis oculi and may spread to involve most of the facial muscles.

Facial myokymia typically signifies intramedullary disease of the pons involving the seventh nerve nucleus or fascicle. It is usually the result of a pontine glioma in children and multiple sclerosis in adults. Rarely, myokymia occurs in Guillain-Barré syndrome. Myokymia may be relieved with carbamazepine (Tegretol), phenytoin sodium (Dilantin), or injection of botulinum toxin.

Intermittent fluttering of the orbicularis *(benign facial fasciculations)* is relatively common. The phenomenon usually lasts for days or weeks.

> Banik R, Miller NR. Chronic myokymia limited to the eyelid is a benign condition. *J Neuroophthalmol.* 2004;24(4):290–292.

Other conditions

Rarely, focal cortical seizures are manifested by gross clonic movements involving 1 side of the face only. The eyes deviate away from the side of the seizure focus during the episode; the patient's ipsilateral hand may also have clonic movements. Frequently, *Todd paralysis,* a transient supranuclear facial paresis, follows the seizure and the eyes may deviate toward the side of the prior seizure focus. The electroencephalogram should be abnormal during the clonic episodes.

Habit spasm such as facial tic or nervous twitch is relatively common, particularly in childhood, and is characterized by stereotyped, repetitive, reproducible facial movements that can be promptly inhibited on command. These movements tend to disappear in time without treatment. Only rarely does Tourette syndrome present with facial twitching alone.

> Coats DK, Paysse EA, Kim D-S. Excessive blinking in childhood: a prospective evaluation of 99 children. *Ophthalmology.* 2001;108(9):1556–1561.

Reflex blepharospasm results from fifth nerve irritation (usually from a severely dry eye), intraocular inflammation, or meningeal irritation (usually associated with photophobia). Treatment of the underlying cause may alleviate the symptoms. Oral facial dyskinesias (tardive dyskinesia) seen after long-term use of major tranquilizers may persist even after the drugs are stopped.

CHAPTER 12

The Patient With Head, Ocular, or Facial Pain

Evaluation of Headache

Headache is a common complaint presented to the ophthalmologist. When pain extends to the orbits, the patient and referring physician may assume that the eyes are in some way responsible for the discomfort. Often the patient may have fears, perhaps unspoken, of a brain tumor.

The history (Table 12-1) is the most important part of a headache evaluation because the ocular examination is normal in the vast majority of patients with headache.

In addition to having a complete ophthalmic examination, the patient complaining of headache should be screened systemically by having the blood pressure and pulse measured and being examined neurologically for meningeal signs (neck stiffness), point tenderness, and symmetry of cranial nerve and motor functions. Any complaint of visual phenomena should prompt careful visual field testing.

In 1988, the International Headache Society published a classification scheme for headaches that includes *primary* headaches (migraine, tension-type, and cluster) and *secondary* headaches (headaches resulting from other causes). In 2004, this classification was revised to incorporate more recent concepts regarding the primary headache syndromes and includes a new category, *chronic migraine,* for patients who have migraine for 15 or more days per month.

Headache Classification Subcommittee of the International Headache Society. The International Classification of Headache Disorders. 2nd edition. *Cephalalgia.* 2004;24(suppl 1):9–160.

Table 12-1 Important Clinical Points of the Headache History

Nature of the headache (sharp or dull, throbbing or constant, "squeezing")
Daily pattern of headache (worse in the morning or later in the day, waking the patient from sleep)
Location of the headache (unilateral or bilateral, localized or diffuse)
Associated phenomena (scintillating scotomata, flashing lights, nausea or vomiting, vertigo, ptosis, tearing, paresthesias, weakness)
Precipitating or alleviating factors (supine position, bending over, coughing, foods)
Overall pattern (when headaches began, chronicity, recent change in pattern)
Family history of headaches

Several clinical features may suggest the need for neuroimaging and additional diagnostic testing:

- sudden onset of severe headache
- unexplained change in headache pattern
- headaches without response to typical therapies
- headaches that are related to physical exertion or change in body position
- new onset of headaches after the age of 50 years
- new headaches in a patient with cancer or immunosuppression
- headaches with focal neurologic signs or symptoms (including papilledema and homonymous hemianopia)
- headaches with a history of fever, neck stiffness, change in mental status, or change in behavior

Medina LS, D'Souza B, Vasconcellos E. Adults and children with headache: evidence-based diagnostic evaluation. *Neuroimaging Clin N Am.* 2003;13(2):225–235.

Patients over age 50 with new headaches should be suspected of having *giant cell arteritis* (temporal arteritis). Other symptoms of this condition include jaw claudication, fever, weight loss, scalp tenderness, polymyalgia, fatigue, and visual complaints. An erythrocyte sedimentation rate (ESR; Westergren method) and C-reactive protein help screen such a patient, but a normal ESR does not exclude the diagnosis (see Chapter 14). Tenderness over the temporal artery (particularly if the artery is enlarged or nodular) may further raise suspicion.

Headache caused by *elevated intracranial pressure,* as with intracranial mass lesions or idiopathic intracranial hypertension, is typically global, constant, and worse in the morning. Bending over or moving the head often worsen it, as do Valsalva maneuvers such as coughing and straining. Vomiting may occur, even without nausea. Other focal neurologic signs, nonlocalizing signs such as sixth nerve palsy, or papilledema may be present. Headaches that awaken patients at night are more likely to have a significant pathologic basis.

A sudden severe headache with stiff neck, changes in mentation, or focal neurologic signs suggests *intracranial hemorrhage.* Neuroimaging is urgently required in these cases. Headache caused by meningitis may be chronic and not associated with focal neurologic deficits. Neck stiffness and pain on flexion, back pain, pain on eye movement, and photophobia may reflect meningeal inflammation.

Diamond ML, Solomon GD, eds. *Diamond and Dalessio's The Practicing Physician's Approach to Headache.* 6th ed. Philadelphia: Saunders; 1999.
Silberstein SD, Lipton RB, Dodick DW, eds. *Wolff's Headache and Other Head Pain.* 8th ed. New York: Oxford University Press; 2007.

Migraine and Tension-type Headache

Migraine is a condition consisting of repetitive bouts of headache. More frequent in women than in men, it is extremely common and may underlie most episodes of headache pain. Familial tendency is strong, and the patient may report having had motion sickness as a child. Onset typically occurs at puberty or young adulthood, and the headaches may decrease after menopause. There may be hormonal variation. Unilaterality, pulsating character, associated nausea or vomiting, photophobia, and aggravation with routine physical activity all support the diagnosis of migraine. Migraine may be exacerbated by menstruation, pregnancy, hunger, stress, certain foods (chocolate, wine, etc), and sleep deprivation.

Spector RH. Migraine. *Focal Points: Clinical Modules for Ophthalmologists.* San Francisco: American Academy of Ophthalmology; 2000, module 1.

Migraine with aura

Previously termed *classic migraine, migraine with aura* (30% of migraine) is heralded by neurologic symptoms that are usually visual. Imagery builds up over minutes with positive phenomena that typically have movement. The classic *fortification spectrum* begins with a small scotoma near fixation that gradually expands (Fig 12-1). The scotoma is bounded by a zigzag, shimmering, colorful or silver visual image that moves temporally into the periphery and then breaks up. Loss of vision may occur (see Chapter 5), most commonly hemianopic but frequently perceived by the patient as monocular (in the eye ipsilateral to the hemianopia). The aura usually lasts less than 45 minutes and is typically followed by a throbbing headache on the contralateral side of the head. Most patients experience associated nausea, photophobia, and phonophobia. When untreated, the attacks typically last from 4 to 72 hours.

Basilar-type migraine (previously classified as *complicated migraine*) is thought to result from transient ischemia within the distribution of the basilar artery and may be

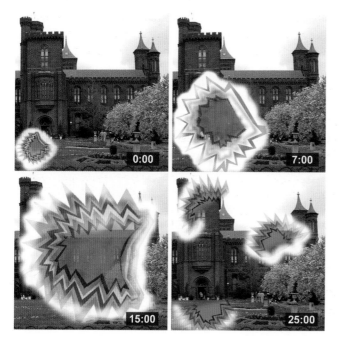

Figure 12-1 Visual aura of migraine. The aura commonly begins in the peripheral visual field, spreads centrally, and fades in the reverse order. The times at bottom right of each image represent minutes from the time the visual aura begins. *(Courtesy of Rod Foroozan, MD.)*

accompanied by bilateral visual loss, diplopia, vertigo, dysarthria, ataxia, and loss of consciousness.

Studies of the pathophysiology of migraine have found evidence for primary dysfunction involving the afferent sensory neurons of the trigeminal nerve and have emphasized genetic factors with a significant familial incidence (familial hemiplegic migraine, a rare autosomal dominant inherited form of migraine, has been mapped to chromosome 19). Activation of the trigeminal nucleus caudalis is thought to cause the release of vasoactive chemokines at the vascular endings of the trigeminal nerve. These neuropeptides are thought to cause dilation of the pial arteries, increase vascular permeability, and induce an inflammatory response that activates trigeminal afferents within the walls of blood vessels.

It has been suggested that migraine is a variant of a channelopathy in which there is increased neuronal excitability. This condition may underlie the spreading depression in the occipital region thought to be responsible for the visual aura and the changes in the blood vessels resulting in pain and other symptoms of basilar-type migraine. These studies have also provided a basis for developing the family of triptans that function by inhibiting release of vasoactive neuromediators.

The typical headache lasts several hours. In basilar-type migraine, a focal neurologic deficit may be part of the aura, or it may occur with the headache and then persist. This deficit is usually transient, but permanent deficits related to intracranial infarction do occur.

Hupp SL, Kline LB, Corbett JJ. Visual disturbances of migraine. *Surv Ophthalmol.* 1989;33(4): 221–236.

Migraine without aura

Previously called *common migraine, migraine without aura* (65% of migraine) has no preceding neurologic symptoms. The headache may be global, not strictly unilateral, and it can last hours to days. Distinguishing between this type of headache and the very common tension-type headache (discussed later in the chapter) is frequently quite difficult.

Migraine aura without headache

Some patients may report only the visual symptomatology of migraine aura without any associated headache. The occurrence of visual symptoms of migraine without headache (*acephalgic migraine*; 5% of migraine) must be differentiated from transient ischemic attacks (TIAs). Visual migraine equivalents include scintillating scotomata, transient homonymous hemianopia without positive visual phenomena, peripheral visual field constriction progressing to tunnel vision or complete visual loss, transient monocular visual loss, and episodic diplopia (usually vertical and accompanied by other neurologic symptoms). Symptoms typically last less than 60 minutes and tend to develop and remit progressively during that time. A positive patient history or family history of migraine with aura is helpful for the diagnosis, as is a description of the deficit. The classic scintillating scotoma with fortification spectrum is suggestive of migraine. Residual visual field defects may indicate another underlying process, such as cerebrovascular disease or a vascular malformation.

Often attributed to migraine, *vasospasm* may, less commonly, affect only 1 eye (sometimes referred to as *retinal migraine*), resulting in monocular visual loss. Transient retinal opacification and narrowing of the retinal arterioles may be seen during symptomatic episodes in some patients.

Winterkorn JM, Kupersmith MJ, Wirtschafter JD, Forman S. Brief report: treatment of vasospastic amaurosis fugax with calcium-channel blockers. *N Engl J Med.* 1993;329(6):396–398.

Evaluation of patients with migraine

If the patient has a typical history of migraine and a normal neurologic and ophthalmic examination, neuroimaging studies are unlikely to show an intracranial abnormality. A history of alternating hemicranial headaches suggests a benign etiology, but most patients with headaches that always occur on the same side of the head are also likely to have migraine. Occasionally, a mass lesion or a large vascular malformation is heralded by typical migraine symptoms (Fig 12-2; also see Chapter 14). In these cases, however, there are often residual visual field defects. This finding underlines the importance of visual field testing in the evaluation of patients with presumed migraine. Referral of patients with suspicious headaches to a neurologist is prudent. The following findings may suggest the need for additional evaluation in patients presumed to have migraine:

- Headache or aura always occurs on the same side.
- Headache precedes the aura.
- Neurologic deficit, including visual field defect, persists after aura resolves.
- Features of aura are atypical (more than 1 aura occurring in a single day, lack of expansion of or change in aura).

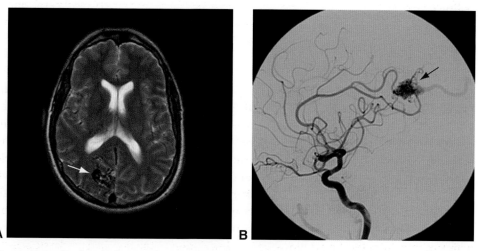

Figure 12-2 Occipital lobe arteriovenous malformation. **A,** Axial T2-weighted MRI showing an irregular hypointense mass *(arrow)* suggestive of a vascular lesion within the right occipital lobe. **B,** Lateral projection cerebral arteriogram confirms that the lesion is an arteriovenous malformation *(arrow)*. *(Courtesy of Rod Foroozan, MD.)*

Silberstein SD. Practice parameter: evidence-based guidelines for migraine headache (an evidence-based review): report of the Quality Standards Subcommittee of the American Academy of Neurology. *Neurology.* 2000;55(6):754–762.

US Headache Consortium. Evidence-based guidelines in the primary care setting: neuroimaging in patients with nonacute headache. Available at: www.aan.com. Accessed 5 February 2008.

Tension-type headache

Tension-type headaches are chronic, described as aching or viselike, typically worse at the end of the day, and often precipitated by stress. The specific pathophysiology and treatment of tension-type headaches remain unclear. They may be associated with depression.

Treatment of migraine and tension-type headache

The specific type of headache and the needs of the patient should guide treatment. Some patients, for example, need only reassurance that they do not have serious intracranial disease. Precipitating or contributing factors should be eliminated as much as possible. Certain foods provoke headaches in some people, and patients should consider avoiding chocolate, nitrates, monosodium glutamate, aged cheese, caffeine, red wine and other alcohol, aspartame (NutraSweet), nuts, and shellfish. The role of estrogens and oral contraceptives is uncertain, but a temporal relationship between initiation of hormone therapy and the development of migraine symptoms indicates that the hormones should be discontinued.

Other environmental migraine triggers include stress or relief from stress (eg, after a final exam or presentation, first day of vacation, weekends), change in sleep patterns, fumes or strong scents such as perfumes and cigarette smoke, and exercise.

Migraine therapy can be divided into acute and prophylactic management. For *acute* relief, various agents can be used, including dihydroergotamine, serotonergic agents, nonsteroidal anti-inflammatory drugs (NSAIDs), and other combined preparations that include caffeine. (*Chronic* caffeine intake, however, worsens headaches.) An antiemetic agent may also be necessary. The "triptans," which are serotonin $5\text{-HT}_{1B/1D}$-receptor agonists, are available in different formulations (oral, injection, nasal spray). They are useful for symptomatic relief of migraine but may be contraindicated in patients with basilar-type migraine. These drugs can, rarely, produce myocardial infarction and are typically not used in patients with suspected or known coronary artery disease. Topiramate, an antiepileptic γ-aminobutyrate (GABA) agonist, has been increasingly used in patients with migraine. Pericranial botulinum toxin injections have been found to be effective for some patients.

Symptomatic treatment has its limitations; in particular, the use of pain medications more than a few times weekly can lead to *analgesic rebound headache.* Patients with migraine may overuse analgesics and develop a constant headache that is relieved only with the continuous use of pain medications. Therefore, a thorough medication history from headache sufferers is important. Analgesic rebound headaches require the withdrawal of analgesics, and hospitalization may be needed.

Goadsby PJ. Recent advances in the diagnosis and management of migraine. *BMJ.* 2006; 332(7532):25–29.

Goadsby PJ, Lipton RB, Ferrari MD. Migraine—current understanding and treatment. *N Engl J Med.* 2002;346(4):257–270.

Prophylactic treatment is warranted if headaches disrupt the functions of daily life beyond what the patient is willing to tolerate. β-Blockers, calcium channel blockers, tricyclic antidepressants, selective serotonin reuptake inhibitors (SSRIs), sodium valproate, and topiramate may be used, as may NSAIDs if their potential for causing analgesic rebound headaches is kept in mind.

Tension-type headaches are more likely to respond to treatment with tricyclic antidepressants and NSAIDs, although the overall success rate is not as high as with migraine. Various forms of biofeedback may be helpful.

Trigeminal Autonomic Cephalgias

The trigeminal autonomic cephalgias include cluster headache, paroxysmal hemicrania, and short-lasting unilateral neuralgiform headache attacks with conjunctival injection and tearing (SUNCT). They are primary headache disorders characterized by unilateral head pain that occurs with ipsilateral cranial autonomic findings.

Cluster headache occurs most frequently in men in their 30s and 40s and is typically precipitated by alcohol use. It is characterized by excruciating bouts of pain localized behind 1 eye, in the distribution of the ophthalmic division of CN V. Associated symptoms include ipsilateral tearing, conjunctival injection, rhinorrhea, and postganglionic Horner syndrome. The pain may wake patients from sleep and cause them to pace with a sense of restlessness, rather than sleep it off. It typically lasts less than 2 hours. Headaches occur in clusters of episodes over days or weeks, then remit for months or years, suggesting that the hypothalamus may play a role in the pathogenesis. Cluster headaches can be difficult to treat. The headache may respond acutely to inhaled oxygen, methysergide maleate (Sansert), subcutaneous sumatriptan, or dihydroergotamine. A 10–14-day tapering dose of prednisone is often successful in aborting the cluster cycle. Verapamil is useful for prophylaxis.

Paroxysmal hemicrania is characterized by short, severe attacks of pain with cranial autonomic features that occur several times per day. The headache typically lasts between 2 and 30 minutes but may continue for hours. A dramatic resolution of the headache occurs with indomethacin, which helps to distinguish this from the other trigeminal autonomic cephalgias.

SUNCT is characterized by unilateral orbital or temporal pain that is severe and throbbing or stabbing. The headache typically occurs more than 20 times per day, lasts 5–240 seconds, and is often associated with conjunctival injection and tearing.

Icepick Pains and Idiopathic Stabbing Headache

Episodic brief, sharp, jabbing pains occur more commonly in those with migraine than in people with other types of headaches. Cluster headache sufferers also have a high incidence of idiopathic stabbing headache, typically located in the same area as the cluster pain. The most common location is in the distribution of the ophthalmic division of CN V: the parietal area, orbit, and temple. The pain lasts less than a second or may occur as a series of stabs. A variant of this entity, the *jabs and jolts syndrome,* consists of knifelike pain lasting less than a minute. Idiopathic stabbing headache often responds to indomethacin, and many patients improve with standard headache prophylactic agents.

Inherited Encephalopathies Resembling Migraine

Mitochondrial myopathy and encephalopathy, lactic acidosis, and strokelike episodes (MELAS) is a mitochondrial disorder that occurs in children and young adults. The symptoms (headache, nausea, vomiting, transient hemianopia, and hemiparesis) suggest migraine, but permanent neurologic disturbance is seen with spongiform cortical degeneration. Serum and CSF lactate levels are elevated, and T2 pathology may be seen on MRI in the temporal, parietal, and occipital lobes. Point mutations may be seen in the mitochondrial DNA.

Headache resembling migraine may occur as the initial symptom of *cerebral autosomal dominant arteriopathy with subcortical infarcts and leukoencephalopathy (CADASIL),* an autosomal dominant angiopathy that has been associated with a mutation in the *NOTCH3* gene on chromosome 19. Headaches occur in 30%–40% of patients with CADASIL and often arise later in life than typical migraine. Recurrent lacunar strokes with neurologic deficits and cognitive decline eventually occur. Widespread leukoencephalopathy, particularly within the temporal and frontal lobes, is seen on MRI.

Bousser M-G, Biousse V. Small vessel vasculopathies affecting the central nervous system. *J Neuroophthalmol.* 2004;24(1):56–61.

Ocular and Orbital Causes of Pain

There is a popular misperception that "eye strain" due to refractive errors and strabismus is a common cause of eye and head pain. Although refractive errors and strabismus should be corrected as appropriate, and such corrections can sometimes ameliorate pain, ocular or orbital pain has many more important causes. The eye is heavily innervated by sensory nerve fibers (see Chapter 1), and inflammatory, ischemic, and even neoplastic involvement of the eye and orbit can produce pain. True ophthalmic causes of eye pain include dry eyes and other forms of keratitis, acute angle-closure glaucoma, and intraocular inflammation. These conditions are most commonly diagnosed through examination of the cornea, anterior segment, and anterior vitreous by slit lamp. Keratitis sicca, or dry eye, is a very common cause of ophthalmic discomfort. Exacerbated by visual tasks that decrease blink frequency, especially work on the computer, it has various causes and results from conditions that either decrease tear production or increase tear evaporation. Keratitis sicca is one of the characteristic features of the autoimmune Sjögren syndrome. Evidence of fluorescein or rose bengal staining, abnormal tear breakup time, or decreased Schirmer test may help confirm dry eye syndrome. Pain on awakening may be related to recurrent erosion syndrome. Angle-closure glaucoma may be confirmed with intraocular pressure measurements and gonioscopy. Posterior segment examination with indirect ophthalmoscopy or slit-lamp biomicroscopy may reveal evidence of choroidal or retinal inflammation or posterior scleritis. Scleritis is usually accompanied by ocular tenderness. These causes of ocular pain are discussed in more detail in BCSC Section 7, *Orbit, Eyelids, and Lacrimal System*; Section 8, *External Disease and Cornea*; and Section 9, *Intraocular Inflammation and Uveitis*.

Idiopathic orbital inflammation usually produces severe eye pain or pain on eye movement, variably accompanied by ocular motility abnormalities, eyelid edema, and proptosis (see the discussion in BCSC Section 7, *Orbit, Eyelids, and Lacrimal System*). Periorbital pain may be the initial manifestation of inflammation within the cavernous sinus *(Tolosa-Hunt syndrome)*. Pain with eye movement commonly accompanies an *inflammatory optic neuropathy* (see Chapter 4), often in association with decreased vision, visual field changes, and an afferent pupillary defect.

Fazzone HE, Lefton DR, Kupersmith MJ. Optic neuritis: correlation of pain and magnetic resonance imaging. *Ophthalmology.* 2003;110(8):1646–1649.

Rapidly expanding tumors of the orbit, orbital apex, and cavernous sinus may also produce eye pain. In these cases, other signs will likely be present, such as a visual field defect, proptosis, pain or resistance with retropulsion of the globe, an afferent pupillary defect, or an abnormal optic nerve appearance.

Harooni H, Golnik KC, Geddie B, Eggenberger ER, Lee AG. Diagnostic yield for neuroimaging in patients with unilateral eye or facial pain. *Can J Ophthalmol.* 2005;40(6):759–763.

Levin LA, Lessell S. Pain: a neuro-ophthalmic perspective. *Arch Ophthalmol.* 2003;121(11):1633.

In addition, periocular pain may actually be referred facial pain, discussed later.

Photophobia

Photophobia occurs most frequently as a result of ocular inflammatory disorders, including keratitis, uveitis (particularly iritis), and less commonly from chorioretinitis. Photophobia may also arise because of meningeal irritation (meningitis and subarachnoid hemorrhage) and migraine.

Facial Pain

Pain associated with ischemia, such as *carotid dissection* or *microvascular cranial nerve palsy,* often localizes around the ipsilateral eye. Most often, pain in the eye area is a manifestation of a headache. Occipital neuralgia produces pain and tenderness over the greater occipital nerve that radiates to the ipsilateral eye area.

Patients may refer localized facial pain to the eye. Common sources of facial pain include dental disorders and sinus disease. Other facial pain syndromes include trigeminal neuralgia, glossopharyngeal neuralgia, temporomandibular joint syndrome (TMJ), carotidynia, and herpes zoster neuralgia. The onset of facial pain in an elderly patient raises the possibility of giant cell arteritis. Facial pain is occasionally a sign of nasopharyngeal carcinoma or metastatic carcinoma affecting the trigeminal nerve or the dura at the base of the brain. In some patients with constant facial pain that is typically deep and boring, no etiology may be identified (sometimes referred to as *atypical facial pain*). Treatment may be difficult and usually requires a combination of anticonvulsants and antidepressants.

Trigeminal Neuralgia

Trigeminal neuralgia, also known as *tic douloureux,* typically occurs during middle age or later. It is most commonly caused (80%–90% of cases) by vascular compression of CN V, although a few reports describe trigeminal neuralgia from demyelinating disease or a posterior fossa mass lesion. The pain is almost always unilateral (95%) and usually involves the maxillary or mandibular distribution of CN V, only rarely (<5%) involving the ophthalmic division alone. Chewing, tooth brushing, or a cold wind may precipitate paroxysmal burning or electric shock–like jabs, lasting seconds to minutes. There may be periods of remission. Sensory function in the face should be normal on testing; any abnormality increases likelihood of a neoplasm. All patients should have neuroimaging of the posterior fossa, preferably with MRI. Treatment options include use of gabapentin (Neurontin), pregabalin (Lyrica), carbamazepine, phenytoin, baclofen, clonazepam, and valproic acid; selective destruction of trigeminal fibers (rhizotomy); or surgical decompression of CN V in the posterior fossa.

Glossopharyngeal Neuralgia

In glossopharyngeal neuralgia, paroxysmal pain occurs unilaterally in the region of the larynx, tongue, tonsil, and ear. Hoarseness and coughing may be present. Pain can be triggered by swallowing and pungent flavors. It is treated with the same medications used for treating trigeminal neuralgia and also may be alleviated by microvascular decompression. *Carotidynia* refers to pain arising from the cervical carotid artery and is typically neck pain that radiates to the ipsilateral face and ear. Carotid dissection should be excluded.

Occipital Neuralgia

Paroxysmal stabbing pain in the distribution of the greater or lesser occipital nerves may be confused with other causes of head and facial pain. Tenderness may be elicited with pressure over the affected nerve. Injection of local anesthetic agents relieves the pain and is helpful in confirming the diagnosis.

Temporomandibular Disease

Pain from the temporomandibular area may arise from either the joint or the muscle. Joint pain exacerbated by chewing or talking suggests joint disease. A click or pop with a limited jaw opening may be present. Pain from the muscle is more difficult to diagnose, as it may be referred to the ear, preauricular area, or neck. Jaw pain or claudication in an elderly patient may be an early symptom of giant cell arteritis.

Carotid Dissection

Carotid dissection often produces pain localized to the face (see Chapter 14). It is often accompanied by sympathetic dysfunction (Horner syndrome) due to involvement of the sympathetic fibers in the wall of the carotid artery (see Chapter 10, Fig 10-4).

Herpes Zoster Ophthalmicus

When *herpes zoster* involves the trigeminal dermatomes, pain may arise in the affected region days before a vesicular eruption is seen (Fig 12-3). The pain is described as aching or burning. Occasionally, no vesicles are apparent *(zoster sine herpete)*. Acutely, the pain may be exacerbated by concomitant iritis (seen on slit-lamp examination). The pain

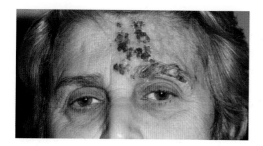

Figure 12-3 Herpes zoster ophthalmicus. This 63-year-old woman developed left-sided scalp pain and a rash in the V_1 distribution on the left side. *(Courtesy of Rod Foroozan, MD.)*

may persist long after resolution of the acute infection *(postherpetic neuralgia),* and it can be extremely discomforting and difficult to treat. Pregabalin (Lyrica), gabapentin (Neurontin), tricyclic antidepressants, and the topical lidocaine patch 5% may be effective in some patients. There is evidence that acute treatment with antivirals may decrease the risk of severe postherpetic neuralgia. A vaccine for herpes zoster may be helpful in reducing the morbidity of postherpetic neuralgia.

Pavan-Langston D. Herpes zoster: antivirals and pain management. *Ophthalmology.* 2008;115 (2 Suppl):S13–S20.

Neoplastic Processes

Pain associated with facial numbness raises the possibility of pathologic involvement of the trigeminal nerve, such as neoplastic processes that affect the nerve in the area of the cavernous sinus and the Meckel cave. Meningiomas affecting only the parasellar region do not generally produce pain. More rapidly growing tumors, such as aggressive undifferentiated malignancies, may produce pain in a larger percentage of patients. Facial cutaneous malignancy, the treatment of which is often not recalled by the patient because it occurred years previously, may be associated with *perineural invasion* and cause progressive pain, numbness, and multiple cranial nerve palsies.

Mental Nerve Neuropathy

An additional form of facial pain associated with numbness is the syndrome of the "numb chin," which most frequently accompanies an inflammatory or a neoplastic process. Sarcoidosis has been associated with a painfully numb chin. The most common neoplastic processes are lymphoma and metastatic breast carcinoma. Rarer causes include osteosarcoma, fibrosarcoma, plasmacytoma, metastatic lung and prostate carcinoma, collagen vascular diseases, trauma, periodontal disease, and sickle cell disease.

CHAPTER 13

The Patient With Nonorganic Ophthalmic Disorders

Visual complaints that have no physiologic or organic basis are called *nonorganic.* There are 4 categories of involvement, including disorders of

1. the afferent visual pathway (acuity, visual field)
2. ocular motility and alignment
3. the pupils and accommodation
4. eyelid position and function

Patients who have ophthalmic problems with no discernible organic cause present a formidable diagnostic challenge. *Malingering* is willful feigning or exaggeration of symptoms, and litigation involving monetary compensation or disability is frequently an issue with these patients. Secondary psychologic gain is often the underlying basis of *Munchausen syndrome,* in which patients intentionally induce physical damage. *Hysteria* is a subconscious expression of nonorganic signs or symptoms; patients with hysteria are often unconcerned about their incapacitating symptoms ("la belle indifference"). Malingering cannot always be clearly differentiated from hysteria, and the terms *functional, nonphysiologic,* and *nonorganic* are used to refer to the entire spectrum of disease. Both types of patients are evaluated with similar techniques to ascertain the validity of the symptoms. It is essential to remember that a significant number of patients with actual organic disease may also exhibit superimposed nonorganic behavior or may exaggerate an organic visual disturbance (so-called nonorganic overlay). Stripping off the overlay from the underlying organic pathology is a challenging, time-consuming task for the clinician. This chapter discusses the most frequently used clinical techniques for assessing and identifying nonorganic visual loss.

The first step in identifying the nonorganic patient is to have a high index of suspicion. The physician's suspicion is often raised during the history when the pattern of visual loss does not fit the common sequence of known diseases. For example, trivial external trauma to the eye would not be expected to cause long-term disabling visual loss. In addition, potential secondary gain factors may become evident during the history. Some patients may be more focused on impending litigation or disability determination than on the diagnosis or treatment of their complaint. Other patients who are naive, worried, and eager to convince the physician of their visual deficit tend to have a "positive" review of ophthalmic symptoms and often are suggestive during the history-taking process.

"Everything counts" is the guiding principle. Each piece of information about the patient, from the time the appointment is made through the completion of the office visit, may help direct the examination. For example, in a tertiary neuro-ophthalmic practice, it was shown that patients who wore sunglasses to their appointments were more likely to have nonorganic visual loss. Throughout the encounter with the patient, the physician should continually observe the patient's general behavior and ocular capabilities. Can the patient successfully ambulate into the room and into the chair? Can he or she find and shake the physician's silently outstretched hand on arrival? Is there a problem with nonvisual tasks such as signing in? The best results are always achieved by avoiding confrontation. The patient's story should be listened to and recorded in an empathetic fashion.

Suspicion increases as the ophthalmic examination progresses without uncovering any objective abnormalities to corroborate subjective visual symptoms. The key issue is the mismatch between objective and subjective examination findings. The examiner must be patient, persistent, and facile with the tests being used so the patient remains unaware of the examiner's goal: demonstrating better function (in acuity, visual fields, ocular motility) than claimed. The concept of *misdirection* is important. In other words, some examination techniques rely on the fact that the patient believes a particular eye or function is being tested as part of the normal eye examination, but in reality the examiner is trying to confirm a nonorganic disorder by demonstrating a nonphysiologic response, improved visual acuity or ocular function.

A diagnosis of a nonorganic component can be confirmed when the patient does something that should not be possible based on the stated symptoms. Other tests may suggest that the patient is not cooperating but do not prove a nonorganic disorder. The examination must be tailored to the individual and the specific complaints. The results of the examination (particularly the patient's response to various testing situations) should be recorded.

The scope and the economic impact of nonorganic ophthalmic disorders are both difficult to measure. Somatic manifestations of psychogenic origins are prevalent in all fields of medicine. One study concluded that they were the basis of at least 10% of visits to family physicians. Currently, no such data are available for visual complaints. In the mid-1980s, Keltner and coworkers estimated that fraudulent disability claims totaled $1 billion for a single year in the state of California, and that did not include the costs of medical evaluation and legal fees. Clearly, extrapolating from these data, the cost to society of nonorganic ophthalmic disturbances is enormous.

Arnold AC. Nonorganic visual disorders. In: Albert DM, Jakobiec FA, eds. *Principles and Practice of Ophthalmology.* 2nd ed. Philadelphia: Saunders; 2000:4317–4324.

Bengtzen R, Woodward M, Lynn MJ, Newman NJ, Biousse V. The "sunglasses sign" predicts nonorganic visual loss in neuro-ophthalmologic practice. *Neurology.* 2008;70(3):218–221.

Keltner JL, May WN, Johnson CA, et al. The California syndrome. Functional visual complaints with potential economic impact. *Ophthalmology.* 1985;92:427–435.

Kline LB. Techniques for diagnosing functional visual loss. In: Parrish RK II, ed. *The University of Miami Bascom Palmer Eye Institute Atlas of Ophthalmology.* Philadelphia: Current Medicine; 2000:493–501.

Miller NR. Neuro-ophthalmologic manifestations of nonorganic disease. In: Miller NR, Newman NJ, Biousse V, Kerrison JB, eds. *Walsh and Hoyt's Clinical Neuro-ophthalmology.* 6th ed. Baltimore: Williams & Wilkins; 2005:1315–1334.

Examination Techniques

A number of different examination techniques are used with patients with nonorganic disorders. These techniques fall into 4 groups, depending on whether the disorders are of the afferent visual pathway, ocular motility and alignment, the pupils and accommodation, or eyelid position and function.

Afferent Visual Pathway

When the afferent visual pathway is involved, examination techniques depend on whether the dysfunction is an acuity loss (complete or partial, bilateral or monocular) or a visual field defect.

Bilateral no light perception

Several tests, both visual and nonvisual, are used when a patient complains of complete bilateral blindness (ie, no light perception).

Nonvisual tasks   Indirect evidence of a nonorganic component to complaints of total blindness may be obtained by a patient's inability to perform nonvisual tasks. These include writing and bringing their fingers together with arms in an extended position. As this latter task is proprioceptive, it does not require visual input. Failure to perform these tasks adequately does not prove a nonorganic disorder, but it should alert the clinician to problems (conscious or unconscious) with patient cooperation.

Pupillary reaction   The presence of a normal pupillary reaction suggests that the anterior visual pathways are intact. However, it does not prove nonorganic loss, as there could be involvement of the bilateral anterior visual pathways or postgeniculate radiations. An aversive reaction to the light by a patient who claims not to see anything establishes at least some level of afferent input.

Optokinetic nystagmus drum   Traditionally, the easiest test to perform with a patient who claims total blindness is to slowly rotate an optokinetic nystagmus (OKN) drum in front of the patient. While doing so, the physician should ask the patient what he or she sees. If the patient claims to see nothing while the eyes move with the drum, a nonorganic component has been established. It is possible for malingerers to purposely minimize or prevent the response by looking around or focusing past the drum.

Mirror test   Although used somewhat less commonly (probably because a large mirror is not available), the mirror test is even more difficult to fool than is the OKN drum test. A large mirror is slowly moved side to side in front of the patient while the examiner observes eye position. If the patient states that he or she sees nothing while the eyes move with the mirror, a subjective–objective mismatch has been documented (Fig 13-1).

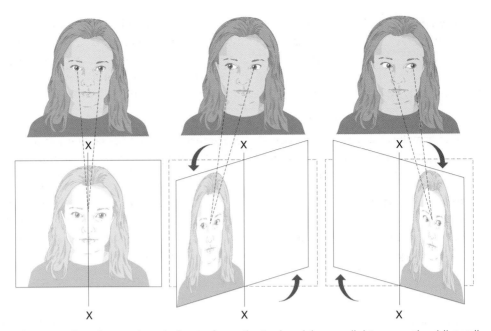

Figure 13-1 Rotating a mirror in front of a patient who claims no light perception bilaterally produces shifts of ocular orientation in the direction of the mirror rotation. Such ocular movement demonstrates that the patient is capable of following his or her own reflection. *(Illustration by C. H. Wooley.)*

Shock value Although perhaps primarily of historical interest (and found in military manuals to detect malingering), tests designed to elicit surprise can still be occasionally employed. Something dropped or an unexpected behavior may elicit evidence of visual activity.

Electrophysiologic testing Visual evoked potentials (VEP) play a limited role in assessing a possible nonorganic disorder. Both false-positives and false-negatives are possible with VEP. The results of VEP are best used to confirm other findings. Increased latency may suggest an organic component to the patient's complaint. Normal VEP in a patient who presents with severe monocular or binocular visual loss and a normal clinical examination supports the diagnosis of nonorganic disturbance of vision. Abnormal pattern-reversal visual evoked response in a patient with a normal neuro-ophthalmic examination should not, by itself, lead to the diagnosis of organic defect. Through a variety of techniques (inattention, lack of concentration, meditation), a patient can willfully suppress a visual evoked response. See also "Visual evoked potential" in Chapter 3 of this volume.

> Morgan RK, Nugent B, Harrison JM, et al. Voluntary alteration of pattern visual evoked responses. *Ophthalmology.* 1985;92:1356–1363.

Monocular no light perception

All of the tests listed under binocular no light perception may be performed unilaterally. In addition, however, several additional approaches are possible. They are based on ocular viewing confusion and tests that require binocularity.

Relative afferent pupillary defect   In the setting of claimed complete visual loss in 1 eye only, other evidence to support optic nerve dysfunction should be present. In most cases this would include the presence of a relative afferent pupillary defect (RAPD) (see Chapter 3). The absence of an RAPD does not confirm a nonorganic disorder, but it substantially increases suspicion in the setting of a normal eye examination.

Base-out prism test   Placing a 4–6 D prism base-out in front of 1 eye with both eyes open should normally elicit an inward shift of that eye (either as a conjugate saccade followed by a convergent movement of the opposite eye or by a convergent movement alone). Movement that occurs when the prism is placed over the "bad" eye indicates vision in that eye.

Vertical prism dissociation test   A 4 D prism is placed base-down in front of the "good" eye of a patient claiming monocular visual loss. If the subject has symmetric vision in both eyes, 2 images should be seen, one above the other. If the subject is able to see the letters only with the "good" eye, then only 1 image should be seen (Fig 13-2).

Golnik KC, Lee AG, Eggenberger ER. The monocular vertical prism dissociation test. *Am J Ophthalmol.* 2004;137(1):135–137.

Confusion tests   Several tests have been devised to confuse the patient as to which eye is actually being used. These tests need to be performed so that they appear to be simply a normal part of the examination. Any suspicion on the part of the patient is likely to lead to closure of 1 eye at a time, which will defeat all of these tests.

In the *fogging test*, a trial frame is placed on the patient. Plus and minus spheres (4–6 D) are placed in front of the "bad" eye, and plus and minus cylinders (4–6 D), with their axes aligned, are placed in front of the other eye. The patient is asked to read the chart while the front lenses are rotated. On the sphere side, rotation will make no difference, but on the cylinder side, vision will become severely blurred as the axes are rotated out of alignment. If the patient continues to read, he or she is doing so with the "bad" eye.

In the *red-green test*, duochrome (Worth 4-dot) glasses are placed over the patient's eyes, with the red lens over the "bad" eye. The red-green filter is then placed over the

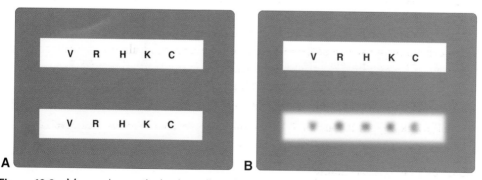

Figure 13-2 Monocular vertical prism dissociation test. In the setting of nonorganic visual loss, the patient will describe seeing 2 images, 1 over the other **(A)**. True organic visual loss will render the patient unable to see the second image or to see only a very blurred second image **(B)**. *(Courtesy of Lanning Kline, MD.)*

Snellen chart, exposing half the letters on a green background and the other half on a red background. The green lens will prevent the good eye from seeing the red background letters. If the red letters are read, the patient is reading with the "nonseeing" eye.

In the *Polaroid slide test,* the patient may wear the Polaroid lenses available with the Titmus stereoacuity test while reading a specially projected chart with corresponding Polaroid filters (Fig 13-3). Letters or lines may be selected that indicate the patient is reading with the "bad" eye.

Stereopsis testing Stereopsis requires binocular vision. Patients may be tested on the standard Titmus test (using their appropriate near correction and the Polaroid glasses). Any evidence of stereopsis demonstrates there is vision in the "bad" eye. It should be noted that patients with vision in only 1 eye may well detect asymmetries in the first several circles on the basis of monocular clues. Drawing a false conclusion can be avoided by asking the patient what he or she sees. If the detection is monocular, the patient will see the circle as shifted to one side. If the circle is "standing out from the page," the patient has binocularity.

Monocular reduced vision

Patients with complaints of decreased but not absent vision are more challenging. The clinician needs to demonstrate convincingly that the patient's actual acuity is better than initially claimed. As patients' acuity is almost always somewhat better when they are pushed, demonstrating a nonorganic component requires a substantial difference between claimed and demonstrated acuity levels. Many of the tests described for patients with binocular or monocular no light perception can be applied to patients with monocular (and binocular) reduced vision.

Confusion tests The confusion tests outlined in the "Monocular no light perception" section are useful if substantial acuity reduction is claimed in 1 eye. The fogging test,

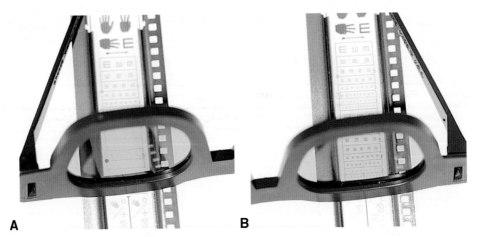

A **B**

Figure 13-3 Specialized polarized projector charts are obscured when a patient looks through 1 lens of the Polaroid glasses **(A)** but are seen when he or she looks through the other lens **(B)**. *(Courtesy of Steven A. Newman, MD.)*

red-green duochrome test, and Polaroid slide test have the potential to give a quantitative acuity measurement if the patient is cooperative enough to continue reading. Unlike assessment of a patient who claims monocular blindness, it is not sufficient to simply demonstrate that the patient can read at all; the physician must determine how far down the chart the patient can read.

Stereopsis   As mentioned earlier, binocular vision is necessary for stereopsis. The presence of stereopsis (as measured by the Titmus test) indicates at least some vision in both eyes. Attempts have been made to equate acuity and quantitative stereopsis (Table 13-1).

Binocular reduced vision

Assessing claims of binocularly reduced vision is the most difficult situation. Proving a nonorganic disorder requires the patient to admit to seeing better than initially claimed. This kind of testing is a contest of wills; sometimes the doctor quits before the patient does. It is imperative not to squeeze the examination into a limited time block. If necessary, the patient should be rescheduled.

Bottom-up acuity   The examination begins with acuity determination on the smallest line on the Snellen chart (20/10). If the patient cannot see these letters, the examiner announces the use of a "larger line" and then goes to the 20/15 line and several different 20/20 lines. The examiner continually expresses disbelief that such "large" letters cannot be identified. If the patient still denies being able to read the letters, he or she is asked to determine the number of characters present and whether they are round, square, and so on. Once the count is established, the examiner might suggest that the characters are letters and the first one is easier to identify than the others. By the time the "very large letters" (ie, 20/50) are reached, the patient often can be cajoled into reading optotypes much smaller than those read on initial acuity testing.

A variation of the bottom-up acuity technique requires time and repetition to demonstrate an improvement in visual acuity. Small (⅛ D) plus and minus lenses are alternately added and subtracted while the patient is asked how many letters are visible and what shape they have. The process may be expanded by using small cylinders. It is sometimes possible to gradually improve the best-recorded acuity with this method (sometimes called "doctor-killing refraction").

Table 13-1 Relationship of Visual Acuity to Stereopsis

Visual Acuity in Each Eye	Average Stereopsis (Arc Seconds of Image Disparity)
20/20	40
20/25	43
20/30	52
20/40	61
20/50	89
20/70	94
20/100	124
20/200	160

Adapted from Levy NS, Glick EB. Stereoscopic perception and Snellen visual acuity. *Am J Ophthalmol.* 1974;78:722–724.

"Visual aids"   The examiner can have the patient wear trial frames with 4 lenses equaling the correct prescription but suggest that they are special magnifying lenses that might allow improved vision. The potential acuity meter can also be presented as a means of "bypassing the visual block." Improvement in either case suggests a nonorganic component.

Use of alternative charts   Often, patients can be persuaded to see substantially better by a switch in optotypes. For example, a patient who refuses to read smaller type than 20/200 using standard optotypes might read much better using tumbling Es or numbers.

Specialty charts   Charts are available with a 50 optotype on top instead of the 400 optotype. Patients who say that they can read only the "top line" immediately improve their resolution by 4 lines. Alternatively, the standard chart may be moved farther away.

Visual field defect

Although less common than acuity loss, complaints of difficulty seeing to 1 side are occasionally made by patients. The problem may be binocular but is more commonly unilateral. The field defects may take many forms but are most commonly nonspecific constrictions.

Automated perimetry   Before discussing techniques that are useful in testing patients with suspected nonorganic visual field defects, it is important to point out what should not be done. Automated perimetry has substantially improved standard visual field testing, but it should not be ordered for patients with suspected nonphysiologic visual fields. Although there may be a high incidence of abnormalities in the reliability indices (false-positives, false-negatives, and fixation losses), completely normal indices are not incompatible with feigned visual field defects. It is actually quite easy to fool these machines. If motivated, a mildly sophisticated observer can reproduce homonymous defects, altitudinal defects, even arcuate and central scotomata. There are no characteristic changes in automated perimetry that would confirm the suspicion of a nonorganic deficit. An unusual situation in which automated perimetry might be pursued is that of a monocular defect that appears to respect the vertical midline. If repeating the field with both eyes open produces a similar, or even incomplete, defect, a nonorganic component is present (Fig 13-4).

> Keane JR. Hysterical hemianopia. The "missing half" field defect. *Arch Ophthalmol.* 1979;97: 865–866.
> Smith TJ, Baker RS. Perimetric findings in functional disorders using automated techniques. *Ophthalmology.* 1987;94:1562–1566.
> Stewart JF. Automated perimetry and malingerers. Can the Humphrey be outwitted? *Ophthalmology.* 1995;102:27–32.

"Non–field testing"   In the setting of a dense field defect, the patient is evaluated with confrontation testing. The area where the patient "can't see" is carefully identified. Later, the patient is tested for "motility." As part of this examination, stimuli are placed in various areas of the patient's peripheral field, including those areas where the patient "couldn't see." Accurate saccades to these nonauditory targets indicates intact visual field.

Confrontation testing   In some cases, confrontation testing ("silent visual fields") might initially appear to confirm a dense visual field defect. The patient is subsequently asked

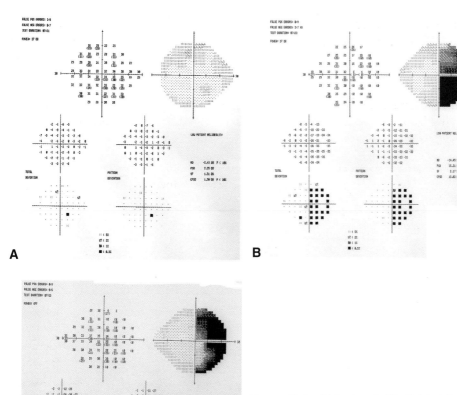

Figure 13-4 "Missing half" field defect. A 33-year-old man complained of decreased vision temporally in the right eye following a motor vehicle accident. Automated perimetry demonstrates a normal field on the left **(A)** and a temporal defect on the right **(B)**. Visual fields performed with both eyes open **(C)** demonstrate persistence of the field defect, indicating a nonorganic basis for the visual complaint. *(Courtesy of Karl C. Golnik, MD.)*

to count fingers in the "nonseeing" field, being instructed to report "none" when none are seen. As the test progresses, the examiner begins showing fingers without saying anything. A response of "none" each time the fingers are put up confirms vision in that area.

Goldmann perimetry The visual field is tested in a continuous fashion in a clockwise or counterclockwise direction starting with the I4e stimulus. A common nonorganic response shows a spiraling isopter getting closer and closer to fixation as testing continues. As larger stimuli (III4e and V4e) are employed, there is often further constriction, resulting in overlapping isopters (Fig 13-5). It is important to make sure there is no step across the vertical or nasal horizontal midline. A step across the midline may indicate that at least some physiologic component is present in the field abnormality.

Tangent screen testing The patient is tested with a 9-mm white stimulus at 1 m. The areas of patient response are marked and the patient is moved back to 2 m. The tangent

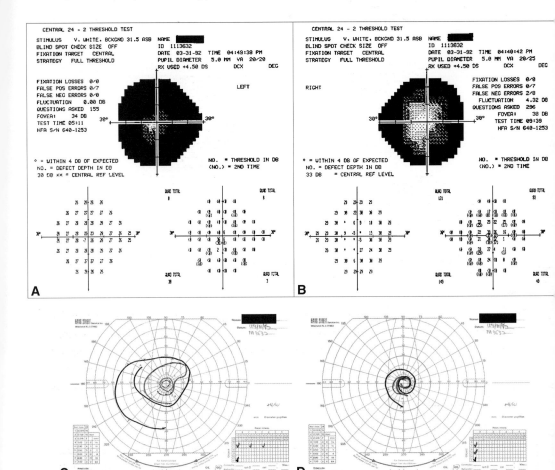

Figure 13-5 A 59-year-old woman complained of 1 year of headaches. **A, B,** Automated static perimetry program 24-2 with a V-sized test object demonstrated severe constriction. **C, D,** Subsequent Goldmann visual fields revealed crossing and spiraling isopters, indicating non-physiologic constriction of the visual fields. *(Courtesy of Steven A. Newman, MD.)*

test is then repeated using an 18-mm white stimulus. The field should expand to twice the original size. Failure to expand (tubular or gun-barrel field) is nonphysiologic and indicates a nonorganic component to the field constriction (Fig 13-6).

Ocular Motility and Alignment

Voluntary nystagmus

Voluntary nystagmus is characterized by irregular, brief bursts of rapid frequency, low amplitude, and pendular eye movements with no slow phase. Most commonly they are horizontal, although on occasion they may be vertical or torsional. The eye movements are bilateral and conjugate and are often associated with convergence, fluttering eyelids,

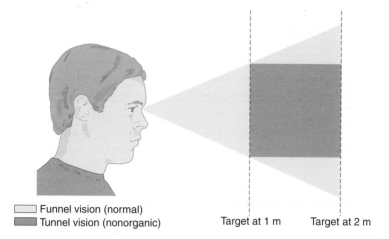

Funnel vision (normal)
Tunnel vision (nonorganic)

Target at 1 m   Target at 2 m

Figure 13-6 Nonphysiologic lack of visual field expansion (tubular or gun-barrel visual fields) is best demonstrated at the tangent screen. *(Illustration by C. H. Wooley.)*

blinking, or strained facial expression. Voluntary nystagmus is difficult to maintain for longer than 10–12 seconds. Patients often complain of oscillopsia and reduced vision. These individuals are identified and differentiated from individuals with ocular flutter by the volitional appearance of the ocular movement disorder, absence of nystagmus when distracted, unsustained movement, and the lack of other neuro-ophthalmic abnormalities (typically cerebellar features).

Gaze palsy

Patients may report inability to move the eyes horizontally or vertically. Such claimed gaze palsies may be overcome by a variety of maneuvers, including oculocephalic testing (doll's head phenomenon), optokinetic testing, mirror tracking, and caloric testing.

Spasm of the near reflex

Spasm of the near reflex is characterized by episodes of intermittent convergence, increased accommodation, and miosis. Patients generally complain of diplopia and, at times, micropsia. The degree of convergence is variable. Some patients demonstrate marked convergence of both eyes, resulting in a large esotropia; others show a lesser degree of convergence, with only 1 eye turning in. This syndrome may be mistaken for unilateral or bilateral sixth nerve palsies, divergence insufficiency, horizontal gaze paresis, or ocular myasthenia. However, the variability of the eye movements, the lack of other neuro-ophthalmic abnormalities, and the occurrence of miosis with convergent eye movements help in reaching the correct diagnosis. Further, when ductions are examined with 1 eye occluded or with oculocephalic testing, both eyes demonstrate full abduction, and the miosis seen with the eyes in an esotropic position immediately resolves. Although spasm of the near reflex is almost always observed in nonorganic patients, it has been associated with Arnold-Chiari I malformation, posterior fossa tumors, pituitary tumors, and head trauma.

Pupils and Accommodation

Fixed, dilated pupil

Few patients provoke more anxiety than those with headaches and a fixed, dilated pupil. The differential diagnosis can be narrowed to 3 basic processes: pharmacologic blockade, oculomotor nerve palsy, and Adie tonic pupil. *Pharmacologic blockade* may occur because of inadvertent or purposeful application of mydriatic or cycloplegic eyedrops or contamination of the fingers from placing a scopolamine patch to prevent motion sickness or postoperative nausea.

The pilocarpine test readily distinguishes parasympathetic denervation from pharmacologic blockade. In the latter, 1% pilocarpine cannot overcome the receptor blockade, and the pupil remains large. A fixed, dilated pupil from injury to the third cranial nerve will constrict briskly in response to 1% pilocarpine, whereas an Adie pupil will constrict with 0.1% pilocarpine because denervation supersensitivity will be present. Pupillary abnormalities are discussed at greater length in Chapter 10.

Changes in pupil size

Widely dilated pupils may be seen in young patients, most likely caused by increased levels of circulating catecholamines. Rare patients are able to voluntarily dilate both pupils. Intermittent miosis occurs in spasm of the near reflex (discussed earlier), accompanied by esotropia and accommodation.

Changes in accommodation

Weakness or paralysis of accommodation sometimes occurs, primarily in children and young adults. Such patients are unable to read unless provided with an appropriate plus lens and, even then, may complain of inability to read clearly. Failure of a patient with normal distance vision to read despite appropriate near vision correction should alert the clinician to the possibility of a nonorganic condition.

Spasm of accommodation is seen with the syndrome of spasm of the near reflex. Patients may complain of blurred distance vision and often can produce 8–10 D of myopia. Refraction without and with cycloplegia during the period of spasm establishes the presence of the induced myopia.

Eyelid Position and Function

Ptosis

Eyelid "droop" from nonphysiologic causes can usually be distinguished by the position of the brow. In the setting of true ptosis, the brow is usually elevated as the patient tries to open the palpebral fissure. With orbicularis overactivity, the brow is lowered.

In addition, patients who feign ptosis cannot simultaneously elevate the eye and maintain a drooping eyelid. Thus, with upward gaze, the ptosis will "resolve." Often the patient will realize this and not cooperate. In such cases, the examiner can use his or her thumb to manually elevate the ptotic lid and the patient will then look upward. The examiner's thumb is then slowly moved away. If the ptosis returns, the condition may well have an organic basis, but if it "resolves," then it is nonorganic.

Blepharospasm

Nonorganic blepharospasm may be unilateral or bilateral. At times, it may cause nonorganic ptosis. Pressure over the supraorbital notch is often useful in inducing a patient with nonorganic blepharospasm to raise the eyelids. Most cases of nonorganic blepharospasm occur in children or young adults and are often triggered by an emotionally traumatic event.

Management of the Nonorganic Patient

In general, patients with nonorganic visual complaints are best managed with an understanding approach and words of encouragement. Confrontation is seldom of benefit to either the patient or the doctor. It is prudent to allow patients a graceful way out of the situation by reassuring them that although their disorder does not suggest underlying damage to the central nervous system, they do, in fact, have a problem that will resolve over time. Often, the symptoms will clear with 1 or 2 follow-up visits, and patients should be reassured of an "excellent prognosis." This is usually more effective in children than adults. Children may be further encouraged through the prescription of "eye rest"—for example, removing "overuse of television."

In patients with combined organic and nonorganic (nonorganic overlay) complaints, it is best to deal with the former problem and attempt to downplay the latter. Frequently, with appropriate management of the organic visual disturbance, the patient's anxiety will be alleviated and the nonorganic complaints will resolve. In some cases, consultation with a psychiatrist or psychologist may be warranted for an underlying psychologic illness. Finally, it is always prudent to follow a patient with what initially appears to be a nonorganic visual disturbance. Occasionally, an organic disorder becomes apparent later and can be dealt with appropriately.

Catalono RA, Simon JW, Krohel GB, Rosenberg PN. Functional visual loss in children. *Ophthalmology.* 1986;93:385–390.

Kathol RG, Cox TA, Corbett JJ, Thompson HS. Functional visual loss. Follow-up of 42 cases. *Arch Ophthalmol.* 1983;101:729–735.

North American Neuro-Ophthalmology Society. 29th Annual Meeting. Controversies session: functional visual loss. Snowbird, Utah. 8–13 February 2003.

Scott JA, Egan RA. Prevalence of organic neuro-ophthalmologic disease in patients with functional visual loss. *Am J Ophthalmol.* 2003;135:670–675.

CHAPTER 14

Selected Systemic Conditions With Neuro-Ophthalmic Signs

Certain neurologic and medical disorders are seen commonly enough and affect vision with such regularity that they deserve separate emphasis. Although the discussion that follows is not comprehensive, it is intended to cover many aspects of diseases with which ophthalmologists should be familiar.

Immunologic Disorders

A variety of immune system–mediated disorders produce neuro-ophthalmic signs and symptoms. Giant cell arteritis, multiple sclerosis, myasthenia gravis, thyroid eye disease, and sarcoidosis are the most common.

Giant Cell Arteritis

Giant cell arteritis (GCA), or *temporal arteritis,* is an inflammatory granulomatous vasculitis that affects large and medium-sized arteries. Incidence increases from age 50 upward, and women are 2–4 times more likely to be affected than men. Early diagnosis and treatment of GCA can limit or prevent permanent visual loss.

Clinical presentation

Systemic symptoms of GCA include headache and tenderness of the temporal artery or scalp. Jaw claudication (pain or weakness worsening with chewing) is the symptom most specific for the disorder, but other symptoms include malaise, anorexia and weight loss, fever, joint and muscle pain, and ear pain. Systemic sequelae can include cerebrovascular ischemia, myocardial infarction, and aortic aneurysm or dissection.

Visual symptoms may include transient or permanent visual loss, diplopia, and eye pain. *Arteritic anterior ischemic optic neuropathy (AAION)* is the most common cause of visual loss (see Chapter 4, Fig 4-8), but central retinal artery occlusion, cilioretinal artery occlusion, posterior ischemic optic neuropathy, and ocular ischemic syndrome also occur. Ocular motor cranial nerve palsies can result in transient or constant diplopia.

Diagnosis

A high level of suspicion of GCA is paramount when encountering patients over age 50 with the visual symptoms just described. Diagnostic evaluation begins with laboratory tests of the erythrocyte sedimentation rate (ESR), complete blood count (CBC), and C-reactive protein. Most cases of GCA show marked elevation of the Westergren ESR (mean 70 mm/hr; often >100 mm/hr), but the level may be normal in up to 16% of cases. The ESR rises with anemia and with age; levels above the laboratory's listed upper limit of normal are common in patients over 70 without arteritis. A more accurate estimate of the upper normal value is obtained by using these formulas: [age]/2 *(males)* or [age + 10]/2 *(females)*. Measurement of C-reactive protein, which may be more specific and less affected by increasing age and anemia, may increase diagnostic accuracy and is currently recommended in conjunction with the ESR. Thrombocytosis (increased platelet count) may suggest active disease. A normochromic normocytic anemia may be present.

Diagnosis is confirmed by temporal artery biopsy, which is recommended whenever clinical suspicion or laboratory studies suggest the possibility of GCA (see BCSC Section 4, *Ophthalmic Pathology and Intraocular Tumors*). Negative biopsy does not rule out arteritis. False-negative results have been estimated at 3%–9%, relating in part to the possibility of discontinuous arterial involvement ("skip areas") and missed lesions; biopsy segments should be 2–3 cm long to minimize the risk of insufficient sampling. If an initial biopsy is negative, a contralateral biopsy should be considered if the clinical picture is highly suspicious. Other imaging strategies (color Doppler ultrasonography, positron emission tomography, and magnetic resonance imaging [MRI]) are being investigated for the diagnosis of GCA, but firm conclusions regarding the accuracy of these techniques cannot be made as yet.

Treatment

When GCA is suspected, early therapy is critical and should begin immediately; confirmational temporal artery biopsy should be done expeditiously to avoid compromising test results. Intravenous methylprednisolone (1 g/day for the first 3–5 days) is often recommended when visual loss is present. For patients with suspected GCA, but without visual loss, oral prednisone 60–100 mg/day is sufficient. The corticosteroids are tapered slowly over 3–12 months or more, depending on response. Corticosteroids do not generally result in visual improvement, but usually they will prevent the occurrence of new ischemic events. The risk of recurrent or contralateral optic nerve involvement on corticosteroid withdrawal has been reported at 7%; thus, tapering must be slow and careful. Recurrent symptoms should prompt reevaluation for disease activity.

Foroozan R, Danesh-Meyer H, Savino PJ, Gamble G, Mekari-Sabbagh ON, Sergott RC. Thrombocytosis in patients with biopsy-proven giant cell arteritis. *Ophthalmology.* 2002;109(7): 1267–1271.

Hayreh SS, Podhajsky PA, Raman R, Zimmerman B. Giant cell arteritis: validity and reliability of various diagnostic criteria. *Am J Ophthalmol.* 1997;123(3):285–296.

Multiple Sclerosis

Patients with *multiple sclerosis (MS)* frequently have visual complaints, and often the ophthalmologist is the first physician consulted. Familiarity with both the ocular and neurologic consequences of MS is important in guiding the ophthalmologist to the appropriate diagnosis.

Epidemiology and genetics

The prevalence of MS in the United States ranges from 6 to 177 per 100,000. Multiple sclerosis is relatively rare throughout Asia and Africa. The disease affects women more often than men (2:1 in some series). It is relatively uncommon in children under 10 years of age, and the incidence is highest among young adults (25–40 years of age). However, examples of onset even after the age of 50 are not rare.

Although the cause of MS remains unknown, multiple factors appear contributory. Epidemiologic studies suggest that genetic factors play a role. The risk of developing MS is approximately 20 times greater in first-degree relatives of patients with the disease. Furthermore, identical twins show a tenfold greater concordance of the disease than do fraternal twins. Population-based concordance studies suggest that 2 or more genes are operative for MS susceptibility, and there is a strong association with HLA-DRB1 antigen.

No specific viral etiology has been identified, but an acquired agent, such as a virus, may precipitate an autoimmune process that attacks myelin.

Kantarci O, Wingerchuck D. Epidemiology and natural history of multiple sclerosis: new insights. *Curr Opin Neurol.* 2006;19(3):248–254.

Mayr WT, Pittock SJ, McClelland RL, Jorgensen NW, Noseworthy JH, Rodriguez M. Incidence and prevalence of multiple sclerosis in Olmstead County, Minnesota, 1985–2000. *Neurology.* 2003;61(10):1373–1377.

Noseworthy JH, Lucchinetti C, Rodriguez M, Weinshenker BG. Multiple sclerosis. *N Engl J Med.* 2000;343(13):938–952.

Course and prognosis

Multiple sclerosis is usually a chronic relapsing disease, but the course of the disease is variable. Spontaneous remissions occur, and 90% of patients have a relapsing course in the early stages. An interval of months or years may precede a clinical relapse (relapsing-remitting MS), although the pathologic disease burden in the central nervous system (CNS) accumulates even in the absence of clinical activity. Within 10 years, approximately 50% of patients with relapsing-remitting disease develop a slow, apparently continuous deterioration of the neurologic status (secondary progressive form). In 10%–20% of patients, the disease progresses inexorably from onset with no recognizable attacks (primary progressive form). Progressive MS is more common when onset occurs in older patients, whose overall disability tends to be greater. Near total disability and, rarely, death within 1–2 years of onset may result after a fulminant course. In contrast, about 20% of patients experience a relatively benign course without serious disability or reduction of life span. As a rule, the longer the interval between the first attack and first relapse, the better the prognosis.

Vukusic S, Confavreux C. Prognostic factors for progression of disability in the secondary progressive phase of multiple sclerosis. *J Neurol Sci.* 2003;206(2):135–137.

Pathology

Although MS is classically considered a demyelinating disease, axonal damage does occur early and is an integral part of the disease process. This axonal loss is manifest as "black holes" on MRI (Fig 14-1). Myelin destruction is seen in association with local perivascular

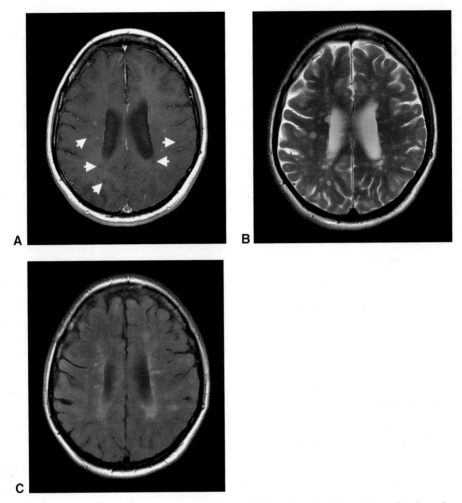

Figure 14-1 Axial MRI scans of a patient with multiple sclerosis show demyelinating plaques. **A,** T1-weighted MRI postgadolinium demonstrates enhancing white matter lesions bilaterally, as well as "black holes" *(arrows).* **B,** T2-weighted MRI shows periventricular multifocal hyperintense white matter lesions consistent with demyelination. **C,** A fluid-attenuation inversion recovery (FLAIR) scan confirms periventricular white matter lesions. *(Reprinted with permission from Slack: Lee AG, Brazis PW, Kline LB.* Curbside Consultation in Neuro-Ophthalmology: 49 Clinical Questions. *Thorofare, NJ: Slack, 2009.)*

mononuclear cell infiltration and is followed by myelin removal by macrophages. The next stage is characterized by astrocytic proliferation with production of glial fibrils. The term *multiple sclerosis* stems from the presence of these numerous gliotic (sclerotic) lesions, which take on spherical, ovoid, or other 3-dimensional configurations but appear as plaques on the surface of brain sections. Plaques are often situated in the white matter at the ventricular margins, the optic nerves and chiasm, the corpus callosum, the spinal cord, and throughout the brainstem and cerebellar peduncles. Peripheral nerves are not involved, and all other organs are normal in uncomplicated cases.

Dutta R, Trapp BD. Pathogenesis of axonal and neuronal damage in multiple sclerosis. *Neurology.* 2007;68(22 Suppl 3):S22–S31.

Clinical presentation

The diagnosis of MS is made by identifying neurologic symptoms and signs that occur over time and that affect different areas of the CNS. Ocular symptomatology is commonly part of the clinical picture of MS, and various ocular complications are discussed in the following sections. Nonocular signs and symptoms attributable to MS may precede, follow, or coincide with the ocular signs. Initially, many symptoms of MS are so transient or benign that the patient may fail to remember previous episodes. Typically, significant episodes last for weeks or months. The physician must ask specifically about transient diplopia, ataxia, vertigo, patchy paresthesias, bladder or bowel dysfunction, and extremity weakness. Fatigue and depression are common and may precede the onset of focal neurologic deficits. Because the symptoms of early MS are often so evanescent and unaccompanied by objective neurologic findings, patients are sometimes considered hysterical.

The cerebellum, brainstem, and spinal cord may be involved singly or simultaneously, thus producing mono- or polysymptomatic complaints. Some of the more common *nonocular* symptoms include

- *Cerebellar dysfunction:* ataxia, dysarthria, intention tremor, truncal or head titubation, dysmetria (sometimes described by the patient as poor depth perception)
- *Motor symptoms:* extremity weakness, facial weakness, hemiparesis, or paraplegia
- *Sensory symptoms:* paresthesias of face or body (especially in a bandlike distribution around the trunk), Lhermitte sign (an electric shock–like sensation in the limbs and trunk produced by neck flexion), pain (occasionally, trigeminal neuralgia)
- *Mental changes:* emotional instability, depression, irritability, fatigue; later in the course, cognitive dysfunction
- *Sphincter disturbances:* frequency, urgency, hesitancy, incontinence; urinary retention leading to urinary tract infection

It has been suggested that infection, trauma, abnormal reaction to certain foreign substances such as drugs or vaccinations, stress, exertion and fatigue, and increased body temperature may induce attacks of MS. No adequately controlled studies have examined these issues. Multiple sclerosis is typically quiescent during the third trimester of pregnancy and may flare up after delivery, suggesting hormonal influences.

Kantarci O, Wingerchuck D. Epidemiology and natural history of multiple sclerosis: new insights. *Curr Opin Neurol.* 2006;19(3):248–254.

Optic neuritis

The clinical signs and symptoms of optic neuritis are discussed in Chapter 4. Even after the recovery of visual loss from demyelinating optic neuritis, transient deterioration of vision may be brought on by exercise and by even small elevations of body temperature (Uhthoff symptom). Some patients with optic neuritis note phosphenes (bright flashes of light) with movement of the affected eye or photisms (light induced by noise, smell, taste, or touch). Optic neuritis is recognized clinically during the patient's course of MS in up to 75% of cases. It is one of the presenting features of MS in approximately 25% of patients. Evidence of optic nerve involvement appears in over 90% of cases at some point, regardless of symptoms, according to visually evoked potential response data. Furthermore, autopsy studies show anterior visual pathway demyelination in virtually all patients with clinical MS.

Patients frequently want to know their risk of developing MS after an episode of optic neuritis. The 15-year follow-up of the Optic Neuritis Treatment Trial (ONTT) showed that the presence or absence of abnormalities on MRI scan of the brain obtained at study entry during an episode of optic neuritis was the strongest predictive factor in determining the likelihood of developing MS. Overall, clinically definite MS developed in 50% of patients in 15 years. However, the probability of developing clinically definite MS based on MRI scan appearance ranged from 25% in patients with no lesions on MRI to 72% with 1 or more lesions. Cerebrospinal fluid (CSF) analysis in a subgroup of ONTT patients showed that oligoclonal banding had predictive value for the development of MS only in patients with a normal MRI scan at study entry. Patients with a prior history of optic neuritis and nonspecific neurologic symptoms were at higher risk of developing MS. (See also "Retrobulbar optic neuritis" in Chapter 4.)

The clinical profile of optic neuritis: experience of the Optic Neuritis Treatment Trial. Optic Neuritis Study Group. *Arch Ophthalmol.* 1991;109(12):1673–1678.

Cole SR, Beck RW, Moke PS, Kaufman DI, Tourtellotte WW. The predictive value of CSF oligoclonal banding for MS 5 years after optic neuritis. *Neurology.* 1998;51(3):885–887.

Optic Neuritis Study Group. Multiple sclerosis risk after optic neuritis: final optic neuritis treatment trial follow-up. *Arch Neurol.* 2008;65(6):727–732.

Funduscopic abnormalities in multiple sclerosis

Nerve fiber layer defects are discussed in Chapter 3. Perivenous sheathing and fluorescein leakage occur along peripheral veins in approximately 10% of patients with MS. Autopsy studies of 47 MS patients confirmed retinitis and periphlebitis in 5%–10%. Anterior or posterior uveitis (including pars planitis) occurs in 0.4% to 26% of MS patients. This reported range is probably due to differences in patient populations, diagnostic criteria, and examination techniques.

Biousse V, Trichet C, Bloch-Michel E, Roullet E. Multiple sclerosis associated with uveitis in 2 large clinic-based series. *Neurology.* 1999;52(1):179–181.

Lightman S, McDonald WI, Bird AC, et al. Retinal venous sheathing in optic neuritis. Its significance for the pathogenesis of multiple sclerosis. *Brain.* 1987;110(pt 2):405–414.

Chiasmal and retrochiasmal abnormalities

The white matter within the optic chiasm, optic tracts, and visual radiations is frequently involved pathologically with MS lesions. Chiasmal or retrochiasmal visual field defects were seen in 13.2% of patients in the ONTT after 1 year of follow-up. Bitemporal and homonymous visual field defects generally follow a course of recovery similar to that seen with optic neuritis (see Chapter 4, Fig 4-32).

Keltner JL, Johnson CA, Spurr JO, Beck RW. Visual field profile of optic neuritis. One-year follow-up in the optic neuritis treatment trial. *Arch Ophthalmol.* 1994;112(7):946–953.

Ocular motility disturbances

Diplopia is a frequent symptom of MS. Attacks of transient diplopia may occur before an observable ocular motor defect becomes clinically apparent. Because MS is a disease of CNS white matter, motility abnormalities are typically localized to the supranuclear, nuclear, and fascicular portions of the ocular motor system. Internuclear ophthalmoplegia, especially when bilateral, is highly suggestive of MS in someone under age 50 years (see Chapter 8, Fig 8-7). Other signs include the complete or partial paralysis of horizontal or vertical gaze or a vertical misalignment (skew deviation) not attributable to single nerve or muscle dysfunction. Although uncommon, MS must be considered in a young adult with an isolated ocular motor cranial nerve palsy and no history of trauma. Because ocular motor palsies most likely reflect fascicular involvement, they are frequently accompanied by other brainstem findings. Sixth nerve involvement is most commonly reported, but partial third or fourth nerve paresis has also been described.

Nystagmus is frequently seen in MS. It may be horizontal, rotary, or vertical. Both pendular and jerk types of nystagmus may occur. Various types of cerebellar eye findings are common, including rebound nystagmus, fixation instability (macrosaccadic oscillations), saccadic dysmetria, and abnormal pursuit movements. Concomitant vertical and horizontal nystagmus occurring out of phase produce circular or elliptical eye movements that are highly suggestive of MS. Occasionally, MS lesions produce dorsal midbrain (Parinaud) syndrome. Patients with eye movement abnormalities typically complain of diplopia, blurred vision, or oscillopsia. Chapters 7, 8, and 9 discuss ocular motility disorders in detail.

Laboratory evaluation

No test unequivocally establishes the presence of MS, which remains a *clinical* diagnosis (Table 14-1). The CSF in patients with definite MS is abnormal in more than 90% of cases. The most common abnormalities are the elevation of immunoglobulin G (IgG), the elevation of the IgG/albumin index, and the presence of oligoclonal IgG bands. None of these findings, however, is specific for demyelinating disease.

McDonald WI, Compston A, Edan G, et al. Recommended diagnostic criteria for multiple sclerosis: guidelines from the international panel on the diagnosis of multiple sclerosis. *Ann Neurol.* 2001;50(1):121–127.

Neuroimaging in multiple sclerosis

An MRI scan with *fluid-attenuated inversion recovery (FLAIR)* sequencing and gadolinium infusion is the neuroimaging study of choice for MS. The MRI scan is particularly sensitive for the identification of white-matter plaques in the CNS, and it is far superior to CT scan for visualizing the posterior fossa and spinal cord (see Fig 14-1; see also Chapter 2, Fig 2-8). The MRI scan shows multiple lesions in 85%–95% of patients with clinically definite MS and in 66%–76% of patients with suspected MS. Although the abnormalities seen on MRI scan are not specific for MS, multifocal lesions that are periventricular and ovoid are most consistent with the condition. The lesions seen with an MRI scan fluctuate over time. Active lesions will enhance with gadolinium-DPTA (diethylenetriamine pentaacetic acid) administration. Hypointense regions on postcontrast T1-weighted scans (black holes) are also a marker of progressive disease. Lesions in the optic nerves of patients with symptomatic optic neuritis may be best visualized on MRI scan with fat-suppression techniques and gadolinium infusion (see Fig 4-22C).

Table 14-1 Criteria for Diagnosis of Multiple Sclerosis

Clinical Presentation	Additional Data Needed for MS Diagnosis
Two or more attacks; objective clinical evidence of 2 or more lesions	None*
Two or more attacks; objective clinical evidence of 1 lesion	Dissemination in space, demonstrated by MRI *or* Two or more MRI-detected lesions consistent with MS plus positive CSF† *or* Await further clinical attack implicating a different site
One attack; objective clinical evidence of 2 or more lesions	Dissemination in time, demonstrated by MRI *or* Second clinical attack
One attack; objective clinical evidence of 1 lesion (monosymptomatic presentation; clinically isolated syndrome)	Dissemination in space, demonstrated by MRI *or* Two or more MRI-detected lesions consistent with MS plus positive CSF† *and* Dissemination in time, demonstrated by MRI *or* Second clinical attack
Insidious neurologic progression suggestive of MS	Positive CSF† *and* Dissemination in space, demonstrated by 1) Nine or more T2 lesions in brain *or* 2) 2 or more lesions in spinal cord *or* 3) 4–8 brain plus 1 spinal cord lesion *or* Abnormal VEP‡ associated with 4–8 brain lesions, or with fewer than 4 brain lesions plus 1 spinal cord lesion demonstrated by MRI *and* Dissemination in time, demonstrated by MRI *or* Continued progression for 1 year

If criteria indicated are fulfilled, the diagnosis is multiple sclerosis (MS); if the criteria are not completely met, the diagnosis is "possible MS"; if the criteria are fully explored and not met, the diagnosis is "not MS."

* No additional tests are required; however, if tests (magnetic resonance imaging [MRI], cerebral spinal fluid [CSF]) are undertaken and are *negative*, extreme caution should be taken before making a diagnosis of MS. Alternative diagnoses must be considered. There must be no better explanation for the clinical picture.

† Positive CSF determined by oligoclonal bands detected by established methods (preferably isoelectric focusing) different from any such bands in serum or by a raised IgG index.

‡ Abnormal visual evoked potential of the type seen in MS (delay with a well-preserved wave form).

Modified from McDonald WI, Compston A, Edan G, et al. Recommended diagnostic criteria for multiple sclerosis: guidelines from the International Panel on the Diagnosis of Multiple Sclerosis. *Ann Neurol.* 2001;50:121–127:Table 3.

Frohman EM, Goodin DS, Calabresi PA, et al. The utility of MRI in suspected MS. Report of the Therapeutic and Technology Assessment Subcommittee of the American Academy of Neurology. *Neurology.* 2003;61(5):602–611.

Diagnosis

The McDonald criteria for diagnosis of MS allow for the use of paraclinical data, including MRI and CSF results (see Table 14-1). Multiple sclerosis can be diagnosed on the basis of 2 or more typical attacks with objective clinical evidence of 2 or more lesions. Alternatively, 2 attacks and 1 objective clinical lesion (an objective physical examination finding, such as a relative afferent pupillary defect or internuclear ophthalmoplegia) or 1 attack and 2 objective clinical lesions in combination with a variety of MRI and/or CSF abnormalities can lead to a diagnosis of definite MS, as described in detail in Table 14-1. Even an insidious neurologic progression suggestive of MS can lead to a definite diagnosis if appropriate paraclinical abnormalities are present. Recurrent optic neuritis, in the absence of other clinical or laboratory manifestations, is not sufficient for diagnosing MS.

McDonald WI, Compston A, Edan G, et al. Recommended diagnostic criteria for multiple sclerosis: guidelines from the International Panel on the Diagnosis of Multiple Sclerosis. *Ann Neurol.* 2001;50(1):121–127.

Treatment

Although there is no cure for MS, several therapies slow the disease and assist specific symptoms. As in the management of optic neuritis, intravenous high-dose corticosteroids are often used to treat acute exacerbations of MS. Immunosuppressant and immunomodulating agents may be useful for long-term treatment. Interferon beta-1b (Betaseron), interferon beta-1a subcutaneous (Rebif), interferon beta-1a intramuscular (Avonex), and glatiramer acetate (Copaxone) all reduce MS exacerbations by approximately one third and demonstrate a positive effect on MRI changes in patients with relapsing-remitting disease.

Current research suggests that early diagnosis and therapy are advantageous; the Controlled High-Risk Subjects Avonex Multiple Sclerosis Prevention Study (CHAMPS) evaluated patients without clinically definite MS who were at high risk for developing the disease as defined by a single demyelinating event (optic neuritis, spinal cord syndrome, or brainstem-cerebellar syndrome) and having 2 or more plaques on MRI scan. Avonex-treated patients were 44% less likely to develop clinically definite MS or to have progression of disability than those treated with placebo over a 2-year period. The BENEFIT (*be*taferon in *ne*wly emerging multiple sclerosis *f*or *i*nitial *t*reatment) study showed similar results for interferon beta-1b.

Mitoxantrone (Novantrone) has been approved for the treatment of secondary progressive MS; however, this agent (and other immunosuppressives) is associated with potentially serious toxicity. Natalizumab (Tysabri) is a recombinant monoclonal antibody that prevents transmigration of leukocytes from the vasculature across the endothelium into the CNS. Tysabri has been associated with 3 cases of progressive multifocal leukoencephalopathy (a serious viral infection of the CNS that is usually fatal) and 2 cases of melanoma; it should be used with caution by physicians experienced in MS therapy. Several additional agents have been used to treat MS, including low-dose oral methotrexate, pulsed corticosteroids, cyclophosphamide, and others. Novel agents and combinations of immunomodulating therapies are being investigated.

Goodin DS, Arnason BG, Coyle PK, Frohman EM, Paty DW; Therapeutics and Technology Assessment Subcommittee of the American Academy of Neurology. The use of mitoxantrone (Novantrone) for the treatment of multiple sclerosis: report of the Therapeutics and Technology Assessment Subcommittee of the American Academy of Neurology. *Neurology.* 2003;61(10):1332–1338.

Hartung HP, Gonsette R, König N, et al. Mitoxantrone in progressive multiple sclerosis: a placebo-controlled, double-blind, randomised, multicentre trial. *Lancet.* 2002;360(9350): 2018–2025.

Interferon beta-1b is effective in relapsing-remitting multiple sclerosis. I. Clinical results of a multicenter, randomized, double-blind, placebo-controlled trial. The IFNB Multiple Sclerosis Study Group. *Neurology.* 1993;43(4):655–661.

O'Connor P; CHAMPS. The effects of intramuscular interferon beta-1a in patients with high risk for development of multiple sclerosis: a post hoc analysis of data from CHAMPS. *Clin Ther.* 2003;25(11):2865–2874.

Rudick RA, Sandrock A. Natalizumab: alpha 4-integrin antagonist selective adhesion molecule inhibitors for MS. *Expert Rev Neurother.* 2004;4(4):571–580.

Myasthenia Gravis

Myasthenia gravis (MG) is an immunologic disorder characterized by weakness. It improves with rest. Most patients with MG develop neuro-ophthalmic abnormalities. Although the disease is usually a systemic disorder, half the affected patients have ocular symptoms and signs at onset, so the ophthalmologist is frequently the first physician encountered. The muscles and nerves are intact in MG, but the acetylcholine receptor sites for neuromuscular transmission are blocked by immune complexes. Myasthenia gravis may be caused, unmasked, or worsened by drugs such as procainamide, quinidine, polymyxin and aminoglycoside antibiotics, monobasic amino acid antibiotics, corticosteroids, β-blockers, calcium channel blockers, chloroquine, lithium, phenytoin, cisplatin, magnesium, and statins.

Drachman DB. Myasthenia gravis. *N Engl J Med.* 1994;330(25):1797–1810.

Purvin V, Kawasaki A, Smith KH, Kesler A. Statin-associated myasthenia gravis: report of 4 cases and review of the literature. *Medicine (Baltimore).* 2006;85(2):82–85.

Smith KH. Myasthenia gravis. *Focal Points: Clinical Modules for Ophthalmologists.* San Francisco: American Academy of Ophthalmology; 2003, module 4.

Clinical presentation

The hallmarks of MG are fluctuation and fatigability (although these are not invariably present). Clinical signs and symptoms usually worsen in the evening and with use of the eyes and may improve with rest. The most common sign of MG is ptosis, which may be unilateral or bilateral. It tends to vary, with the eyelid being more ptotic in the evening, after exertion, or after prolonged upward gaze. Cogan eyelid twitch, elicited by having the patient saccade from downgaze to upgaze, is a brief overelevation of the upper eyelid. Another eyelid sign is enhancement of ptosis; in keeping with Hering's law of innervation, when the more ptotic eyelid is manually elevated, the less ptotic eyelid inevitably falls (see Chapter 11, Fig 11-4). Fatigue of ptosis should be assessed by asking the patient to sustain upgaze for 1 minute or longer.

Myasthenia gravis frequently causes diplopia. The diplopia may be variable, both during the day and from one day to another. The ocular motility pattern may simulate ocular motor cranial nerve paresis (usually sixth or partial pupil-sparing third nerve palsy), intranuclear ophthalmoplegia, supranuclear motility disturbances (eg, gaze palsies), or isolated muscle "palsy" (eg, isolated inferior rectus). Total ophthalmoplegia can occur. Any changing pattern of diplopia, with or without ptosis, should suggest myasthenia gravis. As with ptosis, fatigue of ophthalmoplegia can also be assessed by having the patient sustain gaze in the direction of paresis. Orbicularis oculi weakness is often present in patients with ocular myasthenia gravis and, if present, can be diagnostically crucial in differentiating MG from other causes of ophthalmoplegia.

Pupillary abnormalities and sensory disturbances are not encountered with myasthenia gravis. Their presence should provoke a search for another diagnosis. Systemic symptoms and signs that are encountered in MG include weakness in the muscles of mastication and in the extensors of the neck, trunk, and limbs; dysphagia; hoarseness; dysarthria; and dyspnea. Dysphagia and dyspnea can be life threatening, and they require prompt treatment. Thyroid eye disease occurs in about 5% of MG patients. Its appearance can occasionally complicate the clinical ophthalmic findings.

Diagnosis

The diagnosis of MG is made clinically by identifying typical signs and symptoms, pharmacologically by overcoming the receptor block through the administration of acetylcholinesterase inhibitors, serologically by demonstrating elevated anti–acetylcholine receptor antibody titers or anti–muscle-specific kinase antibody, and electrophysiologically by electromyography (EMG).

If an obvious abnormality is present on examination, an *edrophonium chloride (Tensilon) test,* a *sleep test,* or an *ice-pack test* can confirm the diagnosis of MG. Testing the patient after exercise or when the patient is tired may facilitate the response. Before performing the Tensilon test, the clinician should warn the patient of the short-lived but often discomforting potential side effects of edrophonium, including diaphoresis, lacrimation, abdominal cramping, nausea, vomiting, and salivation. Atropine sulfate (0.4–0.6 mg) should be immediately available, and some physicians treat with atropine (0.4 mg subcutaneously) before administering the edrophonium.

Although major side effects from edrophonium are rare, bradycardia, respiratory arrest, bronchospasm, syncopal episodes, or cholinergic crisis may be precipitated by IV edrophonium administration. The patient's pulse and blood pressure should be monitored throughout the procedure, which should be performed with the patient seated in a chair that can be reclined and with resuscitation equipment on hand. The ophthalmologist must be prepared to deal with severe side effects by injecting atropine sulfate IV and maintaining vital signs. Tensilon can cause severe bradycardia and bronchiolar constriction; thus, for patients with a history of cardiac or pulmonary disease, consultation with the primary physician before performing the Tensilon test is wise.

In most protocols, 2 mg (0.2 cc) of edrophonium are first injected intravenously through a butterfly needle as a test dose. The patient is observed for 60 seconds. If the symptoms disappear or decrease (for example, the eyelid elevates or motility improves), the test is considered positive and can be discontinued. If no response is elicited, another dose of 4 mg edrophonium is given. If there is still no improvement, the final dose of 4 mg is given. Administering the drug in divided doses seems to cause fewer adverse effects. However, many patients develop minor side effects (fasciculations, warmth, nausea) no matter how it is given. When the ocular symptom is significant (such as complete ptosis), the end point (eyelid elevation) is often dramatic. However, a subtle deficit such as minimal diplopia may require that other means be used to better define the end point. Maddox rod tests with prisms or diplopia fields may be performed before and after edrophonium (see Chapter 8). False-positive responses are rare. A negative test does not exclude the diagnosis of MG, and repeat testing at a later date may be needed.

An alternative to the Tensilon test is the *neostigmine methylsulfate (Prostigmin) test*. This test is particularly useful in children and in adults without ptosis who may require a longer observation period for accurate ocular alignment measurements than that allowed by edrophonium. Adverse reactions are similar to those with edrophonium. The most frequent side effects are salivation, fasciculations, and gastrointestinal discomfort. Intramuscular neostigmine and atropine are injected concurrently. A positive test produces resolution of signs within 30–45 minutes.

The *sleep test* is a safe, simple office test that eliminates the need for Tensilon testing in many patients. After having the baseline deficit documented (measurements of ptosis, motility disturbance), the patient rests quietly with eyes closed for 30 minutes. The measurements are repeated immediately after the patient "wakes up" and opens his or her eyes. Improvement after rest is highly suggestive of MG.

The *ice-pack test* is often helpful for diagnosing patients, but only if they have ptosis. An ice pack is placed over lightly closed eyes for 2 minutes. Improvement of ptosis occurs in most patients with MG (Fig 14-2). One exception is the patient with *complete* myasthenic ptosis; the cooling effect may be insufficient to overcome the severe weakness in these patients.

Golnik K, Pena R, Lee A, Eggenberger ER. An ice test in the diagnosis of myasthenia gravis. *Ophthalmology*. 1999;106(7):1282–1286.

Odel JG, Winterkorn JM, Behrens MM. The sleep test for myasthenia gravis. A safe alternative to Tensilon. *J Clin Neuroophthalmol*. 1991;11(4):288–292.

Seybold ME. The office Tensilon test for ocular myasthenia gravis. *Arch Neurol*. 1986;43(8): 842–843.

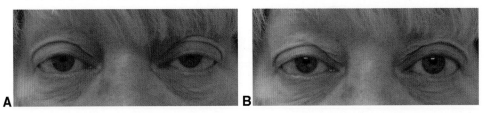

Figure 14-2 **A,** A 57-year-old woman with myasthenia gravis presented with moderate, variable left ptosis. **B,** The left ptosis improved after a 2-minute ice-pack test. *(Courtesy of Karl C. Golnik, MD.)*

Other diagnostic tests for myasthenia gravis include serum assays for anti–acetylcholine receptor antibodies or anti–muscle-specific kinase (MuSK) antibodies and electrophysiologic testing. Three types of *acetylcholine receptor antibody tests* are commercially available. *Binding* antibodies are usually requested, because they are detected in approximately 90% of patients with generalized MG and 50% of patients with ocular MG. *Blocking* antibodies are rarely present (1%) without binding antibodies. *Modulating* antibodies are present as frequently as binding antibodies. Blocking and modulating antibody testing is usually reserved for patients who are negative for the binding antibody and for whom evidence of autoimmune MG is necessary. An assay for anti-MuSK antibodies may detect MG in some patients who do not have anti–acetylcholine receptor antibodies.

Electromyographic repetitive nerve stimulation shows a characteristic decremental response in many patients with systemic myasthenia gravis. Single-fiber electromyography is most sensitive for MG. All myasthenic patients must be investigated radiologically for thymomas, which are visible on a CT scan in 10% of these patients. Malignant thymomas are present in a small percentage of patients. Because there is a high coexistence of myasthenia gravis with other autoimmune disorders, serologic testing should be done for thyroid dysfunction and pernicious anemia.

Evoli A, Tonali PA, Padua L, et al. Clinical correlates of anti-MuSK antibodies in generalized seronegative myasthenia gravis. *Brain.* 2003;126(pt 10):2304–2311.

Weinberg DH, Rizzo JF III, Hayes MT, Kneeland MD, Kelly JJ Jr. Ocular myasthenia gravis: predictive value of single-fiber electromyography. *Muscle Nerve.* 1999;22(9):1222–1227.

Treatment

Medical treatment for myasthenia gravis includes acetylcholinesterase inhibitors, corticosteroids, and other immunosuppressant agents. Thymectomy is the treatment of choice in patients with generalized MG who have thymic enlargement; purely ocular MG is usually not treated by thymectomy. Of course, any patient with a thymoma requires thymectomy. Short-term therapies such as intravenous immunoglobulin or plasmapheresis are occasionally necessary.

Myasthenia gravis is a systemic disease with disastrous potential. Although purely ocular myasthenia gravis does exist, as many as 85% of patients who present with ocular MG will develop systemic MG over the next 2 years. Because MG patients may develop respiratory and other life-threatening manifestations of the disease, it is prudent to manage them in cooperation with a neurologist. If ocular signs remain truly isolated for more than 2 years, the disease is likely to remain clinically ocular; nevertheless, late conversion to generalized MG is possible.

Richman DP, Agius MA. Treatment of autoimmune myasthenia gravis. *Neurology.* 2003;61(12): 1652–1661.

Thyroid Eye Disease

Thyroid eye disease (TED), also known as *thyroid-associated orbitopathy* and *Graves ophthalmopathy,* is an autoimmune inflammatory disorder whose underlying cause remains unknown. The clinical signs, however, are characteristic and may include a combination of eyelid retraction, eyelid lag, proptosis, restrictive extraocular myopathy, and optic neuropathy. The disease activity in the 2 eyes may be remarkably asymmetric. Although typically associated with hyperthyroidism, thyroid eye disease may accompany hypothyroidism or, in rare cases, Hashimoto thyroiditis; in some patients, characteristic eye findings occur without objective evidence of thyroid dysfunction ("euthyroid Graves disease"). The course of the eye disease does not necessarily parallel the activity of the thyroid gland or the treatment of thyroid abnormalities.

Eyelid signs

Upper eyelid retraction is often one of the first clinical signs of TED (Fig 14-3A). When accompanied by eyelid lag (decreased depression of the eyelid when the patient looks downward), it is virtually pathognomonic for thyroid eye disease. Mild asymmetric eyelid retraction is occasionally mistaken for contralateral ptosis. Look at old photographs if there is a question about which eye has the abnormal eyelid position.

Proptosis

The proptosis seen in approximately two thirds of patients with TED tends to be strictly axial without dystopia. Asymmetric amounts of proptosis are not at all uncommon; in some cases, the involvement may appear to be unilateral. Any patient with suspected thyroid eye disease should have exophthalmos measured with a Hertel exophthalmometer. With severe proptosis, incomplete eyelid closure may result in corneal drying accompanied by discomfort and blurred vision.

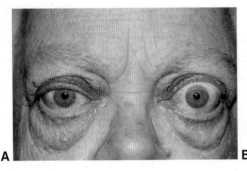
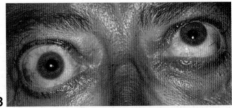
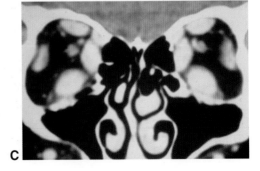

Figure 14-3 Ocular manifestations of Graves disease. **A,** Left eyelid retraction, proptosis, and fat prolapse into upper and lower eyelids. **B,** Marked limitation of elevation of the right eye due to restriction by an enlarged inferior rectus muscle. **C,** Coronal CT scan showing bilateral enlargement of all rectus muscles. *(Part A courtesy of Steven A. Newman, MD; parts B, C courtesy of Karl C. Golnik, MD.)*

Extraocular myopathy

Extraocular muscle enlargement often restricts ocular rotation (Fig 14-3B, C). Most patients with ophthalmoplegia have asymmetric involvement that often leads to ocular misalignment and diplopia. Clinically, the inferior rectus muscle is most commonly involved, followed by the medial rectus and superior rectus. Thus, double vision is most frequently seen when the patient attempts to look up or out, because these affected muscles tether the eye, producing incomplete movement and misalignment. As discussed in Chapter 8, TED is the most common cause of restrictive strabismus.

Compressive optic neuropathy

In 5% of patients with TED, the muscles are sufficiently enlarged at the apex of the orbit to compress the optic nerve (see Chapter 4, Fig 4-23). Optic nerve dysfunction usually results in disturbance of vision (blurred, dim, or dark vision). Signs of optic nerve involvement include decreased Snellen acuity, color vision, and contrast sensitivity, as well as loss of peripheral vision. Visual field defects may include both central scotoma and arcuate visual field defects. Occasionally, the visual field defects are asymptomatic. Asymmetric optic nerve involvement is accompanied by a relative afferent pupillary defect (RAPD), but no RAPD will be seen if the compression is symmetric. Optic disc changes may include disc edema or late optic atrophy. Often, however, the optic disc appears normal (retrobulbar optic neuropathy).

Diagnosis

The diagnosis of TED begins with clinical suspicion. Although abnormal thyroid function tests (quantitative thyroid-stimulating hormone [TSH]), together with the characteristic eye signs, are strong diagnostic indicators, thyroid status may be entirely normal, even in the presence of orbitopathy. Patients with euthyroid TED can present a diagnostic dilemma, but the pathognomonic combination of signs such as eyelid retraction and multiple enlarged extraocular muscles secure the diagnosis in the absence of thyroid dysfunction. In such cases, thyroid-stimulating immunoglobulins, anti–thyroid antibodies, and anti–peroxidase antibodies may help establish the diagnosis. Measurement of the extraocular muscle cross section by B-scan ultrasonography or coronal CT or MRI images is often helpful (see Fig 14-3C). Unlike with inflammatory myositis, the insertions of the muscles into the globe (tendons) are usually spared. The differential diagnosis of proptosis is extensive and includes orbital inflammatory disease, orbital masses, and carotid cavernous fistula. In the setting of eyelid retraction, other conditions to be considered include dorsal midbrain syndrome and aberrant regeneration of the oculomotor nerve.

Treatment

The regulation of thyroid abnormalities is an important part of the care of patients with TED. However, in some studies, treatment with radioactive iodine has been associated with an exacerbation of orbital disease, and some authorities suggest that concurrent corticosteroid therapy may reduce the incidence of this effect. Smoking cigarettes has been identified as a risk factor for the progression of TED, and patients should be encouraged to quit smoking. Corticosteroid therapy (1.0–1.5 mg/kg prednisone) may be effective in decreasing the orbital inflammation, but the side effects of chronic corticosteroid therapy (>2 months) typically outweigh the benefit.

Therapy should be tailored to the signs and symptoms. Many patients require only supportive care for ocular symptoms, such as topical ocular lubricant ointment at night and artificial tears during the day. Taping the eyelids shut at night may also be effective in patients with lagophthalmos. For acute cases with severe corneal problems related to exposure, tarsorrhaphy may be necessary. Recession of the upper and lower eyelid retractors may be done for chronic eyelid retraction. Eyelid surgery should be deferred if orbital surgery or eye muscle surgery is contemplated.

The diplopia associated with TED is related to progressive muscular fibrosis. Although short-term corticosteroid therapy may help control active inflammation, no specific treatment can reverse fibrosis. In acute cases, double vision associated with restrictive strabismus can be eliminated by occlusion. After the deviation becomes stable, eye muscle surgery may achieve realignment. Optical realignment may be possible with spectacle prisms, either prisms ground into the lenses or Fresnel Press-On prisms. Debate exists as to the efficacy of radiotherapy in mild to moderate TED. It is unlikely that radiation will improve proptosis or extraocular motility, although it may help decrease the acute inflammatory symptoms.

The presence of optic nerve dysfunction requires prompt therapeutic intervention. In most cases, a trial of moderately high doses of oral corticosteroids may result in substantial improvement in optic nerve function. Pulsed IV corticosteroids have also been employed. However, the optic nerve dysfunction usually recurs as corticosteroids are tapered. If significant active inflammation is present (conjunctival injection, chemosis), radiation therapy (20 Gy in 2-Gy fractions) may provide some benefit. The definitive treatment is to surgically decompress the optic nerve in the orbital apex. Although any of the 4 orbital walls may be decompressed, removal of the posterior medial wall is usually most effective. This surgical maneuver may be accomplished endoscopically, as an external ethmoidectomy (through the caruncle) or through the maxillary sinus (Caldwell-Luc). When proptosis is the major feature, removal of the orbital floor (by way of an eyelid or conjunctival incision or through the maxillary sinus) and possibly the lateral wall may help decrease the globe prominence. Patients need to be aware that decompression surgery may adversely affect ocular motility and eyelid position. Thus, eyelid and extraocular muscle surgery should be deferred if orbital decompressive surgery is contemplated.

See BCSC Section 7, *Orbit, Eyelids, and Lacrimal System,* for a more extensive discussion of TED; and Section 1, *Update on General Medicine,* for further coverage of thyroid abnormalities.

Bradley EA, Gower EW, Bradley DJ, et al. Orbital radiation for Graves ophthalmopathy: a report from the American Academy of Ophthalmology. *Ophthalmology.* 2008;115(12):398–409.

Sarcoidosis

Sarcoidosis is a multisystem granulomatous disease of unknown origin. Middle-aged adults are most commonly affected; the annual incidence for blacks is about 3 times that for whites (2.4% vs 0.85%). Histopathology shows noncaseating granulomas with accumulation of lymphocytes (CD4). The lungs are involved most frequently, but the eyes, liver, lymph nodes, skin, and musculoskeletal system are commonly affected. Neurologic manifestations occur in 5%–15% of patients and include meningitis, hydrocephalus, parenchymal involvement (hypothalamic most commonly), encephalopathy, seizures, dural venous thrombosis, vasculitis, and peripheral neuropathy.

Gullapalli D, Phillips LH. Neurologic manifestations of sarcoidosis. *Neurol Clin.* 2002;20(1): 59–83.

Rybicki BA, Major M, Popovich J Jr, Maliarik MJ, Iannuzzi MC. Racial differences in sarcoidosis incidence: A 5-year study in a health maintenance organization. *Am J Epidemiol.* 1997;145(3):234–241.

Intraocular manifestations

Iritis, cataract, vitritis, retinal vasculitis ("candlewax drippings"), and chorioretinitis can occur in sarcoidosis. For further discussion of these manifestations, see BCSC Section 9, *Intraocular Inflammation and Uveitis,* and Section 12, *Retina and Vitreous.*

Neuro-ophthalmic manifestations

Facial nerve palsy is the most common cranial neuropathy. Optic neuropathy also occurs and may manifest as either a papillitis or retrobulbar optic neuropathy. Less commonly, a sarcoid granuloma may occur at the optic nerve head (see Chapter 4, Fig 4-13). Infrequently, sarcoid may cause neuroretinitis (disc swelling with a macular star of exudates), optic perineuritis (disc swelling without visual loss or increased intracranial pressure), or papilledema. Visual loss may also occur from chiasmal and retrochiasmal visual pathway involvement. Sarcoidosis can also cause ocular motor cranial nerve palsy, gaze palsy, and a variety of pupillary abnormalities, including tonic pupil, Horner syndrome, and Argyll Robertson pupils.

Frohman LP, Grigorian R, Bielory L. Neuro-ophthalmic manifestations of sarcoidosis: clinical spectrum, evaluation, and management. *J Neuroophthalmol.* 2001;21(2):132–137.

Katz JM, Bruno MK, Winterkorn JM, Nealon N. The pathogenesis and treatment of optic disc swelling in neurosarcoidosis: a unique therapeutic response to infliximab. *Arch Neurol.* 2003;60(3):426–430.

Diagnosis

Although most patients with neurosarcoidosis have abnormalities on MRI scan, about 18% do not. The most common neuroimaging abnormalities found are meningeal and leptomeningeal enhancing lesions. However, none of the abnormalities found on MRI scan are specific. Establishing a definite diagnosis can be difficult. Angiotensin-converting enzyme (ACE) is elevated in 52%–90% of patients if sarcoidosis is active. Gallium scan is not specific, but the combination of positive ACE and gallium scan is reported to be 100% specific and 73% sensitive. Bronchoalveolar lavage, lymph node biopsy, and conjunctival biopsy may be of value. A chest radiograph may direct the biopsy, but CT scan of the chest is indicated if clinical suspicion is high.

Christoforidis GA, Spickler EM, Recio MV, Mehta BM. MR of CNS sarcoidosis: correlation of imaging features to clinical symptoms and response to treatment. *AJNR*.1999;20(4):655–659.

Treatment

Corticosteroids are the mainstay of treatment, but methotrexate, cyclosporine, cyclophosphamide, azathioprine, chlorambucil, and chloroquine are occasionally used in corticosteroid-dependent patients. Radiotherapy has been proposed as an alternate or adjunctive treatment, but the long-term efficacy is not clear.

Inherited Disorders

Numerous inherited disorders result in neuro-ophthalmic signs. Certain myopathies and neurocutaneous syndromes (phakomatoses) are the most common inherited systemic conditions. Inherited optic neuropathies are discussed in Chapter 4 of this volume.

Myopathies

The extraocular muscles are affected by several inherited conditions that result in mitochondrial dysfunction.

Chronic progressive external ophthalmoplegia

Chronic progressive external ophthalmoplegia (CPEO) is an inherited mitochondrial myopathy characterized by slowly progressive, symmetric ophthalmoplegia and ptosis (Fig 14-4). The majority of patients with CPEO have a mitochondrial DNA (mtDNA) point deletion, but nuclear DNA mutations that drive mtDNA mutation can also cause CPEO. Thus, the mode of inheritance can be mitochondrial (maternal), autosomal, or sporadic and the disorder may not be transmissible to the next generation. Patients often present with ptosis and usually do not develop diplopia despite ophthalmoplegia. This

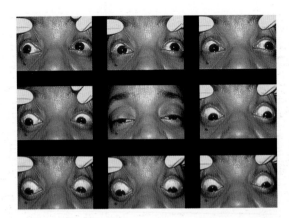

Figure 14-4 A 42-year-old with a 2-year history of progressive ptosis and ophthalmoplegia. Biopsy of the deltoid muscle showed ragged red fibers consistent with CPEO. *(Courtesy of Steven A. Newman, MD.)*

condition is most often mistaken for myasthenia gravis. Family history and old photographs can be helpful in differentiating the 2 conditions. Clinical findings are usually evident by the second decade of life. Systemic symptoms may include generalized muscle weakness. Histopathology of muscle biopsy shows the characteristic "ragged red fibers" (Fig 14-5) and mitochondrial proliferation, and electron microscopic studies show inclusion body abnormalities of the affected mitochondria.

The *Kearns-Sayre syndrome* is also an inherited mitochondrial myopathy. It includes CPEO, pigmentary retinopathy, and cardiac conduction abnormalities, and variably includes cerebellar ataxia, deafness, and elevated CSF protein. Cardiac evaluation is essential to rule out conduction defects.

Bau V, Zierz S. Update on chronic external ophthalmoplegia. *Strabismus.* 2005;13:133–142.

Oculopharyngeal dystrophy

Oculopharyngeal dystrophy is a hereditary condition, usually autosomal dominant, with onset in the fifth and sixth decades of life. The typical presentation is progressive dysphagia followed by proximal muscle weakness and ptosis. Most patients develop CPEO. Pathologic studies show a vacuolar myopathy. The disease is classically seen in patients of French-Canadian ancestry. The only causative mutation described to date is a triplet repeat expansion consisting of 2–7 additional base triplets in a repeat sequence in exon 1 of the polyadenine binding protein nuclear 1 *(PABPN1)* gene.

Myotonic dystrophy

Myotonic dystrophy, a dominantly inherited multisystem disorder, also produces ophthalmoplegia that may mimic CPEO. Two types have been identified: type 1, due to mutation on chromosome 19, and type 2, due to mutation on chromosome 3. Blood tests for these mutations can confirm the diagnosis. Symptoms usually start in late childhood or early adulthood with myotonia that is worsened by excitement, cold, and fatigue. It is easily detected by asking the patient to shake hands; the patient will not be able to quickly

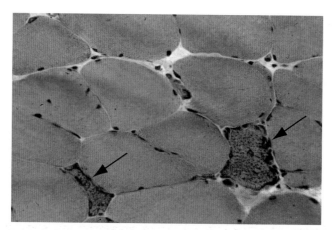

Figure 14-5 Histopathology of muscle in a patient with Kearns-Sayre syndrome shows ragged red fibers *(arrows)*. Specimen stained with modified Gomori trichrome. *(Courtesy of Eric Eggenberger, DO.)*

release his or her grasp. This myopathy is unusual in that it affects distal limb musculature first. Wasting of the temporalis and masseter muscles produces the typical "hatchet face." The myopathic facies, frontal balding, and ptosis cause a distinct and remarkably similar appearance.

Ocular findings include ptosis, pigmentary retinopathy, ophthalmoparesis, and polychromatic lenticular deposits ("Christmas tree" cataracts). The pupils are miotic and respond sluggishly to light. Other features include low intelligence, insulin resistance, hearing loss, cardiomyopathy, cardiac conduction abnormalities, testicular atrophy, and uterine atony. Electromyography provides the definite diagnosis by demonstrating the typical myotonic discharges.

Neurocutaneous Syndromes

Neurocutaneous syndromes, or *phakomatoses,* are disorders characterized by the presence of hamartias and hamartomas involving different organ systems, such as the skin, eyes, CNS, and viscera. Six entities are classically grouped under this category: neurofibromatosis, tuberous sclerosis (Bourneville syndrome), cerebrofacial angiomatosis (Sturge-Weber syndrome), retinal angiomatosis (von Hippel disease), ataxia-telangiectasia (Louis-Bar syndrome), and Wyburn-Mason syndrome (Table 14-2). Klippel-Trénaunay-Weber syndrome has been included by some authors. A syndrome of cavernous hemangioma of the retina associated with CNS angiomas (von Hippel–Lindau) is yet another variant of the phakomatoses. The phakomatoses are discussed at length in BCSC Section 6, *Pediatric Ophthalmology and Strabismus.* In this chapter, we emphasize the neuro-ophthalmic features of these conditions.

These disorders are characterized by tumors formed from normal tissue elements: hamartomas and choristomas. A *hamartoma* is composed of elements normally found at the involved site. The glial retinal tumors of tuberous sclerosis are a type of hamartoma. *Hamartias* are similar to hamartomas histopathologically, but they do not grow. Hamartomas and hamartias differ from true neoplasms in that they seem to be anomalies of tissue formation rather than cellular proliferations arising in previously normal tissue. They lack the capability for limitless proliferation exhibited by true neoplasms. *Choristomas* are tumorlike growths composed of tissue not normally present at the site of growth. All phakomatous lesions are hamartomas, hamartias, or choristomas.

Neurofibromatosis

The 2 most common forms of neurofibromatosis are *von Recklinghausen neurofibromatosis (NF1)* and *bilateral acoustic neurofibromatosis (NF2).* NF1 is the more common form of the disease. It is inherited in an autosomal dominant manner and has been linked to chromosome 17. General features include multiple neurofibromas, pigmented skin lesions, osseous malformations, and associated tumors. The disease is defined by the presence of multiple cutaneous pigmented macules (café-au-lait spots), neurofibromas, and iris (Lisch) nodules (Fig 14-6). Mild cases may show only iris nodules associated with café-au-lait spots.

Neurofibromas are histologically benign and may take the form of either fibroma molluscum or plexiform neurofibromas. They may involve the eyelid and face, occasionally

Table 14-2 The Phakomatoses

Condition	Description	Associated Ocular Conditions	Associated Conditions and Risks	Transmission
von Hippel–Lindau disease (retinal angiomatosis)	Retinal angioma supplied by dilated tortuous arteriole and venule; may be multiple	Retinal exudates, hemorrhages, retinal detachment, glaucoma	Cerebellar capillary hemangiomas, malformation of visceral organs	Autosomal dominant, chromosome 3p25
Sturge-Weber syndrome (encephalofacial angiomatosis)	Capillary hamartia (nevus flammeus) of skin, conjunctiva, episclera, and/or uveal tract, and of meninges	Glaucoma (especially with upper eyelid involvement by nevus flammeus)	Diffuse meningeal hemangioma with seizure disorder, hemiplegia or hemianopia, or mental retardation	Sporadic
Neurofibromatosis type 1 (von Recklinghausen disease)	Occasionally congenital, widespread hamartomas of peripheral nerves and tissue of neural crest derivation	Neurofibromas of eyelid and orbit, uveal melanocytic nevi, retinal glial hamartomas, congenital glaucoma, optic nerve glioma, absence of greater wing of sphenoid with pulsating exophthalmos	Similar hamartomas of CNS, peripheral and cranial nerves, gastrointestinal tract; malignant transformation possible	Autosomal dominant NF1: chromosome 17q11.2
Neurofibromatosis type 2	Bilateral acoustic schwannomas	Posterior subcapsular cataract, combined retinal-RPE hamartoma	Meningioma, glioma, neurofibroma	Autosomal dominant 22q11.2
Tuberous sclerosis (Bourneville syndrome)	Mental deficiency, seizures, and adenoma sebaceum	Angiofibromas of eyelid skin; glial hamartomas of retina and optic disc	Adenoma sebaceum (angiofibromas), cerebral glial hamartomas	Autosomal dominant, chromosome 9q34
Ataxia-telangiectasia (Louis-Bar syndrome)	Progressive cerebellar ataxia, ocular and cutaneous telangiectasis, pulmonary infections	Conjunctival telangiectasis, anomalous ocular movements, and nystagmus	Dysarthria, coarse hair and skin, immunologic deficiency, and mental and growth retardation	Autosomal recessive, chromosome 11q22
Wyburn-Mason syndrome (racemose angioma)	Retinal and midbrain arteriovenous (AV) communication (aneurysms and angiomas) and facial nevi	AV communication (racemose angioma) of retina, with vision loss depending on location of AV communication	AV aneurysm at midbrain; intracranial calcification	Sporadic

Modified from Isselbacher KJ, Braunwald E, Wilson JD, eds. *Harrison's Principles of Internal Medicine.* 13th ed. New York: McGraw-Hill; 1994:2207–2210.

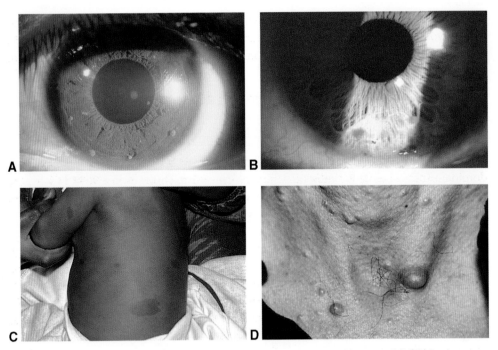

Figure 14-6 The most common ocular finding in neurofibromatosis type 1 (NF1) is the presence of iris Lisch nodules. These are often light-colored in a patient with dark irides **(A)** but may be relatively darker in patients with light irides **(B)**. The diagnosis is often suggested by cutaneous findings, including café-au-lait spots **(C)** or skin neurofibromas **(D)**. *(Part A courtesy of Mark J. Greenwald, MD; parts B–D courtesy of Steven A. Newman, MD.)*

causing marked deformities (see Chapter 11, Fig 11-1). Lisch nodules are pigmented iris hamartomas present in 94%–97% of patients with NF1 who are over the age of 6 years. These nodules do not become symptomatic but may prove helpful in establishing the diagnosis, especially when discovered in asymptomatic relatives.

Other ocular involvement in neurofibromatosis includes congenital glaucoma and retinal astrocytomas. Osseous defects may involve the orbit, commonly the greater wing of the sphenoid, with associated orbital encephalocele. Vertebral and long-bone defects are seen as well. Multiple tumors of the brain, spinal cord, and meninges, as well as of the cranial, peripheral, and sympathetic nerves, may be encountered in these patients. Optic nerve or chiasmal gliomas in children are frequently associated with neurofibromatosis. These lesions cause proptosis and visual loss but are rarely life threatening. Treatment for these lesions is controversial. Additional neoplastic associations include pheochromocytoma and meningioma. See Chapter 4 for a discussion of gliomas and meningiomas of the optic nerve.

Savar A, Cestari DM. Neurofibromatosis type 1: genetics and clinical manifestations. *Semin Ophthalmol.* 2008;23(1):45–51.

Bilateral acoustic neurofibromatosis (NF2) is less common than NF1. Also transmitted as an autosomal dominant trait, NF2 is linked to chromosome 22. Only about 60% of patients with NF2 have café-au-lait spots or peripheral neurofibromas, and Lisch nodules are not a feature of this disease. Bilateral acoustic neuromas usually present symptomatically in young adulthood. Other CNS tumors may occur but not as frequently as in NF1. Other ocular findings may include combined retinal–RPE hamartomas and posterior subcapsular cataracts.

Ferner RE. Neurofibromatosis 1 and neurofibromatosis 2: a twenty-first century perspective. *Lancet Neurol.* 2007;6(4):340–351.

Tuberous sclerosis

Also known as *Bourneville syndrome, tuberous sclerosis* is transmitted as an autosomal dominant trait. There are 2 tuberous sclerosis genes: 1 at chromosome 9q34 *(TSC1)*, the other at 16p13.3 *(TSC2)*. The gene products tuberin (TSC1) and hamartin (TSC2) form a heterodimer that inhibits cell growth and proliferation. The exact mechanism by which mutations in these genes result in tuberous sclerosis is unclear. It has classically been characterized by the triad of adenoma sebaceum, mental deficiency, and epilepsy, although presentation shows great variability. Most patients have seizures, but many have normal mentation. The so-called *sebaceous adenomas* are actually hamartomatous angiofibromas that commonly appear in a butterfly distribution over the nose and cheeks (Fig 14-7). Other skin lesions include periungual fibromas, café-au-lait spots, and shagreen patches (large, leatherlike, hyperpigmented, raised patches that are typically located on the trunk). The *ash-leaf spot,* a leaf-shaped area of skin depigmentation that fluoresces under a Wood lamp, is considered pathognomonic for tuberous sclerosis.

Calcified astrocytic hamartomas *(brain stones)* are frequently evident on plain skull x-ray and CT scan. Other visceral involvement that has been described includes cardiac rhabdomyomas, renal cysts, and angiomyolipomas. The characteristic ocular finding is an astrocytic hamartoma of the retina or optic disc.

Cerebrofacial (encephalotrigeminal) angiomatosis

The inheritance pattern of *cerebrofacial angiomatosis,* or *Sturge-Weber syndrome,* is sporadic. The characteristic skin lesion in Sturge-Weber syndrome is *nevus flammeus (port-wine stain),* an angioma involving skin and subcutaneous tissues that usually follow the distribution of CN V (the trigeminal nerve) (Fig 14-8). This lesion is present from birth, usually unilateral, and commonly associated with a parieto-occipital leptomeningeal hemangioma ipsilateral to the facial vascular hamartoma. Calcification of the cortex underlying the hemangioma can be seen radiographically. A CT scan is best for showing the calcification, but MRI will demonstrate leptomeningeal enhancement typical of this condition. Seizures are a major problem in these patients.

Unilateral congenital open-angle glaucoma is seen in 30%–70% of patients with Sturge-Weber syndrome and is usually associated with an angioma of the upper eyelid. Onset of glaucoma may occur at any time; tonometry should be performed early and repeated periodically. Heterochromia iridis has been described. The characteristic fundus lesion is a choroidal hemangioma, a solitary, yellow-orange, moderately elevated mass seen in the posterior pole of up to 50% of these patients. More diffuse uveal involvement can give the fundus a confluent "tomato catsup" appearance (see Fig 14-8). Exudative retinal detachments may occur in association with these lesions.

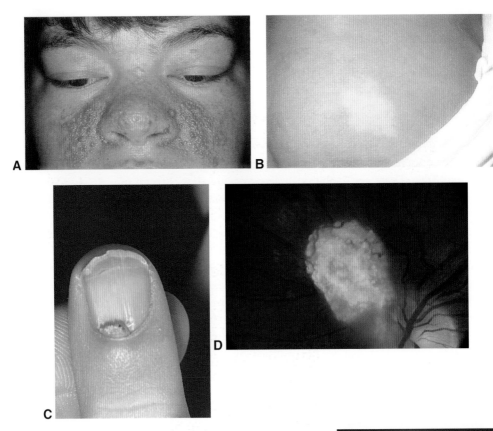

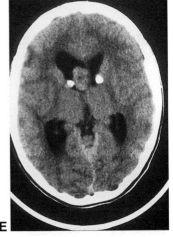

Figure 14-7 A, The hallmark of tuberous sclerosis is adenoma sebaceum involving the cheek, particularly present in the area of the nasolabial fold. Other classic skin findings include the presence of an ash-leaf spot **(B),** best seen with ultraviolet light, and subungual lesions **(C). D,** Ophthalmic findings include the presence of astrocytic hamartomas on funduscopic examination. **E,** Intracranial hamartomas often line the subependymal surface. They frequently calcify, becoming obvious on CT scan. *(Parts A, B courtesy of Mark J. Greenwald, MD; parts C, E courtesy of Steven A. Newman, MD; part D reprinted from Kline LB, Foroozan R, eds. Optic Nerve Disorders. 2nd ed. Ophthalmology Monograph 10. New York: Oxford University Press, in cooperation with the American Academy of Ophthalmology; 2007:164.)*

Klippel-Trénaunay-Weber syndrome may be a variant of cerebrofacial angiomatosis. Nonocular findings include cutaneous nevus flammeus and hemangiomas, varicosities, associated hemihypertrophy of the limbs, and intracranial angiomas. The cutaneous lesions and vascular anomalies are sometimes amenable to laser treatment. Ocular involvement, usually congenital glaucoma and conjunctival telangiectasia, is uncommon.

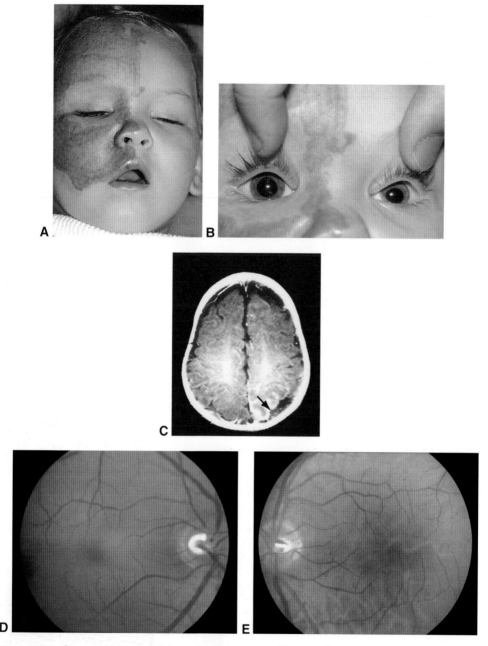

Figure 14-8 Sturge-Weber syndrome. **A,** This 1-year-old was referred for a port-wine stain involving the V_1 and V_2 distributions on the right side, a classic finding in Sturge-Weber syndrome. These patients often have congenital glaucoma. **B,** In an infant with congenital glaucoma, the globe may enlarge significantly (buphthalmos). **C,** Associated cortical vascular malformations following the gyral pattern may also occur *(arrow).* They may be seen on MRI scan. Patients may also have diffuse choroidal hemangiomas causing increased hyperemia and redness of the choroid. **D,** Choroidal hemangioma. **E,** Contralateral normal eye. *(Parts A, B courtesy of Steven A. Newman, MD; part C courtesy of Mark J. Greenwald, MD; parts D, E courtesy of James J. Augsburger, MD.)*

Retinal angiomatosis

Also known as *von Hippel disease, retinal angiomatosis* is transmitted by autosomal dominant inheritance. The disease may also occur sporadically. The characteristic ocular lesion is a retinal capillary angioma: a globular, smooth-surfaced, pink retinal tumor fed by a single dilated, tortuous retinal artery and drained by a similar-appearing vein (Fig 14-9). These lesions are often multiple and are bilateral in 50% of cases. Serous exudation can cause retinal detachment.

Cerebellar hemangioblastomas are seen in approximately 25% of patients with retinal angiomatosis, and this association is known as *von Hippel–Lindau disease.* Hemangioblastomas may also occur in the brainstem or spinal cord and may be associated with syrinxes in these regions.

Patients with cerebellar angiomas may also have renal, pancreatic, hepatic, or epididymal cysts and pheochromocytomas or renal cell carcinoma. Several of these multisystem manifestations are potentially lethal. Early detection of the retinal abnormality by the ophthalmologist should prompt referral of the patient for a thorough systemic investigation.

Ataxia-telangiectasia

Ataxia-telangiectasia, or *Louis-Bar syndrome,* is considered the most common cause of progressive ataxia in early childhood. It is characterized by progressive cerebellar ataxia and oculocutaneous telangiectasia. Thymic hypoplasia, with defective T-cell function and immunoglobulin deficiency, predisposes patients to recurrent sinopulmonary infections. The genetic abnormality is localized to chromosome 11, and the inheritance pattern is generally autosomal recessive. This genetic defect results in inactivation of a critical protein kinase that regulates the response to DNA double-strand breaks. Clinical manifestations of ataxia-telangiectasia occur because of this resultant defective DNA damage signaling. Conjunctival telangiectasia is almost always seen, especially as the child grows older (Fig 14-10). Ocular motility deficits are the classic eye findings—specifically, horizontal and vertical supranuclear gaze palsies. At first, the patient shows an inability to initiate saccades, which may be associated with head thrusting and abnormalities of the fast phase of optokinetic nystagmus. Pursuit becomes impaired, and eventually the disease leads to total ophthalmoplegia. However, oculocephalic responses remain intact. Patients who do not succumb to recurrent infections have a high incidence of malignancy.

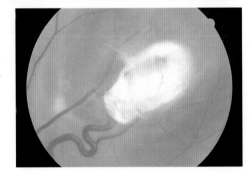

Figure 14-9 Patients with von Hippel syndrome often develop angiomas of the retina. *(Courtesy of Steven A. Newman, MD.)*

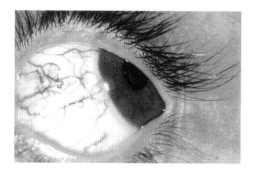

Figure 14-10 Abnormally dilated and tortuous conjunctival vessels in the left eye of a child with ataxia-telangiectasia. *(Courtesy of Mark J. Greenwald, MD.)*

Wyburn-Mason syndrome

Wyburn-Mason syndrome refers to the association of an intracranial arteriovenous malformation (AVM) with an AVM of the ipsilateral retina *(racemose angioma)* (Fig 14-11). The inheritance pattern is sporadic. The AVM consists of direct communications between the arteries and the veins without an intervening capillary bed. The vessels are usually fully developed and may involve any part of the posterior pole. They are usually increased in number, size, and tortuosity. Spontaneous hemorrhage from these lesions may cause decreased vision. Because of the association between retinal and intracranial AVMs, an MRI scan of the brain should be obtained in patients with a retinal AVM. Associated AVMs may be seen in the midbrain, basofrontal region, or posterior fossa, and they may be associated with spontaneous intracranial hemorrhage or convulsions. AVMs can also involve the maxilla, pterygoid fossa, or mandible. Orbital AVMs may be associated with mild proptosis, conjunctival vascular dilation, or a bruit.

Selected Neuro-Ophthalmic Disorders Associated With Pregnancy

Several neuro-ophthalmic abnormalities occur with greater frequency or can be exacerbated during pregnancy or the postpartum period. These include cerebral venous thrombosis, pituitary apoplexy (Sheehan syndrome), posterior reversible encephalopathy

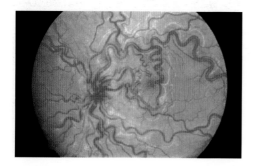

Figure 14-11 Racemose angioma of the retina in Wyburn-Mason syndrome. *(Courtesy of Mark J. Greenwald, MD.)*

syndrome (PRES), and lymphocytic hypophysitis. Venous sinus thrombosis is discussed later in this chapter under cerebrovascular disorders, and pituitary apoplexy is discussed in Chapter 4 (see Chapter 4, Fig 4-31). In addition, preexisting pituitary macroadenomas, meningiomas, and orbital and choroidal hemangiomas can undergo expansion during pregnancy.

Sheth BP, Mieler WF. Ocular complications of pregnancy. *Curr Opin Ophthalmol.* 2001;12(6): 455–463.

Posterior Reversible Encephalopathy Syndrome

Posterior reversible encephalopathy syndrome (PRES) is characterized by headache, altered mental status, seizures, and visual disturbances (transient visual loss, scotomata, photopsias, dimming of vision); MRI shows edema involving the white matter of the cerebral posterior regions, especially parieto-occipital lobes, but frontal and temporal lobes may be involved (Fig 14-12). Causes include acute hypertension, preeclampsia/eclampsia, and immunosuppressive agents (eg, cyclosporine, tacrolimus). The abnormalities seen on neuroimaging are reversible, and the visual prognosis is usually excellent.

Finocchi V, Bozzao A, Bonamini M, et al. Magnetic resonance imaging in posterior reversible encephalopathy syndrome: report of three cases and review of literature. *Arch Gynecol Obstet.* 2005;271(1):79–85.

Lymphocytic Hypophysitis

Lymphocytic hypophysitis is a rare neuroendocrine disorder characterized by autoimmune inflammation of the pituitary gland, with various degrees of pituitary dysfunction, including permanent hypopituitarism. The histopathology consists of an initial monoclonal lymphocytic infiltrate, which can heal with minimal sequelae or progress to fibrosis. Clinical presentation may mimic pituitary tumor, including chiasmal visual field defects and acute-onset diabetes insipidus. Imaging characteristics and endocrine testing are not

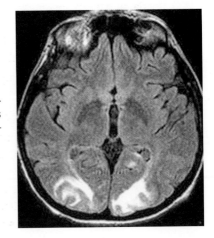

Figure 14-12 Axial FLAIR MRI scan showing reversible bilateral posterior circulation signal abnormalities in a patient with transient cortical blindness and preeclampsia. *(Courtesy of Lanning B. Kline, MD.)*

specific. The diagnosis should be considered if these symptoms and signs occur during pregnancy, but surgical treatment is required if vision is compromised.

Cerebrovascular Disorders

Comprehensive discussion of cerebrovascular disorders is beyond the scope of this text. An overview of common conditions causing neuro-ophthalmic signs and symptoms is given in the following sections.

Transient Visual Loss

Transient neurologic or ophthalmic symptoms in middle-aged or elderly patients suggest a vascular origin. Localization of the symptoms and signs determines whether they result from ischemia in the vertebrobasilar or the carotid artery territory. Although recurrent cerebrovascular ischemia is a concern, the major cause of death in these patients is coronary artery disease. Thus, efforts to control risk factors for cardiovascular disease, such as hypertension, diabetes mellitus, and hyperlipidemias, accompanied by cessation of smoking, should be considered before diagnostic and therapeutic efforts are directed exclusively at the cerebrovascular circulation. Carotid system disorders whose main symptom is transient visual loss are discussed in Chapter 5.

Vertebrobasilar System Disease

The vertebrobasilar arterial system (posterior circulation) is composed of the vertebral, basilar, and posterior cerebral arteries. These blood vessels supply the occipital cortex, brainstem, and cerebellum.

Clinical presentation

Patients with vertebrobasilar insufficiency often present to the ophthalmologist first, because ocular motor and visual symptoms are prominent (Fig 14-13). Nonophthalmic symptoms of *transient ischemic attacks (TIAs)* in the vertebrobasilar system include

- ataxia, imbalance, or staggering
- vertigo combined with other brainstem symptoms such as deafness or vomiting
- transient dysarthria and dysphagia
- hemiparesis, hemiplegia, and hemisensory disturbances
- drop attacks (patient suddenly falls to the ground with no warning and no loss of consciousness)

Bilateral blurring or dimming of vision occurs almost as frequently as vertigo. The patient may complain of the sudden bilateral graying or whiting out of vision. The attacks of dimming last seconds to minutes and may be accompanied by flickering or flashing stars. Photopsias may occur, closely mimicking the scintillating scotomata of migraine. These attacks are frequently repetitive and may occur alone or in combination with the other transient symptoms of vertebrobasilar insufficiency just mentioned. Migraine can produce similar symptoms, with or without an associated headache, and is discussed in Chapter 12.

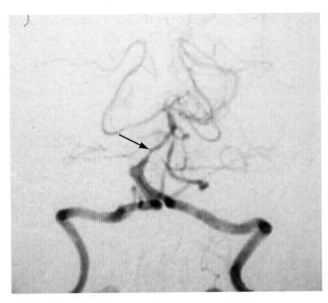

Figure 14-13 A 58-year-old woman had a sudden onset of diplopia and vertigo. On examination, she was found to have a right third nerve palsy and ataxia. Symptoms and signs resolved over 24 hours. The cerebral angiogram showed marked stenosis of the basilar artery *(arrow)*. *(Courtesy of Karl C. Golnik, MD.)*

Homonymous visual field changes without other neurologic symptoms suggest involvement of the posterior circulation. Highly congruous homonymous visual field defects without other systemic symptoms are typical of occipital lobe infarcts. Patients complaining of reading difficulties without obvious cause should have a careful visual field and Amsler grid examination in search of centrally located congruous homonymous visual field defects.

Levin LA. Topical diagnosis of chiasmal and retrochiasmal disorders. In: Miller NR, Newman NJ, eds. *Walsh and Hoyt's Clinical Neuro-Ophthalmology.* 6th ed. Vol 1. Philadelphia: Lippincott Williams & Wilkins; 2005:539–554.

The visual manifestations of cortical infarction are detailed in Chapter 4. Cerebral and cortical blindness, caused by bilateral occipital lobe lesions, is characterized by amaurosis, normally reactive pupils, and an unremarkable fundus appearance. Frequently, patients with cerebral blindness will deny their blindness (Anton syndrome) (see Chapter 6).

Ocular motor disturbances are common with vertebrobasilar insufficiency, and diplopia is a frequent complaint. Examination may reveal horizontal or vertical gaze palsies, internuclear ophthalmoplegia, skew deviation, ocular motor cranial nerve palsies, or nystagmus. An ipsilateral, central Horner syndrome may be present with pontine or medullary infarcts (Wallenberg syndrome).

Etiologies of posterior circulation ischemia

The most frequent causes of vertebrobasilar TIAs and stroke are atheromatous occlusion, hypertensive vascular disease (lacunar infarction), microembolization (either from the vertebrobasilar system or from the heart), fluctuations in cardiac output, and arterial dissection. The following have all been associated with symptoms and signs of vertebrobasilar ischemia: polycythemia, hypercoagulable states, congenital aplasia or hypoplasia of a vertebral or posterior communicating artery, anemia, and vasospasm. Mechanical factors such as cervical spondylosis and chiropractic manipulation of the cervical spine have also been implicated in vertebrobasilar occlusions resulting in severe neurologic deficits. A less common cause of vertebrobasilar dysfunction is a reversal of blood flow in the vertebral artery *(subclavian steal)*, caused by a proximal occlusion of the subclavian artery that produces an unusual alteration in the direction of flow in the ipsilateral vertebral artery. Lowered pressure in the distal segment of the subclavian artery can siphon, or steal, blood from the vertebral artery and produce fluctuating symptoms of vertebrobasilar artery insufficiency.

Clinical and laboratory evaluation

The evaluation of posterior circulation ischemia is similar to the medical workup for carotid system disease. Neuroimaging should be performed on all patients with homonymous visual field defects and other signs of brainstem or cerebellar dysfunction. Magnetic resonance angiography (MRA) and computed tomographic arteriography (CTA) are the best noninvasive methods of evaluating the posterior circulation. Carotid Doppler imaging is not sufficient for evaluating suspected posterior circulation symptoms. Sometimes conventional angiography is necessary to visualize the aortic arch, the configuration of the vertebrobasilar vessels, and the extent of filling from the anterior circulation through the circle of Willis.

The examiner is much less likely to find a treatable structural vascular abnormality with posterior circulation ischemia than with carotid system disease. The evaluation of these patients generally emphasizes a search for underlying cardiac or systemic disorders, including hypercholesterolemia, hypertension, diabetes mellitus, and postural hypotension.

Khan S, Cloud GC, Karry S, Markus HS. Imaging of vertebral artery stenosis: a systematic review. *J Neurol Neurosurg Psychiatry.* 2007;78(11):1218–1225.

Treatment

Most patients with vertebrobasilar TIAs are treated medically with antiplatelet therapy or anticoagulants. Intravascular stent placement can be used in select patients with either carotid or vertebrobasilar stenosis.

Cerebral Aneurysms

Cerebral aneurysms are localized dilations of the vessel wall. They are present in approximately 5% of the population but rarely become symptomatic before age 20. They may be an isolated finding and are commonly associated with hypertension. Less common predisposing conditions include arteriovenous malformations, coarctation of the aorta, polycystic kidney disease, and connective tissue diseases (such as fibromuscular dysplasia, Marfan syndrome, and Ehlers-Danlos syndrome). A familial occurrence is possible, and tobacco use has been shown to be a risk factor.

Figure 14-14 shows possible locations for cerebral aneurysms. The most common type of intracranial aneurysm is the saccular, or "berry," aneurysm that arises at arterial bifurcations. Of these aneurysms, 90% are supratentorial and 10% are infratentorial. Aneurysms arising from the internal carotid artery and basilar artery may produce neuro-ophthalmic manifestations. In general, those >10 mm in size are most likely to rupture. Because high morbidity and mortality result from aneurysm rupture, early detection and surgical intervention can be life-saving. Aneurysms are termed "giant aneurysms" if they are ≥25 mm.

Clinical presentation

Unruptured aneurysms, particularly giant aneurysms, may cause progressive neurologic dysfunction because of their mass effect. An ophthalmic artery aneurysm may cause a

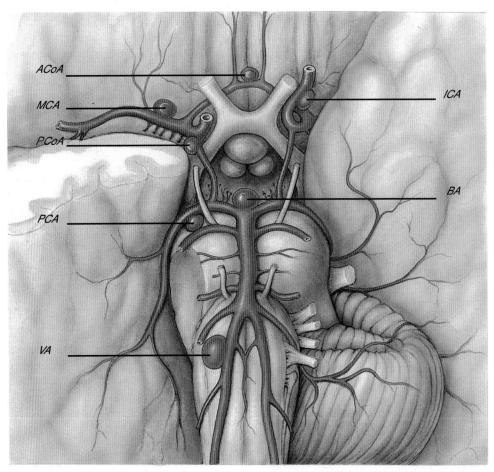

Figure 14-14 Drawing shows locations for intracranial aneurysms arising from cerebral blood vessels. *ACoA* = anterior communicating artery, *BA* = basilar artery, *ICA* = internal carotid artery, *MCA* = middle cerebral artery, *PCA* = posterior cerebral artery, *PCoA* = posterior communicating artery, *VA* = vertebral artery. *(Reprinted from Kline LB, Foroozan R, eds.* Optic Nerve Disorders. *2nd ed. Ophthalmology Monograph 10. New York: Oxford University Press, in cooperation with the American Academy of Ophthalmology; 2007:131.)*

progressive unilateral optic neuropathy and ipsilateral periocular pain. Anterior communicating artery aneurysms produce visual loss by compressing the optic chiasm or optic tract. Aneurysms at the junction of the internal carotid and posterior communicating arteries produce an ipsilateral third nerve palsy. Typically, pain occurs around the ipsilateral eye or the forehead. The combination of headache and a partial or complete third nerve palsy with pupil involvement should raise suspicion of an aneurysm, particularly in persons under age 50. However, pain may be absent with unruptured aneurysms. TIAs, cerebral infarction, and seizures may occur because of flow phenomena or distal embolization.

Intracavernous carotid aneurysms typically produce a cavernous sinus syndrome. These aneurysms often are a fusiform enlargement (dolichoectasia) and not berry type. Cranial nerves III, IV, and VI and the ophthalmic branch of CN V are involved, singly or in combination. Because they are confined by the walls of the cavernous sinus, these aneurysms typically do not rupture but cause progressive neurologic dysfunction. Aneurysms in this location often produce facial pain and should be considered in the differential diagnosis of painful ophthalmoplegia.

A ruptured aneurysm is a neurosurgical emergency. Patients develop symptoms and signs of subarachnoid or intraparenchymal hemorrhage. The headache of a ruptured aneurysm is often described as "the worst of my life" and may be localized or generalized. Nausea, vomiting, and neck stiffness signify meningeal irritation from subarachnoid blood. In rare cases, fever may be present. Elevated intracranial pressure may produce papilledema and sixth nerve palsies. Patients may be disoriented, lethargic, or comatose. Altered mental status is a poor prognostic sign.

Ocular hemorrhage may accompany subarachnoid hemorrhage. Intraretinal, preretinal, subhyaloid, vitreous, subconjunctival, orbital, or optic nerve sheath hemorrhage may be present. Ocular hemorrhages are most likely produced when intracranial pressure in the optic nerve sheath exceeds ocular venous pressure, reducing ophthalmic venous drainage and causing venous rupture. The combination of vitreous and subarachnoid hemorrhage is called *Terson syndrome* (Fig 14-15). Many patients recall symptoms of a "sentinel bleed" before the major rupture. Transient or mild neurologic symptoms with headache are most commonly described.

Laboratory investigation

The definitive diagnostic test for suspected aneurysm is a cerebral arteriogram. A 4-vessel study of both carotid and vertebral arteries is imperative, because 10% of patients have

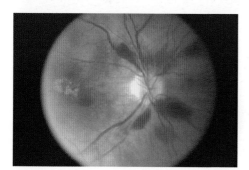

Figure 14-15 A ruptured intracranial aneurysm may produce hemorrhage within the retina, preretinal space, or vitreous (Terson syndrome). *(Courtesy of Steven A. Newman, MD.)*

multiple aneurysms. If the aneurysm has ruptured, vasospasm may prevent its accurate visualization. Likewise, a thrombosed aneurysm might not be visible on arteriography, because its lumen will not fill.

MRI scan demonstrates most aneurysms >5 mm in size. High-quality MRA can detect aneurysms as small as 3 mm. MRA is useful as a screening test for unruptured aneurysms; it is less expensive than angiography and has no associated morbidity (Fig 14-16). CTA can also detect relatively small aneurysms. However, if there is a high level of suspicion for aneurysm, a negative MRA or CTA does not obviate the need for conventional cerebral arteriography.

Computed tomography scanning is useful acutely after aneurysm rupture to detect the presence of intraparenchymal and subarachnoid blood. An enhanced CT scan can demonstrate large aneurysms, but CT scanning is not an acceptable screening test for unruptured aneurysms. If subarachnoid hemorrhage is suspected and the CT scan is negative, lumbar puncture is indicated to confirm the presence of subarachnoid blood. However, a lumbar puncture should not be attempted in the face of midline shift or evidence of cerebral (uncal) herniation.

Prognosis

Modern technology (MRA, CTA) has dramatically increased the detection of unruptured intracranial aneurysms. Their risk of rupture is related to size; aneurysms <10 mm have a rupture rate of <0.05% per year. Giant aneurysms (≥25 mm) have a 6% rupture rate in the first year. Once an aneurysm has ruptured, the morbidity and mortality rate is significant.

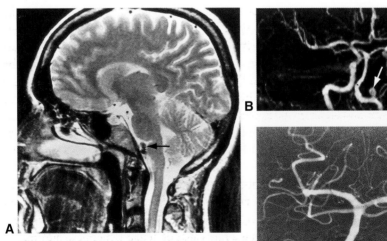
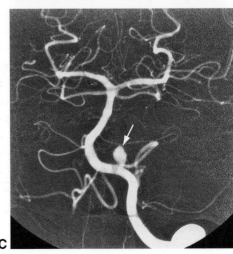

Figure 14-16 **A,** Sagittal view of the brain on a T2-weighted MRI scan shows a low-intensity signal in the subarachnoid space anterior to the medulla *(arrow)*, contiguous with the vertebral artery inferiorly, consistent with flowing blood. **B,** MRA shows a vertebral artery aneurysm *(arrow)*. **C,** The same aneurysm, as demonstrated by conventional arteriography *(arrow)*. *(Courtesy of Leo Hochhauser, MD.)*

The proportion of patients who die at the time of rupture is 30%. If untreated, another 33% die within 6 months of rupture, and 15% more die within 10 years. Many of those who survive suffer severe neurologic deficits.

Unruptured intracranial aneurysms: risk of rupture and risks of surgical intervention. International Study of Unruptured Intracranial Aneurysms Investigators. *N Engl J Med.* 1998; 339(24):1725–1733.

Treatment

Treatment of symptomatic aneurysms prior to rupture is ideal. Supportive treatment to stabilize the patient includes efforts to lower intracranial pressure with hyperventilation or mannitol, treatment of cerebral vasospasm with calcium channel blockers and blood volume expansion, and control of blood pressure.

The definitive treatment is surgical clipping of the aneurysm, but intravascular techniques such as as coil embolization or stent placement are replacing clipping as the preferred treatment of many aneurysms, depending on size, location, and aneurysm anatomy. When aneurysm clipping is technically impossible, ligation of the feeding artery or carotid artery is sometimes necessary.

Arterial Dissection

Dissections may develop in the internal carotid artery or in any of its branches, as well as in the vertebral and basilar arteries. Dissection may arise either extracranially or intracranially and can be traumatic or spontaneous.

Clinical presentation

The clinical features of dissection are variable. Patients may suffer stroke, which typically occurs within the first 30 days of the dissection. The most common presentation of internal carotid artery dissection is headache with ipsilateral ophthalmic signs and contralateral neurologic deficits (see Chapter 10, Fig 10-4). The headache is usually located on the ipsilateral forehead, around the orbit, or in the neck. A bruit may be present. Sometimes symptoms are delayed for weeks or months following trauma. Transient or permanent neurologic symptoms and signs include amaurosis fugax, acute stroke, monocular blindness, and ipsilateral Horner syndrome (see Fig 10-4). If the dissection extends to the intracranial carotid segment, cranial neuropathies can occur, producing diplopia, dysgeusia, tongue paralysis, or facial numbness.

The visual loss associated with carotid dissection may be a result of embolic occlusion of the ophthalmic artery, central retinal artery, short posterior ciliary arteries, or retinal branch arteries. Alternatively, ophthalmic artery occlusion may be caused by the dissection itself. Reduced blood flow from carotid dissection is a rare cause of ocular ischemic syndrome.

Forty percent of dissections affect the vertebral and basilar arteries. General features of these dissections are headache, neck pain, and signs of brainstem and cerebellar dysfunction (Fig 14-17). Ocular motor cranial nerve palsies are commonly seen, and patients may progress to quadriplegia, coma, and death.

Biousse V, Touboul PJ, D'Anglejan-Chatillon J, Lévy C, Schaison M, Bousser MG. Ophthalmologic manifestations of internal carotid artery dissection. *Am J Ophthalmol.* 1998;126(4): 565–577.

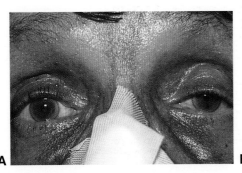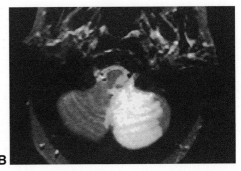

A   B

Figure 14-17 This 75-year-old woman with a 10-year history of hypertension presented with acute onset of left facial pain, double vision, and dizziness. On examination, her visual acuity was 20/30 OU, but she had 2 mm of left ptosis **(A)** and anisocoria, with the left pupil smaller and dilating poorly. Right-beating nystagmus in primary position increased on right gaze and was associated with a torsional component. **B,** MRI scan revealed an infarct of the territory supplied by the left posterior inferior cerebellar artery, producing her central Horner syndrome plus skew deviation and nystagmus (Wallenberg syndrome). *(Courtesy of Steven A. Newman, MD.)*

Diagnosis

An MRI scan is the diagnostic test of choice for extracranial carotid artery dissection. Routine MRI scanning shows a false lumen or an area of clotting in the cervical portion of the carotid artery (crescent moon sign; see Fig 10-4) and may identify areas of brain infarction. Selective arteriography is useful for defining extracranial and intracranial dissection and for visualizing the vertebrobasilar system. Carotid Doppler imaging is not sufficient if dissection is suspected.

Treatment

The treatment of arterial dissection is controversial, depending on the extent and location of the dissection and the patient's overall condition. Extracranial carotid dissections involving the proximal portion of the internal carotid artery may be treated surgically. Anticoagulation therapy is often administered, although recanalization of the artery can occur with or without its use. Vertebrobasilar dissections cannot be approached surgically, but bypass procedures are sometimes employed.

Beletsky V, Nadareishvili Z, Lynch J, Shuaib A, Woolfenden A, Norris JW; Canadian Stroke Consortium. Cervical arterial dissection: time for a therapeutic clinical trial? *Stroke.* 2003;34(12): 2856–2860.

Arteriovenous Malformations

Like aneurysms, AVMs are usually congenital and may be familial. Symptoms typically develop before age 30 with a slight male preponderance, and 6% of patients also have an intracranial aneurysm. Intracranial hemorrhage with or without subarachnoid hemorrhage is the initial presentation in half of the cases. In contrast to patients with saccular aneurysms, those with AVMs are much more likely to become symptomatic before a hemorrhage occurs (Fig 14-18). Seizures are the first manifestation in 30% of affected patients,

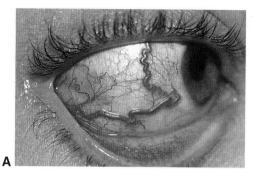

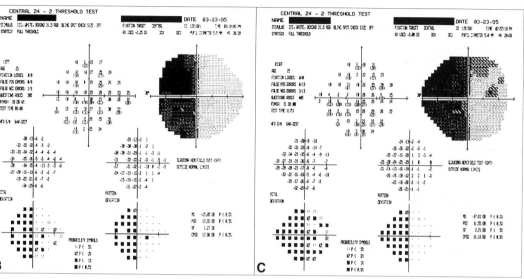

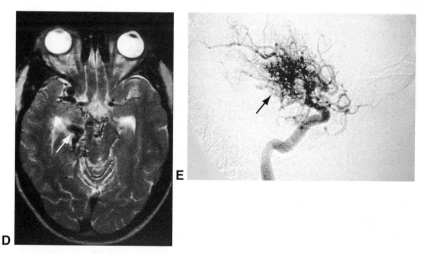

Figure 14-18 **A,** This 24-year-old man was referred with a 2- to 3-year history of prominent blood vessels in the right eye. **B, C,** Visual acuity was 20/20 bilaterally, but visual fields demonstrated a left homonymous hemianopia. **D,** A T2-weighted MRI scan demonstrated a large right basal ganglia arteriovenous malformation (AVM) *(arrow)*. **E,** A right internal carotid angiogram confirmed the basal ganglia AVM *(arrow)*. *(Courtesy of Steven A. Newman, MD.)*

whereas 20% have headaches or other focal neurologic deficits initially. The neurologic symptoms may be progressive or transient.

Of the 90% of AVMs that are supratentorial, about 70% are cortical and 20% are deep. The remaining 10% are located in the posterior fossa or dura mater. Early mortality occurs in up to 20% of cases when bleeding takes place, and the rebleeding rate is 2.5% each year. Most AVMs bleed into the brain, producing headaches and focal neurologic deficits.

The neuro-ophthalmic manifestations of an AVM depend on its location. Cortical AVMs in the occipital lobe may produce visual symptoms and headaches that resemble migraine. The visual phenomena are usually brief and unformed, but typical migrainous scintillating scotomata may, rarely, occur (see Chapter 12, Fig 12-2). Hemispheric AVMs may produce homonymous visual field defects. Signs and symptoms of brainstem AVMs are not specific and may include diplopia, nystagmus, dizziness, ocular motor nerve palsy, gaze palsy, anisocoria, or pupillary light–near dissociation. Reports of transient monocular visual loss caused by a steal phenomenon from an intracranial AVM are rare.

Some patients with AVMs report a subjective intracranial bruit, and occasionally the examiner will detect a bruit with auscultation of the skull over the AVM.

Abnormal arterial communication with one of the dural venous sinuses (dural AVM) results in elevated venous pressure and in turn increased intracranial pressure. Dural AVMs account for 10%–15% of intracranial AVMs. Patients often have tinnitus and an audible bruit in addition to signs and symptoms of increased intracranial pressure. Dural AVMs are difficult to diagnose without catheter angiography and may be mistaken for typical idiopathic intracranial hypertension (IIH) (see Chapter 4). Dural AVMs should be considered in the patient who does not fit the usual IIH demographics and who has no other demonstrable cause of increased intracranial pressure.

Diagnosis

If bleeding is suspected, an unenhanced CT scan will show the hemorrhage. Although unruptured AVMs are typically seen on an enhanced CT scan, MRI scanning is more sensitive for visualizing small AVMs. MRI scan demonstrates the heterogeneous signals representing the various elements of the lesion: blood vessels, brain, flowing and clotted blood, calcium, hemorrhage, or edema. Calcified AVMs are sometimes identifiable on plain radiographs or CT scan. Cerebral angiography is required to clearly show the anatomy and to define the feeding and draining vessels of the AVM.

Treatment

The location of the AVM, the anatomy of feeding and draining vessels, and the size of the lesion all affect the choice of treatment. Surgical resection, ligation of feeding vessels, embolization, and stereotactic radiosurgery can be used alone or in combination. Seizures usually improve with anticonvulsant therapy.

Kupersmith MJ, Vargas ME, Yashar A, et al. Occipital arteriovenous malformations: visual disturbances and presentation. *Neurology.* 1996;46(4):953–957.

Cerebral Venous and Dural Sinus Thrombosis

Occlusion of the cortical and subcortical veins produces focal neurologic symptoms and signs, including neuro-ophthalmic findings. The cavernous sinus, lateral (transverse) sinus, and superior sagittal sinus are most commonly affected. Each produces a distinct clinical syndrome. Lateral and superior sagittal sinus thrombosis are more common in pregnancy and may present with headaches and papilledema and may simulate IIH.

Sloan MA, Stern BJ. Cerebrovascular disease in pregnancy. *Curr Treat Options Neurol.* 2003;5(5): 391–407.

Cavernous sinus thrombosis

Cavernous sinus thrombosis (CST) in the *septic* form results from an infection of the face, sphenoid or ethmoidal sinuses, or oral cavity. Rarely, otitis media or orbital cellulitis is the cause. Patients develop headache, nausea, vomiting, and somnolence. There may also be fever, chills, tachycardia, evidence of meningitis, or generalized sepsis. Ocular signs from anterior infection (facial, dental, orbital) are initially unilateral but frequently become bilateral. They include orbital congestion, lacrimation, conjunctival edema, eyelid swelling, ptosis, proptosis, and ophthalmoplegia. Sixth nerve palsy is the most consistent early neurologic sign. Corneal anesthesia, facial numbness, Horner syndrome, and venous stasis retinopathy can occur. Treatment includes the administration of antibiotics, anticoagulants, or corticosteroids and surgery.

The signs and symptoms of *aseptic* CST resemble those of septic CST, but clinical or laboratory examination shows no evidence of infection. Pain around the eye is common, but orbital congestion is typically less severe than with septic CST. Anticoagulation or antiplatelet therapy is often used.

Lateral (transverse) sinus thrombosis

Lateral sinus thrombosis may be septic or spontaneous (see Chapter 2, Fig 2-11). With the widespread use of antibiotics, septic thrombosis has become rare, but it may result from otitis media.

Patients develop features of systemic infection as well as neck pain, tenderness of the ipsilateral jugular vein, retroauricular edema, and sometimes, facial weakness. Severe facial pain also may occur and when accompanied by sixth nerve palsy is called *Gradenigo syndrome.* The pseudotumor cerebri–like syndrome caused by lateral sinus thrombosis was originally called *otitic hydrocephalus.* Complications include meningitis and extension of the thrombosis. It is treated with antibiotics, mastoidectomy with incision and drainage of the lateral sinus, and intracranial pressure–lowering agents. Prompt treatment yields an excellent prognosis.

Lateral sinus thrombosis is much more likely to be spontaneous and produce a pseudotumor cerebri–like syndrome with increased intracranial pressure. The most common ophthalmic signs are papilledema and sixth nerve palsy.

Superior sagittal sinus thrombosis

Aseptic thrombosis is more common than septic thrombosis in the superior sagittal sinus (SSS). Septic thrombosis is most commonly a result of meningitis. Other causes of septic SSS thrombosis include paranasal sinus infection, pulmonary infections, tonsillitis, dental infections, pelvic inflammatory disease, and otitis media. SSS thrombosis can occur during pregnancy, immediately postpartum, or with oral contraceptive use. Vasculitis and systemic inflammatory disorders predispose to this condition.

The symptoms and signs depend on the extent and location of the occlusion within the SSS. With thrombosis of the anterior third of the sinus, symptoms are mild or absent. Posterior SSS thrombosis may produce a clinical picture similar to pseudotumor cerebri, with headaches and papilledema. It is a diagnosis to consider in atypical pseudotumor cerebri patients, such as slim women and men. If impairment of cerebral venous drainage is marked, altered mental status, seizures, and focal neurologic signs may develop. Cerebral blindness is a rare complication. With increasing intracranial pressure, the condition can be fatal because of intracerebral hemorrhage and brain herniation. Treatment is directed toward the underlying condition. Anticoagulation, fibrinolytic agents, and intracranial pressure–lowering treatments are used.

Diagnosis

Abnormalities can be seen on unenhanced and enhanced CT and MRI scan, although neither test is sensitive enough to be used alone. Standard MRI scan is useful to determine whether a brain abscess, infarction, hemorrhage, or edema is present. Magnetic resonance venography (MRV) is a sensitive and noninvasive method used to visualize the thrombosed vessels directly. Cerebral angiography demonstrates vascular occlusion and is particularly useful for visualizing the internal carotid and ophthalmic arteries.

Neuro-Ophthalmic Manifestations of Infectious Diseases

Myriad infectious diseases may result in neuro-ophthalmic manifestations. This text covers the most common infections encountered in the United States.

Acquired Immunodeficiency Syndrome

Because of the frequency of ophthalmic complaints in human immunodeficiency virus (HIV) infection, ophthalmologists are often the first physicians seen by a patient with acquired immunodeficiency syndrome (AIDS); thus, they must be aware of the different presentations of AIDS. Although considered separately in this text, several factors may be involved in a single patient. Neuro-ophthalmic disorders may result from infection by HIV or from secondary opportunistic infections and malignancy. The eye, afferent visual pathways, and ocular motor system can all be affected. BCSC Section 9, *Intraocular Inflammation and Uveitis,* discusses the following conditions in detail.

Central nervous system lymphoma

High-grade B-cell non-Hodgkin lymphoma is the second most common malignancy in AIDS and the most common neoplasm to affect the CNS. CNS lymphoma can cause diplopia from third, fourth, or sixth nerve involvement. Lymphomatous infiltration of the orbit and optic nerve may lead to disc swelling and visual loss. The diagnosis is made by confirming the presence of neoplastic lymphomatous cells in the spinal fluid or by performing stereotactic brain or meningeal biopsy. Changes shown on MRI scan may resemble those of toxoplasmosis, but they are typically periventricular with subependymal spread. Treatment consists of a combination of radiotherapy and chemotherapy.

Cytomegalovirus

Cytomegalovirus (CMV) is most commonly encountered by the ophthalmologist when the patient develops retinal lesions. CMV retinitis is often the presenting manifestation of AIDS. It is a common opportunistic infection in AIDS patients and a major cause of visual loss. The early lesions are dry, white, granular retinal opacifications that may resemble cotton-wool spots or "crumbled cheese," located at the posterior pole or peripheral retina. Subsequent findings include retinal exudates, vascular sheathing, retinal hemorrhages, choroidal inflammation, and exudative retinal detachment. Untreated CMV retinitis is a potentially blinding condition.

Within the CNS, CMV causes optic neuritis and brainstem encephalitis. Anterior optic nerve infection produces acute visual loss with optic disc swelling. This condition usually occurs in patients with severe CMV retinitis. Others develop anterior optic neuropathy with minimal retinitis (Fig 14-19). Posterior optic neuropathy, which is rare, is characterized by slowly progressive visual loss without disc edema. Brainstem involvement may produce ptosis, internuclear ophthalmoplegia, ocular cranial nerve palsies, horizontal and vertical gaze paresis, and nystagmus.

The diagnosis of CMV infection is made clinically, based on the characteristic ocular findings. Serologic tests and cultures may be inconclusive. CNS disease is often difficult to confirm, and the diagnosis is often made presumptively in the presence of elevated CMV titers in the blood and CSF. See BCSC Section 12, *Retina and Vitreous,* for a complete discussion of CMV diagnosis and treatment.

Herpesvirus

Herpes simplex and herpes zoster can cause infection in patients with AIDS. Acute outer retinal necrosis produces photophobia, ocular pain, floaters, and decreased visual acuity. Ophthalmic findings include panuveitis, vitritis, retinal arteritis, disc edema, and a necrotizing retinitis that initially spares the posterior pole.

CNS encephalitis is the most common manifestation of herpes infection (Fig 14-20). Radiculitis may occur, producing herpes zoster ophthalmicus and Ramsay Hunt syndrome. In general, neuro-ophthalmic findings are uncommon with herpesvirus infection.

Human immunodeficiency virus

HIV infection itself causes acute and chronic CNS manifestations. Acute aseptic meningitis and meningoencephalitis affect 5%–10% of patients, just after HIV infection. Headache, fever, and meningeal signs may accompany a mononucleosis-like syndrome. Occasionally, altered mental status, seizures, optic neuropathy, and cranial neuropathies occur, most commonly seventh nerve paresis.

HIV encephalopathy, or the *AIDS dementia complex,* begins with impaired memory and concentration, behavior changes, and mental slowness. Abnormal pursuit and saccadic eye movements and saccadic intrusions (square-wave jerks) may be present. Late manifestations include profound dementia, behavior changes, psychosis, psychomotor impairment, weakness, visual neglect, visual hallucinations, seizures, and tremor. An optic neuropathy may develop. Ocular signs of HIV infection include cotton-wool spots, perivasculitis, and retinal hemorrhages. MRI scanning demonstrates cerebral atrophy and

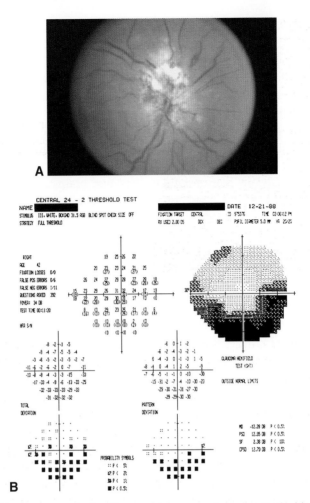

Figure 14-19 A, Disc appearance of a 42-year-old woman who presented with a 3-week history of noticing inferior shadows OD. **B,** Visual acuity was 20/20, but visual field testing demonstrated an inferior arcuate visual field defect. The patient's past medical history was remarkable for transfusion 18 months prior, with evidence of subsequent *Pneumocystis* pneumonia. She was found to be HIV positive, and a diagnosis of CMV optic neuritis was made. *(Courtesy of Steven A. Newman, MD.)*

areas of white matter hyperintensity on T2-weighted images that correspond to areas of demyelination produced by the virus.

Mycobacterium

Mycobacterium tuberculosis and *M avium-intracellulare* can infect the brain and eye. The neuro-ophthalmic manifestations of tuberculous meningitis include photophobia, third and sixth nerve paresis, papilledema, retrobulbar optic neuritis, and anisocoria. Cerebral infarction can result from obliterative endarteritis. Neuroimaging studies may show hydrocephalus, abscess formation, granulomas, and enhancement of the basal meninges with contrast administration.

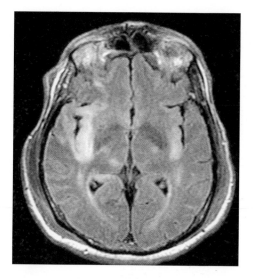

Figure 14-20 Axial FLAIR MRI scan showing bilateral temporal lobe signal abnormalities in a patient with herpes encephalitis. *(Courtesy of Joel Curé, MD.)*

Syphilis

Syphilis frequently accompanies HIV infection, probably because of the shared risk of sexual transmission. Ophthalmic presentations include papillitis, retinal hemorrhages, arterial and venous occlusions, vasculitis, chorioretinitis, necrotizing vasculitis, optic neuritis, and uveitis. Meningovascular syphilis produces visual field defects and ocular motility disorders (ocular motor cranial nerve palsies) in some patients.

The diagnosis of syphilis may be difficult to make in an immunocompromised host. The CSF may show one or more of the following changes: positive syphilis serology, elevated protein, or pleocytosis. However, both false-negative and false-positive serologic results are more common in the patient with HIV. The CSF VDRL alone cannot be relied upon to confirm CNS infection. A course of aqueous penicillin G (12–24 million U/day IV for 10–14 days) is recommended, with reexamination of the CSF to determine the effectiveness of treatment.

Progressive multifocal leukoencephalopathy

Originally described in patients with lymphoproliferative disorders and impaired cell-mediated immunity, *progressive multifocal leukoencephalopathy (PML)* occurs in 1%–4% of patients with AIDS. The disease is caused by the JC virus, a polyomavirus that destroys oligodendrocytes. Gray matter is relatively spared. The central visual pathways and ocular motor fibers can be affected. Neuro-ophthalmic manifestations include homonymous hemianopia, blurred vision, cerebral blindness, prosopagnosia, and diplopia. Other neurologic findings are altered mental status, ataxia, dementia, hemiparesis, and focal deficits.

MRI scan shows areas of demyelination, most frequently in the parieto-occipital region. PML typically involves the subcortical white matter, with focal or confluent non-enhancing lesions (Fig 14-21). Therapy is aimed at correcting the underlying immune deficiency state, and prognosis is poor.

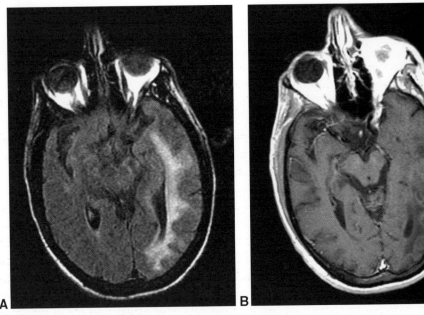

Figure 14-21 Progressive multifocal leukoencephalopathy (PML) in a patient with AIDS. **A,** Axial FLAIR image demonstrates increased signal in the left occipital lobe white matter, sparing the overlying cortex. **B,** Axial gadolinium-enhanced T1-weighted spin echo image (same location as part A) demonstrates a nonenhancing hypointense lesion in the left occipital white matter. T1 hypointensity is typical of PML lesions. Note the absence of mass effect and negligible enhancement. *(Courtesy of Joel Curé, MD.)*

Toxoplasmosis

Ocular toxoplasmosis is not a common complication of AIDS, but CNS toxoplasmosis affects approximately one third of AIDS patients. Retinal lesions are usually found adjacent to blood vessels. Toxoplasmic optic neuritis is rare, characterized by subacute visual loss and optic nerve swelling, at times accompanied by a macular star (neuroretinitis). CNS toxoplasmosis produces multifocal lesions, with a predilection for the basal ganglia and the frontal, parietal, and occipital lobes. Patients develop headaches, focal neurologic deficits, seizures, mental status changes, and fever. Neuro-ophthalmic findings include homonymous hemianopia and quadrantanopia, ocular motor palsies, and gaze palsies. Lifelong antitoxoplasmosis treatment is necessary to prevent recurrences.

MRI scanning typically shows multiple lesions that are isointense with the brain on T1-weighted images and isointense or hyperintense on T2-weighted images. Gadolinium administration reveals enhancement.

Bakshi R. Neuroimaging of HIV and AIDS related illnesses: a review. *Front Biosci.* 2004;9: 632–636.

Currie J. AIDS and neuro-ophthalmology. *Curr Opin Ophthalmol.* 1995;6(6):34–40.

Ormerud LD, Rhodes RH, Gross SA, Crane LR, Houchin KW. Ophthalmologic manifestations of acquired immunodeficiency syndrome–associated progressive multifocal leukoencephalopathy. *Ophthalmology.* 1996;103(6):899–906.

Lyme Disease

Lyme borreliosis is caused by infection with *Borrelia burgdorferi,* a spirochete transmitted by deer ticks. The disease typically occurs in 3 stages and can produce ocular and neuro-ophthalmic manifestations. Lyme disease is discussed further in BCSC Section 1, *Update on General Medicine,* and Section 9, *Intraocular Inflammation and Uveitis.*

In *stage 1,* 60%–80% of patients develop a localized infection characterized by a skin rash *(erythema chronicum migrans)* that is sometimes associated with fever, regional lymphadenopathy, and minor constitutional symptoms (Fig 14-22). This stage typically occurs within days or weeks of infection. The ocular findings include conjunctivitis, photophobia, periorbital edema, diffuse choroiditis, exudative retinal detachment, and iridocyclitis.

Stage 2 follows within days or weeks and represents disseminated infection through the blood or lymphatic system. Stage 2 is associated with symptoms in the skin, nervous system, or musculoskeletal sites. Annular or malar rash, arthralgia, pancarditis, lymphadenopathy, splenomegaly, hepatitis, hematuria, proteinuria, malaise, and fatigue may be present. Neuro-ophthalmic findings at this stage consist of keratitis, panophthalmitis, papilledema (pseudotumor cerebri–like syndrome), granulomatous iritis, vitritis, pars planitis, and orbital myositis. Two thirds of patients have ocular findings at this stage.

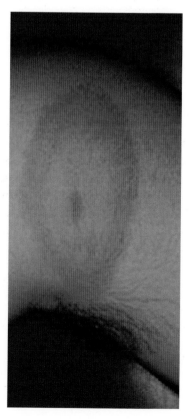

Figure 14-22 Erythema chronicum migrans, the characteristic skin rash of stage 1 Lyme disease. *(Courtesy of Robert L. Lesser, MD.)*

Cranial neuropathies can occur, most commonly facial nerve palsy, optic neuritis, meningitis with headache and neck stiffness, and radiculopathies.

Stage 3 represents persistent infection. Arthritis and scleroderma-like skin lesions are prominent. Keratitis and neurologic conditions predominate, including chronic encephalomyelitis, spastic paraparesis, ataxic gait, subtle mental disorders, and chronic radiculopathy. The neurologic picture may resemble MS, clinically and radiographically.

The diagnosis is made clinically when the patient has been exposed to an endemic area (the patient might not recall a tick bite) and shows the typical rash of erythema chronicum migrans. The presence of an elevated Lyme antibody titer in the serum or CSF is helpful. The ELISA is typically used for screening, but the Western blot technique confirms the diagnosis.

Treatment should be orchestrated by an infectious disease specialist.

Balcer LJ, Winterkorn JM, Galetta SL. Neuro-ophthalmic manifestations of Lyme disease. *J Neuro-ophthalmol.* 1997;17(2):108–121.

Fungal Infections

Fungal infections are caused by species that proliferate either with polymorphonuclear leukocyte deficiencies (aspergillosis, mucormycosis, blastomycosis, candidiasis) or with defective T-cell function (cryptococcosis, histoplasmosis, coccidioidomycosis). The 2 main types of fungi are molds and yeasts, although some fungi can have characteristics of both.

Molds (filamentous fungi) are composed of hyphae, which extend and branch to form a mycelium, enabling the mold to grow. Molds reproduce when a portion of the hyphae breaks off. Aspergillosis and mucormycosis are CNS infections caused by molds.

Yeasts are round, with outpouchings called buds or pseudohyphae. Yeasts are septated and reproduce by budding: the parent cell divides and one of the daughter nuclei migrates into a bud on the surface of a cell. Coccidioidomycosis, cryptococcosis, and histoplasmosis are caused by yeasts. *Candida* can grow as a yeast or a mold.

Weinstein JM. Viruses (except retroviruses) and viral diseases. In: Miller NR, Newman NJ, eds. *Walsh and Hoyt's Clinical Neuro-Ophthalmology.* 6th ed. Vol 3. Philadelphia: Lippincott Williams & Wilkins; 2005:2775–2825.

Aspergillosis

The *Aspergillus* fungus grows in hay, grain, decaying vegetation, soil, and dung. It is contracted by inhaling or chewing grain, breathing in a building during renovation, or eating contaminated foods (pepper). The most frequent mode of transmission is inhalation of spores. Many species of *Aspergillus* infect humans. The 3 main types of infections are allergic aspergillosis, aspergillomas, and invasive aspergillosis.

Allergic aspergillosis affects the bronchopulmonary system and the paranasal sinuses. Neuro-ophthalmic findings are rare; they occur secondarily with sphenoid sinus involvement. Signs and symptoms include optic neuropathy, proptosis, diplopia, and headache.

Aspergillomas, or *fungus balls,* may arise in the orbit, paranasal sinuses, or brain. They can occur in either immunocompromised or immunocompetent patients. Orbital aspergillomas produce symptoms of orbital masses, with proptosis, visual loss, diplopia, and pain. Orbital lesions also typically involve the sinuses or brain. Extension to the optic canal, cavernous sinus, optic nerves, and optic chiasm produces neuro-ophthalmic findings (Fig 14-23). Intracranial aspergillomas act like mass lesions in causing progressive neurologic deficits.

Invasive aspergillosis typically occurs in immunocompromised patients. Most patients initially have pulmonary involvement, although the skin, orbit, or sinuses may be the nidus of infection. CNS infection occurs secondarily by either direct or hematogenous spread of organisms. Ophthalmic manifestations include acute retrobulbar optic neuropathy, endophthalmitis, orbital apex syndrome, and cavernous sinus syndrome. Vascular invasion produces cerebral infarction or hemorrhage. Meningitis, intracranial abscess, epidural and subdural hematoma, mycotic aneurysm formation, and encephalitis are serious sequelae of invasive aspergillosis.

Treatment includes systemic corticosteroids and antifungal agents such as amphotericin B. New azoles such as voriconazole and posaconazole may be superior to amphotericin B in the management of invasive aspergillosis. Surgical intervention is necessary to treat aspergillomas and invasive aspergillosis. The mortality rate for invasive aspergillosis is extremely high (>90%).

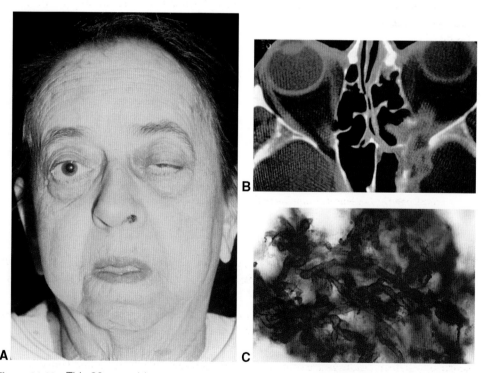

Figure 14-23 This 82-year-old woman presented with a 6-week history of left brow and orbital pain. **A,** 4 weeks prior to evaluation she suddenly lost vision in her left eye and 1 week later she developed ptosis and proptosis. **B,** CT scan revealed a destructive lesion at the orbital apex, which on fine-needle aspiration biopsy **(C)** proved to be an aspergilloma.

Levin LA, Avery R, Shore JW, Woog JJ, Baker AS. The spectrum of orbital aspergillosis: a clinicopathological review. *Surv Ophthalmol.* 1996;41(2):142–154.

Metcalf SC, Dockrell DH. Improved outcomes associated with advances in therapy for invasive fungal infections in immunocompromised hosts. *J Infect.* 2007;55(4):287–299.

Mucormycosis

Mucormycosis is caused by several different mold fungi of the Zygomycetes class. These fungi, which inhabit decaying matter, are ubiquitous but of such low virulence that infection occurs only in debilitated hosts. The mold enters the body through the respiratory tract and proliferates, causing hyphal invasion of tissues. It grows rapidly, producing a more acute infection than other fungi. These organisms have a predilection for blood vessels; and hemorrhage, thrombosis, and ischemic necrosis are hallmarks of the disease. Aneurysm and pseudoaneurysm formation in the intracranial vasculature can produce devastating consequences when rupture occurs. The 2 types of mucormycosis producing ophthalmic involvement are rhinocerebral and CNS mucormycosis.

Rhinocerebral mucormycosis usually occurs in patients with diabetes, patients taking corticosteroids, or neutropenic patients receiving antibiotics. The initial infection spreads from the facial skin, nasal mucosa, paranasal sinuses, or the hard palate (Fig 14-24). The fungus spreads to the nearby blood vessels, affecting the orbital vessels, carotid arteries, cavernous sinuses, or jugular veins. Orbital and neurologic signs are produced by infarction, thrombosis, or hemorrhage. Untreated, rhinocerebral mucormycosis may bring about rapid deterioration, leading to death within days. A few patients develop a chronic course with little indication of systemic illness.

Most patients have headache or facial pain. Other symptoms and signs depend on the location of the infection. Orbital involvement produces orbital swelling, pain on eye movement, conjunctival injection and chemosis, corneal ulceration, ophthalmoplegia, and visual loss. Retinal infarction, ophthalmic artery occlusion, and optic nerve infiltration are mechanisms of blindness. Other common presentations are painful diplopia and cranial neuropathy. An orbital apex, cavernous sinus, or chiasmal syndrome may be present. Neurologic signs include hemiparesis, aphasia, seizures, and altered mental status.

Central nervous system mucormycosis is very rare. The fungus usually gains access to the CNS from the nose or paranasal sinus, but there is no nasal, sinus, ocular, or orbital disease when the neurologic manifestations appear. Infection of the orbit, palate, nose,

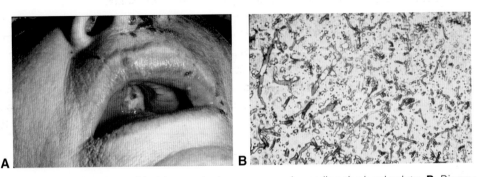

Figure 14-24 **A,** A patient with rhinocerebral mucormycosis eroding the hard palate. **B,** Biopsy demonstrated typical nonseptate hyphae. *(Courtesy of Lanning B. Kline, MD.)*

and sinuses typically occurs secondarily. Meningitis, abscesses, cranial nerve involvement, and seizures are common.

The diagnosis of mucormycosis requires a high index of suspicion, because many of the laboratory investigations are nonspecific. Computed tomography scan may demonstrate bone destruction, soft-tissue alteration in the paranasal sinuses and orbit, air–fluid levels in the sinuses and orbits, or brain abscess formation. MRI scan, MRA, and arteriography may be helpful for showing vascular thrombosis. The definitive test is a biopsy that demonstrates vascular invasion, tissue necrosis, eschar formation, inflammatory cells, and nonseptate hyphae.

Mucormycosis has a mortality rate of about 50%. The underlying systemic disease should be treated and immunosuppressant agents eliminated, if possible. Therapy includes aggressive surgical debridement of necrotic tissue and administration of amphotericin B. The new triazole, posaconazole, shows promise in the treatment of mucormycosis. Hyperbaric oxygen may be helpful.

Spellberg B, Edwards J, Ibrahim A. Novel perspectives on mucormycosis: pathophysiology, presentation and management. *Clin Microbiol Rev.* 2005;18(3):556–569.

Cryptococcosis

Cryptococcus neoformans, the most common fungus causing cryptococcosis, is found in pigeon droppings and contaminated soil. Although it is ubiquitous, it rarely causes infection in otherwise healthy people. However, infection does occur in approximately 10% of patients with AIDS, and it is the most common life-threatening mycosis in these patients.

The most common neuro-ophthalmic abnormality is papilledema from cryptococcal meningitis. The onset of symptoms is usually insidious, with a waxing and waning course. Headache, nausea, vomiting, dizziness, and mental status changes are the most common complaints. Diplopia from unilateral or bilateral sixth nerve palsies may occur as a false localizing sign of increased intracranial pressure. Inflammation at the base of the brain produces other cranial neuropathies. Photophobia, blurred vision, retrobulbar pain, homonymous visual field defects, or nystagmus may occur.

Optic nerve involvement manifests as a retrobulbar neuritis, producing gradual visual loss over hours to days. It is postulated that adhesive arachnoiditis is one cause of visual loss with cryptococcal infections. The infiltration of organisms within the visual pathways and the perioptic meninges has been shown postmortem. Other ophthalmic complications include papilledema, retinochoroiditis, and cotton-wool spots.

The diagnosis is confirmed by demonstrating the *C neoformans* capsular antigen or by isolating the yeast in the CSF. Most patients with CNS cryptococcosis have disseminated disease, with evidence of infection in the blood, lungs, bone marrow, skin, kidneys, and other organs. Serum antigen titers are helpful for this reason.

Antifungal treatment consists of amphotericin B and flucytosine. Intrathecal amphotericin treatment may be necessary. Fluconazole or itraconazole is used for maintenance therapy. Visual loss caused by papilledema can be prevented with CSF shunting or optic nerve sheath fenestration. The mortality rate of patients with treated CNS cryptococcosis is 25%–30%. The prognosis is worse in patients with an underlying malignancy or AIDS.

Perfect JR, Casadevall A. Cryptococcosis. *Infect Dis Clin North Am.* 2002;16(4):837–874.

Prion Diseases

Prion diseases, also known as *transmissible spongiform encephalopathies,* include kuru in New Guinea; sporadic Creutzfeldt-Jakob disease (CJD), which is found worldwide; and a new variant of CJD (vCJD) found mostly in the United Kingdom and France. Variant CJD has been linked to bovine spongiform encephalopathy ("mad cow" disease), which is a prion disease in cattle.

Prions are infectious agents formed by the conversion of a normal cell surface protein (PrP^C) to a misfolded cell surface protein called PrP^{CJD} or PrP^{SC} (for the animal prion disease scrapie). Upon association with a normal PrP^C molecule, an abnormal PrP^{CJD} induces a conformational change in the normal protein, resulting in propagation of the abnormal form. The resulting accumulation of the abnormal prion protein alters neuronal function, causing the symptoms of CJD. Sporadic CJD may result from somatic mutation in the prion protein gene or, more likely, from the spontaneous, random conversion of a normal prion protein to an abnormal prion protein and the subsequent expansion of the altered form. About 10% of CJD cases are familial and due to inherited mutations in the *PrP* gene.

Creutzfeld-Jakob disease (CJD) is uniformly fatal, presenting as a rapidly progressive dementia that results in death, usually in 8 months. The most commonly reported visual symptoms include diplopia, supranuclear palsies, complex visual disturbances, homonymous visual field defects, hallucinations, and cortical blindness. Occasionally, in the Heidenhain variant of CJD, patients present primarily with isolated visual symptoms.

Diagnostic testing includes MRI, electroencephalogram (EEG), lumbar puncture, and possibly brain biopsy. MRI diffusion-weighted images show typical high-intensity cortical and basal ganglia lesions. The EEG shows typical periodic sharp wave complexes (PSWCs). Cerebrospinal fluid usually contains the 14-3-3 protein. Brain histopathology shows a spongiform degeneration. No treatment is currently available.

Buono LM. Prion disease. *Int Ophthalmol Clin.* 2007;47(4):121–129.

Radiation Therapy

Several types of radiation therapy (RT) are currently available, and techniques continue to evolve and emerge with scientific advances. Traditional whole-brain RT, which is used to treat cerebral malignancies, is delivered in fractions over approximately 1 month. More recent advances, such as 3-dimensional conformal RT, use a computer to help concentrate radiation in a precise area; this is accomplished through the use of complex asymmetric 3-dimensional shapes. Radiation surgery (radiosurgery) refers to linear accelerator or gamma knife techniques, which are distinct from traditional radiation therapy. Radiosurgery is typically given in a single sitting, using computer-based techniques to focus radiation at the desired regions. These techniques may treat malignancies, occasional inflammatory lesions, and vascular malformations.

Complications of RT directed at the nervous system may take several forms and can occur years after therapy. Immediate complications include transient swelling of the involved tissue. Later complications of neuro-ophthalmic interest include radiation necrosis,

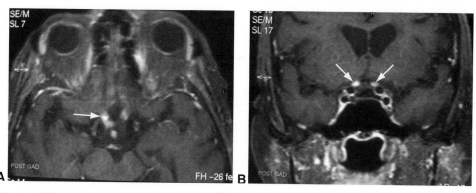

Figure 14-25 **A,** Axial and **(B)** coronal T1-weighted fat-suppressed MRI of a patient with radiation optic neuropathy. Radiation was performed for a pituitary adenoma, and the patient developed visual loss OD > OS months after the radiation. MRI demonstrates enhancing optic nerves *(arrows)* in the prechiasmal region. *(Photographs courtesy of Eric Eggenberger, DO.)*

cranial neuropathies, and ocular neuromyotonia (see Chapter 8). Radiation necrosis involves death of nervous system tissue with attendant edema. This may simulate the imaging appearance of recurrent neoplasm on traditional MRI or CT imaging. Occasionally, functional imaging techniques such as PET or magnetic resonance spectroscopy (MRS) are required to separate these entities radiographically; neoplasms generally display a hypermetabolic profile, whereas radiation necrosis is hypometabolic in nature.

Of greater concern to the neuro-ophthalmologist is radiation optic neuropathy. This rare complication typically occurs months after radiation administration and produces subacute optic neuropathy. Radiation optic neuropathy is in part dose-related, being more likely to occur with higher doses (often >5000 cGy). MRI scan of radiation optic neuropathy usually demonstrates an enhancing optic nerve (Fig 14-25). Treatment is often ineffective, but anticoagulation, hyperbaric oxygen, and corticosteroids have all been used. Ocular neuromyotonia occurs months to years after radiation treatment. This uncommon syndrome produces episodic "spasms" of CN III, IV, or VI, causing recurrent short-lived episodes of diplopia. Although rare, this entity is important for the ophthalmologist because it responds to carbamazepine.

Barnett GH, Lindsey ME, Adler JR, et al; American Association of Neurological Surgeons; Congress of Neurological Surgeons Washington Committee Stereotactic Radiosurgery Task Force. Stereotactic radiosurgery—an organized neurosurgery-sanctioned definition. *J Neurosurg.* 2007;106(1):1–5.

Basic Texts

Neuro-Ophthalmology

Brodsky MC, Baker RS, Hamed LM. *Pediatric Neuro-Ophthalmology.* New York: Springer-Verlag; 1996.

Burde RM, Savino PJ, Trobe JD. *Clinical Decisions in Neuro-Ophthalmology.* 3rd ed. St Louis: Mosby; 2002.

Glaser JS. *Neuro-Ophthalmology.* 3rd ed. Philadelphia: Lippincott; 1999.

Gold DH, Weingeist TA. *Color Atlas of the Eye in Systemic Disease.* Philadelphia; Lippincott Williams & Wilkins; 2001.

Harrington DO, Drake MV. *The Visual Fields: Textbook and Atlas of Clinical Perimetry.* 6th ed. St Louis: Mosby; 1990.

Kline LB, Bajandas FJ. *Neuro-Ophthalmology Review Manual.* 6th ed. Thorofare, NJ: Slack; 2008.

Lee AG, Brazis PW, Kline LB, eds. *Curbside Consultation in Neuro-Ophthalmology.* Thorofare, NJ: Slack; 2009.

Leigh RJ, Zee DS. *The Neurology of Eye Movements.* 3rd ed. New York: Oxford University Press; 1999.

Liu GT, Volpe NJ, Galetta SL. *Neuro-Ophthalmology: Diagnosis and Management.* Philadelphia: Saunders; 2001.

Loewenfeld IE. *The Pupil: Anatomy, Physiology, and Clinical Applications.* 2 vols. Oxford: Butterworth-Heinemann; 1999.

Miller NR, Newman NJ, Biousse V, Kerrison JB, eds. *Walsh and Hoyt's Clinical Neuro-Ophthalmology.* 6th ed. 3 vols. Philadelphia: Lippincott Williams & Wilkins; 2005.

Trobe JD. *The Neurology of Vision.* New York: Oxford University Press; 2001.

Wong AMF. *Eye Movement Disorders.* New York: Oxford University Press; 2008.

Related Academy Materials

Focal Points: Clinical Modules for Ophthalmologists

For information on Focal Points modules, go to http://one.aao.org/CE/EducationalProducts/
FocalPoints.aspx.

Arnold AC. Optic nerve meningioma (Module 7, 2004).
Farris BK. Temporal artery biopsy (Module 7, 2003).
Lee MS. Diplopia: diagnosis and management (Module 12, 2007).
Lee AG, Brazis PW. Giant cell arteritis (Module 6, 2005).
Lee AG, Brazis PW, Curry RC. Neuro-ophthalmic complications of cardiac surgery (Module 6, 2001).
Pardo G. Multiple sclerosis and optic neuritis (Module 12, 2003).
Patel AD. Optic atrophy (Module, 2006).
Smith KH. Myasthenia gravis (Module 4, 2003).
Torun N, Ing E. Neuro-ophthalmologic emergencies (Module 9, 2008).
Vaphiades MS, Kline LB. Functional visual disorders (Module 1, 2005).
Volpe NJ, Liu GT, Galetta SL. Idiopathic intracranial hypertension (IIH, pseudotumor cerebri) (Module 3, 2004).

Print Publications

Arnold AC, ed. *Basic Principles of Ophthalmic Surgery* (2006).
Fishman GA, Birch DG, Holder GE, Brigell MG. *Electrophysiologic Testing in Disorders of the Retina, Optic Nerve, and Visual Pathway.* 2nd ed. Ophthalmology Monograph 2 (2001).
Kline LB, ed. *Optic Nerve Disorders.* 2nd ed. Ophthalmology Monograph 10 (2007).
Rockwood EJ, ed. *ProVision: Preferred Responses in Ophthalmology.* Series 4. Self-Assessment Program (2007).
Wilson FM II, ed. *Practical Ophthalmology: A Manual for Beginning Residents.* 5th ed. (2005).

Online Materials

For Preferred Practice Patterns, Complementary Therapy Assessments, and Ophthalmic Technology Assessments, go to http://one.aao.org/CE/PracticeGuidelines/default.aspx.

Basic and Clinical Science Course (Sections 1–13); http://one.aao.org/CE/Educational Products/BCSC.aspx
Clinical Education Cases; http://one.aao.org/CE/EducationalContent/Cases.aspx

Clinical Education and Ethics Courses; http://one.aao.org/CE/EducationalContent/Courses.aspx.

Focal Points modules; http://one.aao.org/CE/EducationalProducts/FocalPoints.aspx

Maintenance of Certification Exam Study Kit, version 2.0 (2007); http://one.aao.org/CE/MOC/default.aspx

Rockwood EJ, ed. *ProVision: Preferred Responses in Ophthalmology.* Series 4. Self-Assessment Program, 2-vol set (2007); http://one.aao.org/CE/EducationalProducts/Provision.aspx

CDs/DVDs

Chung SM, Gordon LK, Lee MS, Odel JG, Purvin VA. *LEO Clinical Update Course on Neuro-Ophthalmology* (CD-ROM, 2005).

Wilson ME Jr. *Ocular Motility Evaluation of Strabismus and Myasthenia Gravis.* From *Strabismus Evaluation and Surgery* (DVD, 1993; reviewed for currency 2007).

To order any of these materials, please order online at www.aao.org/store or call the Academy's Customer Service toll-free number 866-561-8558 in the U.S. If outside the U.S., call 415-561-8540 between 8:00 AM and 5:00 PM PST.

Credit Reporting Form

Basic and Clinical Science Course, 2009–2010
Section 5

The American Academy of Ophthalmology is accredited by the Accreditation Council for Continuing Medical Education to provide continuing medical education for physicians.

The American Academy of Ophthalmology designates this educational activity for a maximum of 40 *AMA PRA Category 1 Credits*™. Physicians should only claim credit commensurate with the extent of their participation in the activity.

If you wish to claim continuing medical education credit for your study of this Section, you may claim your credit online or fill in the required forms and mail or fax them to the Academy.

To use the forms:

1. Complete the study questions and mark your answers on the Section Completion Form.
2. Complete the Section Evaluation.
3. Fill in and sign the statement below.
4. Return this page and the required forms by mail or fax to the CME Registrar (see below).

To claim credit online:

1. Log on to the Academy website (www.aao.org/cme).
2. Select Review/Claim CME.
3. Follow the instructions.

Important: These completed forms or the online claim must be received at the Academy by June 2012.

I hereby certify that I have spent _____ (up to 40) hours of study on the curriculum of this Section and that I have completed the study questions.

Signature: _____

Date

Name: _____

Address: _____

City and State: _____   Zip: _____

Telephone: (_____) _____   Academy Member ID# _____
          area code

Please return completed forms to: **Or you may fax them to:** 415-561-8575
American Academy of Ophthalmology
P.O. Box 7424
San Francisco, CA 94120-7424
Attn: CME Registrar, Customer Service

375

2009–2010
Section Completion Form

Basic and Clinical Science Course

Answer Sheet for Section 5

Question	Answer	Question	Answer
1	a b c d	21	a b c d
2	a b c d	22	a b c d
3	a b c d	23	a b c d
4	a b c d	24	a b c d
5	a b c d	25	a b c d
6	a b c d	26	a b c d
7	a b c d	27	a b c d
8	a b c d	28	a b c d
9	a b c d	29	a b c d
10	a b c d	30	a b c d
11	a b c d	31	a b c d
12	a b c d	32	a b c d
13	a b c d	33	a b c d
14	a b c d	34	a b c d
15	a b c d	35	a b c d
16	a b c d	36	a b c d
17	a b c d	37	a b c d
18	a b c d	38	a b c d
19	a b c d	39	a b c d
20	a b c d	40	a b c d

Section Evaluation

Please complete this CME questionnaire.

1. To what degree will you use knowledge from BCSC Section 5 in your practice?

   ☐ Regularly

   ☐ Sometimes

   ☐ Rarely

2. Please review the stated objectives for BCSC Section 5. How effective was the material at meeting those objectives?

   ☐ All objectives were met.

   ☐ Most objectives were met.

   ☐ Some objectives were met.

   ☐ Few or no objectives were met.

3. To what degree is BCSC Section 5 likely to have a positive impact on health outcomes of your patients?

   ☐ Extremely likely

   ☐ Highly likely

   ☐ Somewhat likely

   ☐ Not at all likely

4. After you review the stated objectives for BCSC Section 5, please let us know of any additional knowledge, skills, or information useful to your practice that were acquired but were not included in the objectives. [Optional]

5. Was BCSC Section 5 free of commercial bias?

   ☐ Yes

   ☐ No

6. If you selected "No" in the previous question, please comment. [Optional]

7. Please tell us what might improve the applicability of BCSC to your practice. [Optional]

Study Questions

Although a concerted effort has been made to avoid ambiguity and redundancy in these questions, the authors recognize that differences of opinion may occur regarding the "best" answer. The discussions are provided to demonstrate the rationale used to derive the answer. They may also be helpful in confirming that your approach to the problem was correct or, if necessary, in fixing the principle in your memory.

1. The medial orbital wall is composed of all of the following bones *except:*
   a. ethmoid
   b. palatine
   c. maxilla
   d. sphenoid

2. The brainstem horizontal saccadic generator is the
   a. nucleus reticularis tegmenti pontis
   b. paramedian pontine reticular formation
   c. interstitial nucleus of Cajal
   d. rostral interstitial nucleus of the medial longitudinal fasciculus

3. The test least likely to be helpful in determining nonorganic visual loss is
   a. Goldmann perimetry
   b. automated perimetry
   c. confrontation visual field testing
   d. vertical prism dissociation test

4. A 20-year-old, previously healthy, man complains of headache and has a fixed, dilated left pupil. His examination is otherwise normal. Which of the following is least likely to be helpful in the initial evaluation?
   a. dilute (0.1%) pilocarpine test
   b. 1% pilocarpine test
   c. cocaine test
   d. observation

5. A 54-year-old woman reports visual loss in the right eye occurring over 3 days. Vision is no light perception in the right eye. What finding would suggest nonorganic visual loss?
   a. direct pupillary light reaction
   b. no eye movements when a mirror moves over the right eye
   c. no eye movements when a 6 D base-out prism is placed over the right eye
   d. no monocular optokinetic nystagmus when the OKN drum is rotated from the patient's left to right

6. Which of the following characterizes the vestibular ocular reflex?
   a. It conveys information concerning angular head acceleration.
   b. It subserves pursuit eye movements.
   c. It is concerned with the accuracy of saccadic eye movements.
   d. It conveys auditory input to the brain.

7. Which of the following is characteristic of saccadic eye movements?
   a. They always travel at a constant high rate of speed.
   b. They vary their speed in accord with the intended amplitude of the movement.
   c. They are rarely used to explore environmental space visually.
   d. They often overshoot their target in normal individuals.

8. A horizontal gaze palsy is indicative of which of the following?
   a. a lesion of the ipsilateral frontal lobe
   b. a lesion of the contralateral frontal lobe
   c. damage to the pontine gaze centers
   d. carotid territory cerebral infarction

9. A pupil-sparing third (oculomotor) nerve palsy with aberrant regeneration
   a. may rarely be due to diabetes
   b. often indicates a structural lesion compressing the oculomotor nerve
   c. is best evaluated with CT
   d. may be "microvascular" in origin and requires assessment of stroke risk factors

10. Which of the following is true of fourth (trochlear) nerve palsies?
    a. They are a common cause of diplopia posttrauma.
    b. They can generally be diagnosed by observation of the ductions.
    c. They are associated with abducting nystagmus.
    d. They are commonly related to compressive lesions, such as aneurysms.

11. Which of the following is a form of jerk nystagmus?
    a. ocular flutter
    b. oculopalatal myoclonus
    c. opsoclonus
    d. downbeat

12. Downbeat nystagmus often localizes to which area?
    a. parasellar region
    b. dorsal midbrain
    c. cerebral hemispheres
    d. cervicomedullary junction

13. Which of the following statements regarding the pupils is true?
    a. Dense amblyopia can cause an ipsilateral afferent pupillary defect.
    b. Dense macular scars of age-related macular degeneration typically produce afferent pupillary defects.

c. Optic tract lesions cannot produce afferent pupillary defects because the fibers are post-chiasmal.

d. Bilateral afferent pupillary defects are seen with bilateral optic neuropathies.

14. Which of the following statements regarding perimetry is false?

a. The automated visual field is the best perimetric means of quantitating visual field loss.

b. The Amsler grid is the best visual field test for assessing metamorphopsia.

c. Goldmann perimetry is the best visual field test for those who require active interaction with the examiner.

d. The tangent screen is the best visual field test for patients with multiple sclerosis.

15. A 35-year-old woman presents with sudden painful loss of vision of her right eye. Her examination reveals vision of 20/80 OD and 20/20 OS. Pupils demonstrate an afferent pupillary defect of the right eye. A dense inferior altitudinal defect encroaches on central fixation OD, and the left visual field is normal. The remainder of the examination is normal, including the fundus examination. How would you counsel this patient?

a. She is unlikely to have optic neuritis because the optic nerve on examination is normal; however, she needs an MRI scan of the orbits to rule out a tumor.

b. She has optic neuritis and should begin one of the proven treatments for multiple sclerosis (MS) to prevent its onset.

c. She has optic neuritis and should have an MRI scan of the brain to assess her risk for MS.

d. She should have an MRI scan to rule out a tumor, as well as take oral corticosteroids to assess the benefit.

16. A 28-year-old obese woman complains of transient visual loss lasting seconds in the right eye when rising from a bent position. Examination reveals normal acuity OU with bilateral disc edema. What is the best course of action?

a. medical therapy for intracranial hypertension; no need for neuroimaging

b. CT of the brain, then medical therapy for intracranial hypertension

c. MRI, MRV, lumbar puncture, then medical therapy for intracranial hypertension

d. CT of the brain, then a shunting procedure for intracranial hypertension

17. A 77-year-old hypertensive man complains of sudden loss of vision in the left eye. He is found to be 20/25 OD and light perception OS, with a dense left afferent pupillary defect. Right fundus examination demonstrates a normal optic disc but a number of cotton-wool spots. Examination of the left eye shows pallid disc edema and cotton-wool spots as well. What is the appropriate sequence of evaluation in this patient?

a. immediate erythrocyte sedimentation rate (ESR) and C-reactive protein; the office to call patient with results

b. immediate ESR and C-reactive protein, then the institution of corticosteroids, followed by a temporal artery biopsy

c. immediate ESR and C-reactive protein, then a temporal artery biopsy, followed by the institution of corticosteroids, depending on biopsy results

d. immediate ESR and C-reactive protein, then the institution of corticosteroids; no biopsy necessary if clinical suspicion is high

18. Which of the following would be the best imaging study in a patient with a right optic neuropathy and third nerve palsy?

    a. MRI of the brain and orbits with contrast and fat suppression

    b. MRA of the head and neck

    c. cerebral arteriography

    d. MRI of the brain with contrast

19. Which of the following clinical findings would make CT preferable to MRI in a patient with optic neuropathy?

    a. history of multiple sclerosis and optic neuritis

    b. history of cochlear implantation

    c. history of allergic reaction to iodinated contrast

    d. history of pituitary adenoma

20. Which of the following conditions involving the facial muscles is most likely to be unilateral?

    a. apraxia of eyelid opening

    b. essential blepharospasm

    c. hemifacial spasm

    d. Guillain-Barré syndrome

21. A lesion causing facial palsy and ipsilateral decreased hearing and nystagmus is most likely

    a. a pontine stroke

    b. a cerebellopontine angle tumor

    c. Bell's palsy

    d. a parotid gland tumor

22. Which of the following clinical findings is most likely to suggest the need for additional diagnostic testing in a patient with headaches?

    a. headaches that alternate sides

    b. family history of headaches

    c. change in the pattern of headaches

    d. headaches precipitated by certain foods

23. A patient with unilateral pain with eye movement, a relative afferent pupillary defect, and normal ocular motility most likely has

    a. inflammation within the cavernous sinus (Tolosa-Hunt syndrome)

    b. optic neuritis

    c. trigeminal neuralgia

    d. myositis

24. Visual hallucinations may occur as a result of all of the following *except:*

    a. bilateral visual loss (Charles Bonnet syndrome)

    b. sildenafil citrate (Viagra)

    c. cancer-associated retinopathy

    d. parietal lobe lesions

25. A patient with a normal eye examination, including visual field testing, is unable to see both a pen and bottle held in front of him. This is known as

    a. optic ataxia

    b. prosopagnosia

    c. simultanagnosia

    d. Anton syndrome

26. Which of the following characterizes alexia without agraphia?

    a. It results from a disconnection between hemispheres.

    b. It is a form of visual-spatial relationship disruption.

    c. It occurs when the dominant parietal lobe is damaged.

    d. It is part of Balint syndrome.

27. A previously healthy 24-year-old woman complains of blurred vision and mild pain around the right eye for 2 days. Visual acuity is 20/100 OD with a right RAPD. Funduscopy is normal. An MRI shows 2 ovoid periventicular white matter lesions. Which of the following statements is true?

    a. She should be treated with intravenous methylprednisolone to ensure visual recovery.

    b. Her risk of developing multiple sclerosis is 25% over the next 15 years.

    c. Immunotherapy (eg, interferon beta-1b) should be considered to decrease the risk of developing multiple sclerosis.

    d. It is unlikely her vision will improve.

28. A 67-year-old woman developed variable double vision 1 month ago and appears to have fatigable ptosis. She has no systemic symptoms. Which of the following statements is true?

    a. A normal anti-acetylcholine receptor antibody level effectively rules out myasthenia gravis.

    b. Her risk of developing generalized myasthenia is about 20%.

    c. The 30% occurrence of concomitant thyroid eye disease may complicate the diagnosis of myasthenia.

    d. An improvement of 2 mm in ptosis following a 2-minute ice application to the eyelid confirms the diagnosis of myasthenia.

29. Which of the following conditions does not predispose an individual to specific intracranial lesions?

    a. ataxia-telangiectasia (Louis-Bar)

    b. racemose angioma (Wyburn-Mason)

    c. retinal angiomatosis (von Hippel–Lindau)

    d. tuberous sclerosis (Bourneville)

30. A 78-year-old man with ischemic heart disease and hypertension experiences a single 10-minute episode of painless visual loss in his left eye. He describes the episode as a "gray window shade" being pulled down and then released. Which is the most likely etiology of his visual loss?

    a. migraine

    b. vertebrobasilar circulation insufficiency

    c. Uhthoff phenomenon

    d. retinal artery embolus

31. The main finding of the North American and European trials (NASCET 1991 and ECST 1995) that compared medical therapy to carotid endarterectomy in patients with symptomatic carotid stenosis was that

    a. there is no difference between medical and surgical therapy in preventing stroke

    b. medical treatment is superior to surgical treatment for reducing the risk of ipsilateral stroke in patients with severe (≥70%) carotid stenosis

    c. surgical treatment is superior to medical treatment for reducing the risk of ipsilateral stroke in patients with severe (≥70%) carotid stenosis

    d. surgical treatment is superior for reducing the risk of ipsilateral stroke, regardless of the degree of carotid stenosis

32. A healthy 50-year-old woman acutely develops a painful, postganglionic Horner syndrome. Imaging should be directed to find what pathology?

    a. brainstem stroke

    b. apical lung tumor

    c. carotid dissection

    d. multiple sclerosis

33. All of the following are features of Adie tonic pupil *except:*

    a. segmental contraction of the iris sphincter

    b. poor light reflex

    c. predilection for children and adolescents

    d. cholinergic denervation supersensitivity

34. Dyschromatopsia and a relative afferent pupil defect in a patient with 20/20 visual acuity most likely indicates a disorder of the

    a. retina

    b. optic nerve

    c. optic radiation

    d. visual cortex

35. In a 78-year-old woman with sudden loss of vision and a history of malaise, weight loss, and earache, which of the following is most appropriate?

    a. CT scan of brain and orbits

    b. MRI of brain

    c. immediate referral to a neurologist

    d. evaluation of erythrocyte sedimentation rate and C-reactive protein

36. The most important factor in determining the workup of a patient with acute third nerve palsy is

    a. age of patient

    b. pupil involvement

    c. presence or absence of pain

    d. visual acuity

37. Leber hereditary optic neuropathy is associated with

    a. sex-linked recessive transmission

    b. autosomal recessive transmission

    c. a pathognomonic optic nerve appearance

    d. a mitochondrial DNA mutation

38. The most likely cause of transient binocular loss of vision in a 21-year-old woman is

    a. migraine

    b. thromboembolism

    c. pseudotumor cerebri

    d. cerebral arteriovenous malformation

39. A patient with sudden onset of severe headache, sixth nerve palsy, and a bitemporal visual field defect likely has

    a. a ruptured ophthalmic artery aneurysm

    b. pituitary apoplexy

    c. meningeal carcinomatosis

    d. multiple sclerosis

40. An isolated sixth nerve palsy in a patient older than 50 years is most often due to

    a. demyelinating disease

    b. traumatic brain injury

    c. microvascular ischemia

    d. brain tumor

Answers

1. **b.** The medial wall of the orbit is composed of the maxillary, lacrimal, sphenoid, and ethmoidal bones. The palatine bone forms a small area of the orbital floor.

2. **b.** The excitatory burst neurons for generating horizontal saccades are located in the paramedian pontine reticular formation (PPRF). Horizontal smooth pursuit eye movements arise from the nucleus of the sixth nerve. The nucleus reticularis tegmenti pontis contains the long-lead burst cells within the brainstem. Located within the midbrain, the interstitial nucleus of Cajal contains inhibitory burst neurons for vertical saccades and is the vertical integrator for vertical gaze. The rostral interstitial nucleus of the medial longitudinal fasciculus, which is also located in the midbrain, is the vertical and torsional saccadic generator.

3. **b.** Visual field abnormalities with automated perimetry can often be feigned by patients with nonorganic visual field loss, even in the setting of reliable testing indices. In nonorganic visual field loss, Goldmann perimetry can demonstrate spiraling or overlapping (reversal) of isopters. Confrontation visual field testing can be used to show nonorganic peripheral visual field loss when the patient responds correctly to the number of fingers held in the previously unseen visual field. Patients with nonorganic unilateral visual loss will indicate double vision with the vertical prism dissociation test.

4. **c.** The cocaine test is helpful when evaluating a patient with a miotic pupil suspected of having a Horner pupil. The dilute (0.1%) and 1% pilocarpine tests should be considered in a patient with a fixed and dilated pupil possibly due to an Adie pupil or pharmacologic mydriasis, respectively.

5. **a.** Any direct pupillary light reaction indicates some level of afferent visual function. A negative mirror test, negative monocular OKN response, and negative base-out prism test are all indicative of organic and profound visual loss.

6. **a.** The vestibular ocular reflex (VOR) is primarily involved in sensing angular head acceleration and conveys this information to the ocular motor centers to facilitate rapid and compensatory eye movements, allowing the fovea to remain on the target of regard. Although the eighth cranial nerve transmits both cochlear (hearing) and vestibular information, the VOR is not concerned with auditory information.

7. **b.** Saccades follow a "main sequence" pattern, with increasing velocity in proportion to the intended amplitude of the movement; accordingly, larger saccadic eye movements travel at a faster rate of speed than do small saccades. Saccades are the primary method used when exploring space visually. Hypermetric, or saccades that overshoot their target, are always abnormal, generally indicating cerebellar dysfunction. Saccades are easily tested at the bedside by having the patient direct his or her gaze between targets.

8. **c.** A horizontal gaze palsy typically indicates damage to the ipsilateral pontine horizontal gaze center (eg, a right pontine horizontal gaze center lesion produces a right gaze palsy; the eyes will be deviated to the left and unable to move fully rightward). Gaze preferences indicate a supranuclear lesion of the frontal eye fields; a right frontal lobe lesion produces a tendency for the eyes to be deviated to the right, but this can be overcome by the vestibular ocular reflex (hence the supranuclear nature of the lesion). Carotid territory infarctions would not be expected to affect the pontine horizontal gaze centers.

9. **b.** Aberrant regeneration indicates compression of the outside of the oculomotor nerve; the most common pathologic entities producing this are aneurysm, tumor (meningioma), or trauma (easily seen in the history). Depending on the individual case features, this is often best evaluated by MRI or angiography (contrast or noninvasive angiography such as CTA or MRA). Aberrant regeneration never results from a microvascular (eg, diabetic) third nerve palsy or myasthenia gravis.

10. **a.** Fourth nerve palsy is the most common cause of posttraumatic diplopia. It requires alternate cover testing in all positions of gaze to determine if the pattern conforms to the Parks-Bielschowsky 3-step test. Although internuclear ophthalmoplegia is commonly associated with abducting nystagmus, it is not a feature of fourth nerve palsies. Aneurysmal compression rarely causes a fourth nerve palsy.

11. **d.** Downbeat is the only form of jerk nystagmus among this group. In order to be classified as nystagmus, a slow phase is required; accordingly, flutter, square waves, and opsoclonus are saccadic intrusions because they have only fast phases and no slow phases. Oculopalatal myoclonus is a form of pendular nystagmus, which has only slow phases. Downbeat nystagmus has a fast and a slow phase, thus qualifying as a form of jerk nystagmus.

12. **d.** Downbeat nystagmus often localizes to a lesion in the cervicomedullary junction.

13. **a.** Dense amblyopia has been reported to cause a mild relative afferent pupillary defect (RAPD). Macular scars, despite the profound central loss of acuity, do not cause an afferent pupillary defect. Optic tract lesions may result in an RAPD of the eye contralateral to the lesion because each tract contains more crossed fibers than uncrossed fibers. Because RAPD measures the afferent input of 1 optic nerve versus the other, there is no such thing as bilateral RAPDs.

14. **d.** Automated visual fields offer significant advantages over manual perimetry, but quantitative analysis is more uniform, comparable, and useful for scientific studies. The Amsler grid allows the patient to explain the distortion he or she sees. Goldmann perimetry offers an advantage for children and the elderly, who need more interaction with the examiner, but it requires a skilled technician or examiner. The tangent screen is most useful in testing for nonorganic visual loss.

15. **c.** This is the most common clinical presentation of optic neuritis: acute painful loss of vision in a woman between 18 and 45 years of age. The Optic Neuritis Treatment Trial (ONTT) recommendations include an MRI scan of the brain to assess the risk of multiple sclerosis. If the patient has 1 or more white matter lesions, her risk is 72% in a 15-year period, whereas the patient with a normal MRI (zero lesions) has a 25% risk of MS; the highest rate of conversion falls within the first 5 years. The overall rate of conversion of all patients to MS is 50% at 15 years. Patients with abnormal MRIs should be referred to a neurologist to determine if the patient should begin one of the established treatments to delay the onset and progression of MS.

16. **c.** Although idiopathic intracranial hypertension (IIH) is a leading cause of papilledema, it remains a diagnosis of exclusion. Before establishing the diagnosis of IIH, all patients with papilledema should undergo emergent neuroimaging to rule out a mass lesion, subsequent lumbar puncture with documentation of the opening pressure, and a determination of spinal fluid composition. The majority of patients respond favorably to medical therapy. Surgical treatment should be reserved for patients who fail maximal medical therapy.

17. **b.** This patient has suffered ischemic optic neuropathy. Given his age, profound degree of visual loss, bilateral cotton-wool spots, and pallid disc edema, giant cell arteritis should be considered likely. The risk of contralateral visual loss is imminent (within days), and therefore corticosteroids should be instituted immediately, followed by a temporal artery biopsy. A biopsy is important to support long-term corticosteroid use in older patients, who often have other medical problems that place them at high risk for corticosteroid-induced complications.

18. **a.** The combination of an optic neuropathy and third nerve palsy suggests that the problem involves the orbital apex. MRI is better than CT in delineating soft-tissue disease detail. Fat suppression should be used to eliminate the hyperintense (bright) signal created by orbital fat, which would obscure the anatomical contents of the orbit.

19. **b.** Cochlear implants are metallic and a contraindication for MRI.

20. **c.** Hemifacial spasm is characteristically unilateral, whereas apraxia of the eyelid opening, essential blepharospasm, and Guillain-Barré syndrome cause bilateral abnormalities.

21. **b.** The cerebellopontine angle lies in close proximity to the eighth (vestibuloacoustic) nerve and the seventh (facial) nerve. A pontine stroke would not cause decreased hearing. Bell's palsy causes a facial palsy without nystagmus.

22. **c.** A family history of headaches is often seen in patients with primary headache disorders such as migraine and tension headache. Some known precipitants of migraine include red wine, monosodium glutamate, and caffeine. Recurrent unilateral headaches, especially if they alternate sides, are characteristic of migraine. A change in the pattern of headaches may indicate a structural lesion.

23. **b.** Pain with eye movement and a relative afferent pupillary defect are clinical hallmarks of optic neuritis. Processes isolated to the cavernous sinus are not associated with optic neuropathy and are often associated with ocular motor cranial nerve palsy resulting in diplopia. Isolated myositis and trigeminal neuralgia are not associated with an optic neuropathy.

24. **b.** Sildenafil citrate (Viagra) may cause perception of a blue tinge (an illusion). Formed and unformed visual hallucinations may occur secondary to severe bilateral visual loss (Charles Bonnet syndrome). Cancer-associated retinopathy frequently causes flashing lights (unformed hallucinations), and parietal lobe lesions may produce either formed or unformed hallucinations.

25. **c.** Simultanagnosia is a failure to integrate multiple elements of a scene. A patient with optic ataxia will reach for an object and miss it. Prosopagnosia is the inability to recognize faces. Anton syndrome is the denial of visual loss; it usually occurs with cortical blindness due to bilateral parieto-occipital lesions.

26. **a.** Alexia without agraphia results from a disconnection between hemispheres (occipital lobe to dominant angular gyrus). It is not a form of visual-spatial relationship disruption (eg, simultanagnosia). Damage to the dominant parietal lobe produces alexia with agraphia. Balint syndrome comprises the triad of simultanagnosia, optic ataxia, and acquired oculomotor apraxia.

27. **c.** Several studies have shown that patients at high risk for developing MS (1 neurologic episode and 2 or more plaques) have less risk if treated with immunotherapy. Intravenous methylprednisolone may hasten visual recovery but does not alter the ultimate recovery

of vision. Her risk of developing MS is 72% over the next 15 years (1 or more plaques and 1 episode of optic neuritis). Vision usually improves over 3 months.

28. **d.** The ice test is safe and confirmatory when improvement of at least 2 mm of ptosis occurs. Anti-acetylcholine receptor antibodies are positive in only about 60% of patients with ocular myasthenia. As many as 85% of patients who present with ocular myasthenia go on to develop systemic myasthenia. If the patient has ocular myasthenia for only 2 years, the conversion rate is about 10%. Concomitant thyroid eye disease occurs in about 5% of patients.

29. **a.** Ataxia-telangiectasia. Wyburn-Mason syndrome includes midbrain arteriovenous malformations; retinal angiomatosis includes cerebellar hemangioblastomas; and tuberous sclerosis is named for the intracranial hamartomas (tubers) that occur.

30. **d.** The historical description is particularly important in the evaluation of a patient with transient visual loss. Migrainous visual loss typically progresses to a maximal deficit over 20 minutes, is often accompanied by positive visual phenomena, and usually affects both eyes. Vertebrobasilar insufficiency causes a transient homonymous hemianopic deficit. Uhthoff phenomenon is visual loss associated with increased body temperature and indicates demyelinating disease, an unlikely disorder for a 78-year-old man. Retinal artery embolus produces acute, painless, monocular visual loss that usually lasts for less than 5 minutes and often has an altitudinal pattern described as a "curtain" descending over vision.

31. **c.** NASCET prospectively compared the effectiveness of carotid endarterectomy with medical management in patients with symptomatic carotid artery stenosis. Patients with amaurosis fugax, carotid TIAs, or mild strokes were randomized to either medical management, which included daily aspirin, or carotid endarterectomy followed by medical management. Subsequent stroke was significantly reduced in patients with 70%–99% carotid stenosis who underwent surgery, provided that the morbidity and mortality rates for angiography and surgery at the treating facility were acceptable (<4%). Surgery was not better than medical therapy in patients with moderate (50%–69%) carotid stenosis.

32. **c.** Acute, painful Horner syndrome is an emergency and should be considered a carotid dissection until proven otherwise, particularly if accompanied by other neurologic deficits, such as visual loss, hemispheric dysfunction, difficulty swallowing (dysphagia), or distorted sense of taste (dysgeusia). Most cases can be diagnosed from noninvasive imaging (head and neck MRI with and without contrast). The reason for such urgency in these patients lies with the high risk of embolization to the eye or brain within the first 2 weeks following a dissection. Early anticoagulation is generally recommended.

33. **c.** A tonic pupil represents injury to the postganglionic parasympathetic pathway. Most cases of unilateral tonic pupil are idiopathic, called Adie pupil; occur in women between the ages of 20 and 50 years; and do not require neuroimaging.

34. **b.** Although dyschromatopsia and a relative afferent pupillary defect might occur with extensive retinal disease, these findings are characteristically seen with optic nerve disorders. Lesions of the optic radiations or visual cortex do not cause pupil abnormalities.

35. **d.** This patient has a history strongly suggestive of giant cell arteritis. Erythrocyte sedimentation rate and C-reactive protein elevations further support the diagnosis, which is confirmed histologically with a temporal artery biopsy. The ophthalmologist should initiate treatment and take steps to confirm the diagnosis without delay.

36. **b.** The status of the pupil in a patient with acute third nerve palsy, regardless of age, presence or absence of pain, or level of visual acuity, is critically important. A patient with pupil involvement should be considered to have an intracranial aneurysm until proven otherwise.

37. **d.** Leber hereditary optic neuropathy is related to a mitochondrial DNA mutation, most frequently at the 11778 position, less commonly at the 3460 and 14484 locations. The mutation is transmitted by mitochondrial DNA inherited from the mother. Thus, only women transmit the disease.

38. **a.** Thromboembolism, pseudotumor cerebri, and cerebral arteriovenous malformations can cause transient loss of vision, but they are much less likely to do so than migraine, which occurs in approximately 20% of women and is often associated with transient monocular or binocular visual disturbances, with or without headache.

39. **b.** Sudden loss of vision, headache, and ocular motor nerve palsies occur with rapid expansion of a pituitary tumor into the suprasellar and cavernous sinus regions. Prompt neuroimaging and emergency management are essential in these cases.

40. **c.** Sixth nerve palsies can occur with demyelinating disease, traumatic brain injury, and brain tumor, but they most commonly occur in adults with vasculopathic risk factors and are thought to be due to microvascular ischemia. Spontaneous recovery within 3 months typically occurs in these patients.

Index

(*f* = figure; *t* = table)